Handbook of
Mental Health Services for Children, Adolescents, and Families

Issues in Clinical Child Psychology

Series Editors: **Michael C. Roberts**, *University of Kansas—Lawrence, Kansas*
Lizette Peterson,[‡] *University of Missouri—Columbia, Missouri*

[‡]Deceased.

A Continuation Order Plan is available for this series. A continuation order will bring delivery of each new volume immediately upon publication. Volumes are billed only upon actual shipment. For further information please contact the publisher.

Handbook of
Mental Health Services
for Children,
Adolescents, and
Families

Edited by

Ric G. Steele
University of Kansas
Lawrence, Kansas

and

Michael C. Roberts
University of Kansas
Lawrence, Kansas

Kluwer Academic / Plenum Publishers
New York, Boston, Dordrecht, London, Moscow

Library of Congress Cataloging-in-Publication Data

Handbook of mental health services for children, adolescents, and families / edited by Ric
    G. Steele and Michael C. Roberts.
        p. cm.—(Issues in clinical child psychology)
    Includes bibliographical references and index.
    ISBN 0-306-48560-5 (hbk.)—ISBN 0-306-48561-3 (eBook)
        1. Child mental health services—United States.   2. Teenagers—Mental health services—
United States.   3. Youth—Mental health services—United States.   4. Family—Mental health
services—United States.   I. Steele, Ric G.   II. Roberts, Michael C.   III. Series.

RJ501.A2H36 2004
362.2′083′0973–dc22

2004042177

ISBN 0-306-48560-5

© 2005 by Kluwer Academic/Plenum Publishers
233 Spring Street, New York, New York 10013

http://www.kluweronline.com

10 9 8 7 6 5 4 3 2 1

A C.I.P. record for this book is available from the Library of Congress

To Carol, for her love and support

—RGS

To my wife and children

—MCR

Contributors

Gerald J. August, Department of Psychiatry, University of Minnesota Medical School, Minneapolis, Minnesota 55454

Beth A. Auslander, University of Texas Medical Branch at Galveston, Galveston, Texas 77555

Barrie E. Berquist, Department of Psychiatry, University of Minnesota Medical School, Minneapolis, Minnesota 55454

Leonard Bickman, Department of Psychology, Peabody College, Vanderbilt University, Nashville, Tennessee 37212

Michael L. Bloomquist, Department of Psychiatry, University of Minnesota Medical School, Minneapolis, Minnesota 55454

Barbara L. Bonner, Center on Child Abuse and Neglect, Department of Pediatrics, University of Oklahoma Health Sciences Center, Oklahoma City, Oklahoma 73164

Keri J. Brown, Department of Psychology, Columbus Children's Hospital, Columbus, Ohio 43215

Bryan D. Carter, Kosair Children's Hospital, University of Louisville School of Medicine, Louisville, Kentucky 40202

Bruce F. Chorpita, Department of Psychology, University of Hawaii at Manoa, Honolulu, Hawaii 96822

Ann M. McGrath Davis, University of Kansas Medical Center, Kansas City, Kansas 66160

Artemio de Dios Brambila, Division of Child and Adolescent Psychiatry, Department of Psychiatry, University of New Mexico School of Medicine, Albuquerque, New Mexico 87131

Christina Donkervoet, Child and Adolescent Mental Health Division, Hawaii Department of Health, Honolulu, Hawaii 96813

Glen Dunlap, Department of Child and Family Studies, Florida Mental Health Institute, University of South Florida, Tampa, Florida 33612

Rebecca Ettelson, Department of Psychiatry, University of Tennessee Health Science Center, Memphis, Tennessee 38105

David L. Fenell, Counseling and Human Services Program, University of Colorado at Colorado Springs, Colorado Springs, Colorado 80933

Jerry Flanzer, National Institute on Drug Abuse, Bethesda, Maryland 20892

Patricia A. Graczyk, Institute for Juvenile Research, Department of Psychiatry, University of Illinois at Chicago, Chicago, Illinois 60612

E. Wayne Holden, Applied Research Division, ORC Macro, Atlanta, Georgia 30329

Alan J. Hovestadt, Counselor Education and Counseling Psychology, Western Michigan University, Kalamazoo, Michigan 49008

Julie Heim Jackson, Department of Counseling, Developmental, and Educational Psychology, Boston College, Chestnut Hill, Massachusetts 02467

Anne K. Jacobs, Clinical Child Psychology Program, University of Kansas, Lawrence, Kansas 66045

T. Rene Jamison, School Psychology Program, University of Kansas, Lawrence Kansas 66045

Michelle R. Kees, Center on Child Abuse and Neglect, University of Oklahoma Health Sciences Center, Oklahoma City, Oklahoma 73104

Bernadette M. Landolf, Behavior Therapy Center of Greater Washington, Silver Spring, Maryland 20901

Steven W. Lee, School Psychology Program, University of Kansas, Lawrence, Kansas 66045

Susanne S. Lee, Department of Psychiatry, University of Minnesota Medical School, Minneapolis, Minnesota 55454

Heidi J. Liss, National Rural Behavioral Health Center, University of Florida, Gainesville, Florida 32610

Robin Mathy, Department of Psychiatry, University of Minnesota Medical School, Minneapolis, Minnesota 55454

Trisha T. Miller, Disaster Mental Health Institute, University of South Dakota, Vermillion, South Dakota 57069

Shelagh Mulvaney, Department of Psychology, Peabody College, Vanderbilt University, Nashville, Tennessee 37212

William D. Murphy, Department of Psychiatry, University of Tennessee Health Science Center, Memphis, Tennessee 38105

Joseph E. Nyre, Department of Child and Adolescent Psychiatry, University of Chicago, Chicago, Illinois 60637; Department of Pediatrics, Southern Illinois University Medical School, Springfield, Illinois

Jacqueline Page, Department of Psychiatry, University of Tennessee Health Science Center, Memphis, Tennessee 38105

Diane Powell, Department of Child and Family Studies, Florida Mental Health Institute, University of South Florida, Tampa, Florida 33612

Beverly Pringle, National Institute on Drug Abuse, Bethesda, Maryland 20892

Camille Randall, Clinical Child Psychology Program, University of Kansas, Lawrence, Kansas 66045

Gilbert Reyes, Disaster Mental Health Institute, University of South Dakota, Vermillion, South Dakota 57069

Michael C. Roberts, Clinical Child Psychology Program, University of Kansas, Lawrence, Kansas 66045

Susan L. Rosenthal, University of Texas Medical Branch at Galveston, Galveston, Texas 77555

Rolando L. Santiago, Center for Mental Health Services, Substance Abuse, and Mental Health Services Administration, Rockville, Maryland 20857

Merritt D. Schreiber, Terrorism and Disaster Branch, National Center for Child Traumatic Stess, David Geffen School of Medicine at UCLA, Los Angeles, California

Mary B. Short, University of Texas Medical Branch at Galveston, Galveston, Texas 77555

Julianne M. Smith-Boydston, Bert Nash Center, Lawrence, Kansas 66044

Terry Stancin, Department of Pediatrics, MetroHealth Medical Center, Case Western Reserve University School of Medicine, Cleveland, Ohio 44109

Ric G. Steele, Clinical Child Psychology Program, University of Kansas, Lawrence, Kansas 66045

Robert L. Stephens, Applied Research Division, ORC Macro, Atlanta, Georgia 30329

Beth Todd-Bazemore, Disaster Mental Health Institute, University of South Dakota, Vermillion, South Dakota 57069

Patrick H. Tolan, Institute for Juvenile Research, Department of Psychiatry, University of Illinois at Chicago, Chicago, Illinois 60612

Luis A. Vargas, Division of Child and Adolescent Psychiatry, Department of Psychiatry, University of New Mexico School of Medicine, Albuquerque, New Mexico 87131

Eric M. Vernberg, Clinical Child Psychology Program, University of Kansas, Lawrence, Kansas 66045

Renee T. von Weiss, Children's Hospital of Minneapolis, Minneapolis, Minnesota 55404

Ngan Vuong, University of Kansas Medical Center, Kansas City, Kansas 66160

Mary E. Walsh, Department of Counseling, Developmental, and Educational Psychology, Boston College, Chestnut Hill, Massachusetts 02467

Contents

1

Mental Health Services for Children, Adolescents, and Families

Trends, Models, and Current Status

RIC G. STEELE and MICHAEL C. ROBERTS

In 1999, the American Psychiatric Association reported that approximately 13 million children (or about 18% of children in the United States) were in need of mental health or substance abuse services. This estimate is consistent with other recent reports of psychiatric or psychosocial morbidity (e.g., Costello et al., 1996; R. E. Roberts, Attkisson, & Rosenblatt, 1998), with reports of children with diagnosable or distressing conditions ranging from 16% to 22%, depending on type of condition, diagnostic specificity, and demographic characteristics. Although variations in measurement may account for some of the differences, the current estimates of children in need of services are significantly higher than those reported by Jane Knitzer (1982) in her landmark publication, *Unclaimed Children*. In this first comprehensive report on the state of child and adolescent mental health and services, Knitzer noted that, although the need is great, as many as two thirds of the children with mental health problems did not receive services.

Since the early 1980s, public and private initiatives have exerted considerable efforts toward meeting these needs. Nevertheless, the U.S. Surgeon General's Office recently reported that less than one third of the children with diagnosable mental disorders receive services in a given year (Department of Health and Human Services, 1999). The purpose of

RIC G. STEELE and MICHAEL C. ROBERTS • Clinical Child Psychology Program, University of Kansas, Lawrence, Kansas 66045.

1

this chapter is to introduce the historical and contemporary influences on mental health service delivery, and to characterize the range of services that are available to children, youth, and families—many of which are represented in the chapters of this volume.

BRIEF HISTORY OF SERVICE DELIVERY TO CHILDREN

Parenting, education, and treatment of children and adolescents have evolved over recorded history (Peterson & Roberts, 1991). Early "interventions" with children, who exhibited disordered behavior frequently, were harsh and were aimed at eliminating innate evil tendencies or the influences of evil forces (e.g., demons, or Satan), and the treatments designed to remedy the condition often resulted in harm or greater impairment to the child. It was not until the mental hygiene movement of the late 19th and early 20th centuries that changes in attitudes and social policy resulted in observably better treatment for children and youth with mental health needs. Reforms were made toward more humane and enlightened treatment of adults (and to some degree, children) with mental disorders in hospital settings and treatment centers of a variety of types.

As part of this movement, Lightner Witmer established what many consider to be the first psychology clinic at the University of Pennsylvania in 1896—interestingly, mandated to serve the needs of the public while training graduate students in the new field of "clinical psychology" (Witmer, 1907/1996). Indeed, the field of school psychology also traces its origins to Witmer because of his orientation to education interventions (French, 1990). As noted by Witmer, a specific objective of the University of Pennsylvania Psychological Clinic was "the offering of practical work to those engaged in the professions of teaching and medicine, and to those interested in social work, in the observation and training of normal and retarded children" (Witmer, 1996, p. 249).

Another significant change in treatment came in the social reform efforts resulting in the first Juvenile Psychopathic Institute in Chicago (now Institute for Juvenile Research) and later the Judge Baker Guidance Center in Boston. These centers provided more intense psychiatric and psychological assistance to children and families than had been provided in the past. Douglas Thom's Habit Clinic was established shortly thereafter to apply behavioral principles to discrete problematic behaviors. These types of child treatment centers were replicated and adapted into a number of child guidance clinics across the country.

Since then, various theoretical orientations have guided the contexts of psychotherapeutic interventions, and have also led to a diverse range in the organization of service delivery systems (Peterson & Burbach, 1988; Peterson & Roberts, 1991). However, these influences (i.e., theoretical orientation and therapeutic context) have not been the only forces in the evolution of mental health service delivery. Various financing arrangements (M. C. Roberts & Alexander, 1990) as well as public and private policies have frequently dictated the nature and availability of mental health services for youth. As we describe below, these influences have not always acted in concert with professional, theoretical, or therapeutic goals.

FEDERAL INFLUENCES ON SERVICE DELIVERY

With the apparently changing appreciation for the mental health needs of children and adolescents, a number of federally initiated programs began to facilitate the development and implementation of services for youth and families, some of which continue to exert influence. Among the first federal influences on mental health service needs of children was the Joint Commission on the Mental Health of Children (JCMHC, 1969; Dougherty, Saxe, Cross, & Silverman, 1986). This commission, established in 1965, was specifically mandated to assess the prevalence of "emotional disorders" in children, including those with specific psychiatric diagnoses as well as those with impairments in social and educational functioning (JCMHC, 1969). Although earlier federal reports had suggested the need to develop new programs for emotionally disturbed children (e.g., White House Conference on Children in 1909), the 1969 report of the Joint Commission was the first to assess the degree to which children's mental health needs were being meet, and to detail specific recommendations to improve service delivery. These recommendations included the development of child advocacy systems, prevention and remediation services, integrated mental and physical health care systems, family-based treatment models, and mechanisms for increasing research into diagnosis and treatment (Dougherty et al., 1986). Although some of these recommendations have subsequently been implemented, the Joint Commission's 1969 report did not lead to any specific federal action.

A more focused federal initiative in 1975, the *Project on the Classification of Exceptional Children*, had more tangible results for specific subsets of children with mental health needs (cf. Hobbs, 1975). Perhaps building upon the earlier Joint Commission's findings, the Project recommended the establishment of advisory groups at the local, state, and federal levels that would provide input to agencies that coordinated mental health services for "exceptional" children. In addition to advocating specific attention to family support, improved residential care, and better organization and coordination of services, the Project also recommended that all children, regardless of ability, should have access to free and appropriate public education. These recommendations resulted in the passage of Public Law 94-142, the Education for All Handicapped Children Act of 1975.

Following closely on the heels of PL 94-142, the President's Commission on Mental Health (1978) and its Panel on Infants, Children, and Adolescents returned to the recommendations of the 1969 Joint Commission, reporting that little had been done to address several of the deficits in mental health coverage for youth and families. In particular, the Commission found that children of minority ethnic group membership and adolescents were particularly at risk for suboptimal mental health care. The President's

Commission made a number of recommendations that were consistent with the original report of the Joint Commission, including mandates to more fully integrate mental health care into overall health care, to realize the development of prevention services, to provide services to families of children with identified mental health needs, and to fund more basic and evaluation research.

However, unlike its predecessor, the 1978 Commission's report called attention to the mental health needs of minority populations, recognizing that some intervention or prevention efforts might need to be adapted with respect to differences across ethnic groups. Further, the President's Commission recommended the organization of services along a continuum of intensiveness, matching the needs of individual clients to specific levels of care, noting a particular deficit in adequate residential services for children and adolescents. It also called for the development of an integrated network of mental health services in schools, juvenile courts, neighborhood centers, and occupational centers that would address some of the specific needs of adolescents, such as depression and suicide, teenage pregnancy, delinquency, and substance abuse (Dougherty et al., 1986).

Although the President's Commission report resulted in the *Mental Health Systems Act of 1980*, specifically authorizing many improvements in the organization, coordination, and delivery of mental health services for children with severe emotional problems, the act was repealed in 1981 before it was implemented—being replaced by the Alcohol, Drug Abuse, and Mental Health (ADM) block grant (PL 97-35; Dougherty et al., 1986). The ADM block grant program moved the funding of children's mental health systems, including the monies allocated for funding community mental health centers, to the purview of state governments (Lourie, 2003). States were (and are) to use the grants to fund community mental health centers, emphasizing the specific programs that are most needed. Although PL 97-35 was well intended, some have suggested that the act was a step backward in terms of children's mental health care, on the grounds that there were no provisions specifically allocating funds to children's services (Knitzer, 1982; Lourie, 2003). This federal act represented a significant loss of targeted funds that had been allocated under the Mental Health Systems Act of 1980, and made no requirements of the State Mental Health Agencies to provide for specific services for youth or families.

In approximately the same time frame as the President's Commission on Mental Health (i.e., 1979–1982), the Children's Defense Fund commissioned Jane Knitzer, a psychologist, to survey federal and state agencies and provide a report on the current state of children's mental health services. The resulting document, *Unclaimed Children* (Knitzer, 1982), represented the most comprehensive assessment of services for children to date, and was the first empirically derived report dealing with youth and family mental heath care (Dougherty et al., 1986). In addition to providing estimates of the number of children in need of services, Knitzer noted current deficits in the organization and delivery of mental health services. Similar to the 1969 Joint Commission report, Knitzer highlighted inequitable service delivery across demographic groups, such that children of minority ethnic group membership and children of lower socioeconomic status were more likely to receive no or inappropriate care. With regard to continua of services, she noted that the most expensive and restrictive level of care (i.e., psychiatric hospitalization) was the most accessible resource for children, and that alternatives to inpatient care were remarkably scarce. Knitzer also noted disorganization among state mental health service systems, as well as inadequate levels of child specialization in a majority of state mental health systems.

Based on her findings, Knitzer (1982) made six key recommendations that included changes in the organization, incentives, and regulation of state mental health agencies. In particular, she recommended that ADM block grant funds be specifically targeted for the development of programs for children and other underserved populations, that a federal child advocacy system be established that would help coordinate services for children, and that incentives be developed for creating and maintaining coordinated services for children.

As one important result of Knitzer's report, the National Institute of Mental Health funded the Child and Adolescent Service System Program (CASSP) as a means of coordinating service systems within the states. Under the encouragement of CASSP, states developed interagency *systems of care*, which would bring together mental health, special education, juvenile justice, and child welfare agencies. Consistent with the recommendations of several previous commissions, initial efforts were made to determine how these various systems could communicate with one another at the state (administrative) level. Subsequent efforts focused on creating community level systems of care that could provide youth and families with integrated and coordinated services. Much of the current understanding of and emphasis on systems of care in mental health service delivery is a direct result of CASSP (Day & Roberts, 1991; Knitzer, 1993). A second goal of CASSP was to enhance child and adolescent mental health policy focus and funding at the state level. In one sense, CASSP was mandated to reinstate the funds and policy focus that were done away with by the repeal of the Mental Health Systems Act of 1980.

The 1990s witnessed relatively few federal initiatives that would have a general impact on mental health service delivery to children and families. Rather, the Individuals with Disabilities Education Act (IDEA) of 1990, which was revised in 1997, would have a specific impact on mental health service delivery in the school environment. Under the provisions of IDEA (which was passed to amend PL 94-142), the U.S. Department of Education is mandated to assist states in providing all children with disabilities appropriate public education, and to prepare them for independent living and/or employment. As part of this mandate a number of mental health services may be provided, including psychological services, counseling and social work services, and parent counseling and training. Consistent with the previous calls for action, IDEA provided federal incentives for the integration of mental health and special education services for at least some youth and families.

Two additional federally initiated reports (i.e., *Report of the Surgeon General on Children's Mental Health* and *Healthy People 2010*) also have significantly highlighted child and adolescent mental health needs with potential influence on mental health service organization and delivery. However, because so little time has passed since their publication, their full impact has yet to be determined.

With regard to the first of these, in 2000, the U.S. Surgeon General David Satcher convened a meeting of experts from various disciplines and agencies involved with youth and family mental health service provision. In the ensuing report, the first of its kind from this federal office, the Surgeon General highlighted mental health promotion, early detection and assessment, and equal and universal access to mental health care as issues in need of continued attention (U.S. Public Health Service [US PHS], 2000). Specifically, he outlined a national action agenda with four guiding principles: promotion of mental health as an essential part of child health, integration of mental health into all systems that serve children and youth, encouragement of family and youth participation in planning and evaluation of mental health services, and development of public-private health infrastructures to support these efforts. These principles shaped the development of eight specific goals endorsed by the panel and the US PHS, which included provisions for eliminating racial/ethnic/economic barriers to mental health services, continuing efforts to coordinate services across agencies and professions, monitoring of access to and coordination of services, and training of competent providers.

Among the specific concerns evidenced by the Surgeon General's report is the movement of child and family mental health services toward a community health model that balances "health promotion, disease prevention, early detection and universal access to care" (US PHS, 2000, p. 14). Not surprisingly, this goal is echoed by the U.S. Department of Health and Human Services (US DHHS, 2000) in its most recent objectives for health promotion and illness prevention, *Healthy People 2010*. This document specifies a number of youth and family mental health objectives that are consistent with the general movement of integrating systems of mental health services (e.g., juvenile justice and mental health), as well as providing appropriate and competent services to a greater proportion of children in need. Although the *Healthy People* report is consistent with previous editions (e.g., *Healthy People 2000*), the emphasis appears to be slowly changing toward greater attention to the psychological service needs of children.

The recent history of federal initiatives regarding mental health service provision is complicated. On the one hand, similar recommendations have been repeatedly made since 1965, suggesting that more needs to be done in terms of *acting* on the many insightful reports that have been generated. On the other hand, although the language of the various reports is similar, some evolution of the calls for change in mental health service provision is evident. For example, the Surgeon General's report (US PHS, 2000) called for improvements in the systems of care to include systems of preventive care. This is an obvious advance over earlier calls for the creation of systems of care, which were primarily oriented to remediation or therapeutic interventions for existing problems. Nevertheless, even as some hurdles are overcome, others must be met. For example, as one of the Surgeon General's panelist (Jane Knitzer) commented "...access to mental health services too often hinges on a child having the SED label. This is inconsistent with the emerging science of risk and resilience and makes it difficult to develop meaningful prevention" (US PHS, 2000, p. 43).

PROFESSIONAL/PRIVATE INFLUENCES ON SERVICE DELIVERY

In addition to the federal initiatives to improve the quality and accessibility of mental health services for children, adolescents, and families, there have been a number of private and professional influences on mental health care. Among these have been the sometimes interrelated effects of the American Psychological Association (APA), the American Academy of Pediatrics, and managed care organizations.

A number of initiatives sponsored by or affiliated with the APA already have had both direct and indirect effects on the provision of mental health service delivery. For example, in 1992, Section 1 of Division 12 (then the section on Clinical Child Psychology of the Division of Clinical Psychology of APA) and Division 37 (Child, Youth, and Family Services of APA) commissioned a joint task force to identify and characterize model programs in mental health service delivery. The resulting report (M. C. Roberts, 1996) identified 23 such programs as well as six characteristics common to the service programs. These characteristics (e.g., youth-centered philosophies and missions; contextual/ecological view of the child; collaborative, interagency approaches to problems; attempts to diminish barriers; accountability) appear consistent with the spirit of several earlier federal recommendations, and suggest that (1) some mental health programs had begun to respond to early federal communications regarding children's services, and (2) professional organizations had taken up the challenge to improve upon mental health service delivery.

More recently, Division 12 (the Society of Clinical Psychology of the APA) articulated a statement on the need for and evaluation of empirically supported treatments (Task Force on Promotion and Dissemination of Psychological Procedures, 1995). This report went beyond earlier meta-analyses of treatment efficacy and proposed a method for establishing the degree to which specific treatments have empirical support. Chambless and colleagues (1996, 1998) further articulated criteria for establishing empirical support, and Kazdin and Weisz (1998) specifically applied the resulting criteria to child and adolescent populations. Divisions 53 (Society of Clinical Child and Adolescent Psychology) and 54 (Society of Pediatric Psychology) have dedicated a number of special articles to the identification and evaluation of empirically supported interventions (see, e.g., Lonigan, Elbert, & Johnson, 1998; Spirito, 1999).

Although still new and relatively controversial (see Steele & Roberts, 2003, for review), the movement toward empirically supported therapies (ESTS; or evidence-based therapy) has already provided an impetus for additional research into the effectiveness of interventions, as well as examination of cultural and economic moderators of treatment efficacy, as have been called for by federal reports for sometime. Perhaps, engendering some or much of the controversy, the EST initiative has also increased the accountability of service providers by providing regulatory and reimbursing agencies a benchmark by which to judge the success of programs and services. For example, implementation of the Felix Consent Decree in Hawaii (see Chorpita & Donkervoet, this volume) has resulted in a mandated reliance on ESTS as well as more systematic evaluation of mental health services.

Finally, the EST movement has had an effect on the availability and prioritizing of public research and training funds: Recent funding opportunities have been authorized with the specific intent of demonstrating the effectiveness of evidence-based therapies in the "real world" of the clinic (Foxhall, 2000). This is most evident in the National Institute of Mental Health's prioritization of research that translates findings from tightly controlled laboratory conditions (efficacy studies), to wider, more homogeneous populations (effectiveness studies), to clinics (practice), and finally to policy and financial decision making (systems research; Clinical Treatment and Services Research Workgroup, 1998). The proposed Child HealthCare Crisis Relief Act (HR 1359 and S 1223) also incorporates language to prioritize reimbursement of graduate loans to new mental health professionals who "have familiarity with evidence-based methods in child and adolescent mental health services" (lines 16–18, p. 6). Although the eventual impact of this legislation is uncertain (at the time of this writing, HR 1359 had been referred to the House Energy and Commerce Committee, Subcommittee on Health; see http://thomas.loc.gov for an update), it nevertheless represents a national recognition of the value of evidence-based practices that has been provided (in part) by professional organizations.

Ongoing APA efforts continue to work on a number of fronts to improve youth and family mental health services. In concert with the Surgeon General's report on children's mental health care (US PHS, 2000), the APA has chaired or participated in a number of consortia, coalitions, and work groups to find ways to specifically advocate for the mental health needs of children (Anderson, 2004). These have included the National Consortium for Child and Adolescent Mental Health, the President's New Freedom Commission on Mental Health, and the APA Working Group on Children's Mental Health. These various initiatives have been intended to incorporate evidenced-based interventions into integrated mental health systems for children, increase research and training funds that are specifically targeted for developmental and clinical child issues, and promote a primary mental health care system for children and adolescents. Consistent with these initiatives, the APA Council of Representatives recently adopted a resolution in support of the further development and dissemination of evidence-based interventions—including specific development of culturally relevant services—for children and adolescents (American Psychological Association [APA], 2004).

Beyond the efforts outlined above, APA and the American Academy of Pediatrics (AAP), along with several other related organizations issued a joint consensus statement in 2000 regarding mental health and substance abuse services for children, adolescents, and families (AAP, 2000). In it, the professional organizations noted the current shortage of mental health services for youth and families, the lack of coordination across systems of mental health services, barriers to adequate service delivery, and problems with the current quality assurance measures. In addition to noting these deficits, the task force proposed a number of recommendations that could be implemented by the professional organizations themselves (e.g., training in and use of empirically supported therapies), as well as those that would require partnership with health management organizations (e.g., compensation for case management, elimination of mental health restrictions) or federal government agencies (e.g., increased support of training programs, mechanisms for dovetailing multiple funding streams for complicated cases).

As suggested above, a recent influence on the provision of mental health services for children has been the emergence of managed care. Although some commentators have suggested positive results of the business model on mental health services (e.g., increased accountability, reliance on ESTs; Stroul, Pires, Armstrong, & Meyers, 1998), many have been concerned that any gains that child services have made over the past several decades may be jeopardized (M. C. Roberts & Hurley, 1997; Stroul et al., 1998; Yanos, Garcia, Hansell, Rosato, & Minsky, 2003). Of particular importance is the impact of managed care on the range of services available to children, clinical decision making, and access to and quality of services.

A recent survey conducted by Stroul et al. (1998) attempted to address such questions. Specifically, they queried 10 state mental health systems regarding the impact of managed care on mental health service delivery to youth. Perhaps surprisingly, the results of the survey indicated little, if any, influence of managed care on quality of care or on accountability. However, Stroul et al. noted that the development and use of quality measurement or outcome data were "rare" (p. 131). This observation is consistent with a more recent review of the impact of managed care on children's mental health services: Hutchinson and Foster (2003) reported that no study was located that assessed the effect of managed care on quality of mental heath services for children and adolescents.

With regard to the impact of managed care on "systems of care," Stroul et al. (1998) reported that 6 of the 10 states surveyed indicated that managed care had improved the availability of case management, perhaps improving continuity of care. This effect seems to have been more pronounced among states with "carve-out" plans for mental health services. Dickey, Normand, Norton, Rupp, and Azeni (2001) have presented opposing data, indicating that continuity of care appeared to decline, at least in one sample of children with disabilities.

Stroul et al. (1998) reported that there had been mixed results with regard to access to services. Overall, they reported that more children had accessed mental health services under managed care, but children with serious emotional disorders had more difficulty obtaining appropriate services and placements. The authors linked this finding to the trend of children with serious emotional disturbance (SED) requiring services from multiple agencies, and at varying levels of intensity for longer periods of time. In particular, children with SED may be more likely to require inpatient services, which seem to have become more difficult to obtain under managed care.

Finally, the survey suggested that managed care may have a deleterious effect on the development of new services for children and families. Although states with "carve-out" plans had a more diverse array of services at different levels of intensity, interviewees reported that managed care organizations "expected providers to develop [new] services on their own initiative, but that providers were not willing to take such risks without knowing which services would ultimately be purchased by [managed care organizations]" (p. 128). If uncorrected, this trend could have a negative impact on the range of services provided to youth and families.

More recently, Stroul, Pires, Armstrong, and Zaro (2002) provided a qualitative case study, which prompted some speculation regarding the circumstances under which managed care might facilitate the systems-of-care philosophy that has come to represent the "ideal" held by many mental health professionals. Among the circumstances outlined, Stroul et al. specifically noted the utilization of stakeholder input in the planning and implementation of the managed care organization. Furthermore, Stroul et al. noted that the system-of-care philosophy was more likely to prevail when a broad array of services were available within the behavioral health system, and when provisions were made to encourage service coordination and interagency service planning activities. Finally, the authors noted the necessity of educating managed care organizations about the needs of children and adolescents (and their families) as well as how the system-of-care philosophy addresses those needs.

RANGE OF CURRENT SERVICES AVAILABLE TO CHILDREN, YOUTH, AND FAMILIES

Perhaps as a result of the federal, professional, and private influences just outlined, both the breadth and the depth of mental health services for youth and families have increased over the past several decades. Although some evidence suggests that the availability of inpatient care for youth with SED is still lacking (US PHS, 2000), the development of a range of outpatient services—including specialized and innovative programs—suggests that children and youth may now be better able to access appropriate services than ever before, but this is not a clear-cut or indisputable conclusion.

As characterized by Lyman and Wilson (2001), services available to youth and families vary along a number of dimensions, including restrictiveness or disruptiveness, effectiveness (including cost-effectiveness), and child-program compatibility. From least restrictive to maximally restrictive, programs may be characterized as *outpatient*, *day treatment* (or *partial hospitalization*), *shelter* or *respite care*, *foster care*, *group home*, *residential*, *inpatient hospitalization*, and *institutional*. Variables that define this progression include the degree to which daily routines are disrupted by the intervention itself, as well as the degree to which the programs focus on reentry into the community. Certainly, one of the challenging and ultimately vital aspects of service coordination and delivery is the selection of appropriate level (or levels) of care.

Although this volume is not organized along this continuum, the services and programs presented here represent interventions from across the spectrum of mental health settings. Chapters in the first section of this handbook are specific to a particular modality of service delivery. For example, Jacobs, Randall, Vernberg, Roberts and Nyre (chapter 4) provide coverage of a specific school-based intervention for children with SED, whereas Vargas and de Dios Brambila (chapter 9) outline the services subsumed under the heading of "inpatient and residential treatments." Each of the chapters in this section provides a perspective on how services are organized and delivered as well as how they are (or could be) evaluated.

Chapters in the second section outline an array of services for particular populations, and cover a range of service settings. For example, Kees and Bonner (chapter 10) focus on a range of prevention and intervention services for children who have been abused, and their families. Similarly, Murphy, Page, and Ettelson (chapter 15) address services for adolescent sex offenders, detailing the strengths of various service settings (e.g., outpatient, residential) and components of interventions. Both types of chapters demonstrate the variety and organization of various services among different populations. We anticipate that these chapters may generate creativity with regard to coordination of services within and across settings.

We devote the third section of the handbook to innovative or novel forms of service delivery. These chapters deal with specific services that are just emerging (e.g., Liss, chapter 19; Brown, chapter 20), as well as recent developments that have altered the ways in which services are delivered or evaluated (Chorpita & Donkervoet, chapter 21). Despite concerns that current funding strategies are not encouraging of the development of novel programs for youth, the selections for this handbook suggest that a number of talented people continue to expand the range of services that are available. How widespread are these innovations? The fact that they are considered innovative—oftentimes unique—and that they stand out from the other service delivery methods suggests that there remains room for them to develop in more locales.

Consistent with the system-of-care model, the final section of this book concerns the evaluation of mental health services. After a general overview of program evaluation approaches and methods (Roberts & Steele, chapter 23), we present two chapters on specific large-scale program evaluations that, in addition to providing valuable conclusions regarding the targets of their respective evaluations, provide a useful guide for the subsequent conduct of program evaluations. We conclude with a brief look to the future organization of mental health service delivery, and proposal for areas of research.

CONCLUSION

Mental health services for children, adolescents, and families are expanding and changing due to the range of problems now presenting, and the recognition that traditional services and models have been relatively inadequate at addressing the needs. This handbook attempts to fairly comprehensively, but succinctly, present the range of services in a variety of settings for multiple problems presenting in childhood. Page limits preclude a fully comprehensive presentation of services for specific problems, so the particular service programs for a problem or population were selected for illustration. This organization reflects our ultimate goal of presenting these services in such a way as to encourage collaboration and coordination within and across mental health service systems. Further, the empirical basis of the handbook is designed to encourage further research that will have a maximum impact on service delivery (i.e., efficacy, effectiveness, practice, and systems research).

REFERENCES

American Academy of Pediatrics. (2000). *Insurance coverage of mental health and substance abuse services for children and adolescents: A consensus statement (RE0090)*. Retrieved November 7, 2000 from http://www.aap.org/policy/re0090.html

American Psychiatric Association. (1999). *Issues affecting mental health coverage for children*. Washington, DC: American Psychiatric Association.

American Psychological Association. (2004, February). *Resolution on children's mental health*. Passed by Council of Representatives.

Anderson, N. B. (2004). Running commentary: Childhood mental health advocacy efforts. *Monitor on Psychology, 35*(1), 9.

Chambless, D. L., Baker, M. J., Baucom, D. H., Beutler, L. E., Calhoun, K. S., Crits-Christoph, P. (1996). Update on empirically validated therapies II. *The Clinical Psychologist, 51*, 3–16.

Chambless, D. L., & Hollon, S. (1998). Defining empirically supported therapies. *Journal of Consulting and Clinical Psychology, 66*, 7–18.

Clinical Treatment and Services Research Workgroup of the National Institute of Mental Health, National Advisory Mental Health Council. (1998). *Bridging science and service*. Bethesda, MD: National Institutes of Health. Retrieved July 15, 2003, from http://www.nimh.nih.gov/research/bridge.htm#br8

Costello, E. J., Angold, A., Burns, B. J., Erkanli, A., Stangl, D. K., & Tweed, D. L. (1996). The Great Smoky Mountains Study of Youth: Functional impairment and serious emotional disturbance. *Archives of General Psychiatry, 53*, 1137–1143.

Day, C., & Roberts, M. C. (1991). Activities of the Child and Adolescent Service System Program for improving mental health services for children and families. *Journal of Clinical Child Psychology, 20,* 340–350.

Department of Health and Human Services (1999). *Mental health: A Report of the Surgeon General.* Rockville, MD: U.S. Department of Health and Human Services, Substance Abuse and Mental Health Services Administration, Center for Mental Health Services, National Institutes of Health, National Institute of Mental Health.

Department of Health and Human Services. (2000). *Healthy People 2010.* Retrieved January 18, 2004, from http://www.healthypeople.gov

Dickey, B., Normand, S. L., Norton, E. C., Rupp, A., & Azeni, H. (2001). Managed care and children's behavioral health services in Massachusetts. *Psychiatric Services, 52,* 183–188.

Dougherty, D. M., Saxe, L. M., Cross, T., & Silverman, N. (1986). *Children's mental health: Problems and services—A background paper.* Washington, DC: Office of Technology Assessment.

Foxhall, K. (2000). Research for the real world. *Monitor on Psychology, 31,* 28–36.

French, J. L. (1990). History of school psychology. In T. B. Gutkin & C. R. Reynolds (Eds.), *Handbook of school psychology* (2nd ed., pp. 3–20). New York: Wiley.

Hobbs, N. (1975). *The futures of children: Categories, labels, and their consequences.* San Francisco: Jossey-Bass.

Hutchinson, A. B., & Foster, E. M. (2003). The effects of Medicaid managed care on mental health care for children: A review of the literature. *Mental Health Services Research, 5,* 39–54.

Joint Commission on the Mental Health of Children. (1969). *Crisis in child mental health: Challenge for the 1970's.* New York: Harper & Row.

Kazdin, A. E., & Weisz, J. R. (1998). Identifying and developing empirically supported child and adolescent treatments. *Journal of Consulting and Clinical Psychology, 66,* 19–36.

Knitzer, J. (1982). *Unclaimed children: The failure of public responsibility to children and adolescents in need of mental health services.* Washington, DC: Children's Defense Fund.

Knitzer, J. (1993). Children's mental health policy: Challenging the future. *Journal of Emotional and Behavioral Disorders, 1,* 8–16.

Lonigan, C. J., Elbert, J. C., & Johnson, S. B. (1998). Empirically supported psychosocial interventions for children: An overview. *Journal of Clinical Child Psychology, 27,* 138–145.

Lourie, I. S. (2003). A history of community child mental health. In A. J. Pumariega & N. C. Winters (Eds.), *The handbook of child and adolescent systems of care* (pp. 1–16). San Francisco: Jossey-Bass.

Lyman, R. D., & Wilson, D. R. (2001). Residential and inpatient treatment of emotionally disturbed children and adolescents. In C. E. Walker & M. C. Roberts (Eds.), *Handbook of clinical child psychology* (3rd ed., pp. 881–894). New York: Wiley.

Peterson, L., & Burbach, D. J. (1988). Historical trends. In J. L. Matson (Ed.), *Handbook of treatment approaches in childhood psychopathology* (pp. 3–28). New York: Plenum.

Peterson, L., & Roberts, M. C. (1991). Treatment of children's problems. In C. E. Walker (Ed.), *Clinical psychology: Historical and research foundations* (pp. 313–342). New York: Plenum.

President's Commission on Mental Health. (1978). *Report to the President from the President's Commission on Mental Health,* vol. 1 (Commission Report) and vol. 3 (Task Panel Reports). Washington, DC: U.S. Government Printing Office.

Roberts, M. C. Ed. (1996). *Model programs in child and family mental health.* Mahwah, NJ: Lawrence Erlbaum Associates.

Roberts, M. C., & Alexander, K. (1990). Programs and services for children's health care. *Child, Youth, and Family Services Quarterly, 13*(2), 13.

Roberts, M. C., & Hurley, L. K. (1997). *Managing managed care.* New York: Plenum.

Roberts, R. E., Attkisson, C. C., & Rosenblatt, A. (1998). Prevalence of psychopathology among children and adolescents. *American Journal of Psychiatry, 155,* 715–725.

Spirito, A. (1999). Introduction to special series on empirically supported treatments in pediatric psychology. *Journal of Pediatric Psychology, 24,* 87–90.

Steele, R. G., & Roberts, M. C. (2003). Therapy and interventions research with children and adolescents. In M. C. Roberts & S. S. Ilardi (Eds.), *Handbook of research methods in clinical psychology* (pp. 307–326). Oxford, UK: Blackwell.

Stroul, B. A., Pires, S. A., Armstrong, M. I., & Meyers, J. C. (1998). The impact of managed care on mental health services for children and their families. *Future of Children, 8*(2), 119–133.

Stroul, B. A., Pires, S. A., Armstrong, M. I., & Zaro, S. (2002). The impact of managed care of systems of care that serve children with serious emotional disturbances and their families. *Children's Services: Social Policy, Research, and Practice, 5*, 21–36.

Task Force on Promotion and Dissemination of Psychological Procedures. (1995). Training in and dissemination of empirically validated treatments: Report and recommendations. *The Clinical Psychologist, 48*(1), 3–23.

U.S. Public Health Service. (2000). *Report of the Surgeon General's Conference on Children's Mental Health: A National Action Agenda.* Washington, DC: Department of Health and Human Services.

Witmer, L. (1996). Clinical psychology. *American Psychologist, 51*, 248–251. (Original work published in 1907 in *Psychological Clinic, 1*, 1–9)

Yanos, P. T., Garcia, C. I., Hansell, S., Rosato, M. G., & Minsky, S. (2003). Managed care and clinical decision-making in child and adolescent behavioral health: Provider perceptions. *Administration and Policy in Mental Health, 30*, 307–321.

2

Mental Health Services for Young Children[†]

DIANE POWELL and GLEN DUNLAP

In recent years, the national emphasis on school readiness has been accompanied by an increased appreciation for the crucial role assumed by healthy social and emotional development. It is now well understood that the foundations are laid during the earliest years for children to accomplish the developmental tasks of establishing emotional and behavioral self-regulation and social competency (Shonkoff & Phillips, 2000). Although most children proceed through this process smoothly, evidence has accumulated that significant numbers of young children experience social, emotional, and behavioral challenges and, without intervention, these problems are likely to persist. Increasingly, the importance of early mental health and behavioral services is recognized (New Freedom Commission on Mental Health, 2003); however, the multiple pathways and systems through which young children enter into and receive mental health services have developed largely in a haphazard manner, in isolation from each other, and with little attention to coordination or effectiveness. Furthermore, there is little research on utilization and service systems for young

DIANE POWELL and GLEN DUNLAP • Department of Child and Family Studies, Florida Mental Health Institute, University of South Florida, Tampa, Florida 33612.

[†] This chapter was prepared with support from the Center for Evidence-Based Practice: Young Children with Challenging Behaviors, Grant No. H324Z010001, funded by the Office of Special Education Programs, U.S. Department of Education. However, no endorsement of the authors' statements by the supporting agency should be inferred. Much of the content described herein, as well as additional sources of information, can be found on the Center's web site, www.challengingbehavior.org, work. In particular, the reader is referred to two documents posted on the web site: (1) Pathways to Service Utilization: A Synthesis of Evidence Relevant to Young Children with Challenging Behavior, by Diane Powell, Dean Fixson, and Glen Dunlap, and (2) Systems of Service Delivery: A Synthesis of Evidence Relevant to Young Children at Risk of or Who Have Challenging Behavior, by Barbara J. Smith and Lise Fox.

children with mental health needs to provide guidance for the systemic delivery of effective practices and strategies (Powell, Fixsen, & Dunlap, 2003;
Smith & Fox, 2003).

This chapter provides a review of the ways in which children from
birth to kindergarten are identified, referred, and receive mental health
services. The scope and topography of mental health problems in infants
and preschool age children are briefly explored, and information on the
prevalence, course, and correlates of early emotional and behavior problems is presented. The pathways by which children with behavioral health
problems are identified and enter into services, including the relevant evidence base, are described together with the national policies and funding
streams within which these pathways are embedded. A description of the
existing services and the mechanisms and strategies through which they
are delivered completes this section. A final section is included to discuss
recent policy, funding, and programmatic initiatives and innovations that
contribute to the emergence of a more comprehensive system of care for
young children.

SOCIAL/EMOTIONAL/BEHAVIORAL PROBLEMS
IN YOUNG CHILDREN

The development of social competence during the early years is dependent on acquiring emotional, behavioral, and attentional self-regulation
within the context of secure and nurturing relationships. However, determining what is developmentally normative behavior is not always easy.
The persistence, intensity, and pervasiveness of problematic behavior, as
well as the degree to which it interferes with other developmental tasks,
are critical considerations in discriminating children who will grow out of
emotional and behavioral difficulties from those whose behavior warrants
intervention.

In infants and toddlers, disruptions of healthy social and emotional
development are most often manifested as difficulties in establishing wake
and sleep rhythms and feeding routines, attachment difficulties, and ex-
cessive crying and resistance to soothing. These processes are embedded
in relationships and interactions between the child and caregivers, and
disruptions may be a function of child factors, such as temperament, or
caregiver factors that affect the ability to provide responsive nurturing care.
In preschool age children, extremes of withdrawal and shyness, and of
acting-out behaviors such as physical and verbal aggression, destruction,
self-injury, and noncompliance, are indicators of problematic development
(Smith & Fox, 2003).

Numerous studies have investigated the prevalence of social, emotional, and behavioral problems in young children. Though results vary
depending on the methods, instruments, and populations used, studies of
children aged 2–5 years within pediatric and preschool settings have found
the rates of psychosocial problems to be between 9% and 23% (Campbell,
1995; Lavigne et al., 1996; Webster-Stratton & Hammond, 1998). These

findings validate the anecdotal reports of preschool teachers and childcare providers that increasing numbers of the young children display behavior problems of increasing severity (Yoshikawa & Knitzer, 1997).

For many young children, psychosocial problems are not transient, but rather persist over time. Approximately 50% of the children identified with problems as preschoolers continue to have problems into the school years (Campbell, 1995) and children whose disruptive behavior begins early are most likely to exhibit serious and intransigent antisocial problems in adolescence and adulthood (Campbell, Shaw, & Gilliom, 2000). However, despite such high prevalence and persistence rates, data for 1998 indicate that only 1–2% of preschoolers used any mental health specialty services during the year (Sturm et al., 2000).

Many circumstances in the lives of young children have been associated with psychosocial problems and poor outcomes, notably persistent poverty and chronic family adversity. These conditions act through direct effects on children and through contributions to family stress, and researchers have only recently begun to develop models that sort out relationships and interactions among these and other variables (Sameroff & Fiese, 2000). However, attention has increasingly turned to identifying those risk factors that are potent, causal, and amenable to change and thus should be the targets of intervention. These appear to be predominantly relationship-based factors, such as problematic parenting, parental mental health problems, poor bonding with parents, difficulties with teachers, and poor peer relationships (Huffman, Mehlinger, & Kerivan, 2000).

PATHWAYS TO SERVICES: IDENTIFICATION, REFERRAL, AND THE ROLE OF NATIONAL POLICIES AND FUNDING STREAMS

Children with social and emotional problems are most commonly identified through the various systems and programs that serve them. These include the primary systems of healthcare, and early care and learning programs. In addition, specific populations of young children may be identified through specialized service programs including early intervention, home visiting, and child welfare programs. A number of state and federal funding streams support these systems, and the laws and policies governing the funding streams influence the scope and configuration of identification and referral opportunities and, thus, the rates at which children are identified and receive services. These funding streams are spread across the areas of healthcare, early care and learning, child welfare, mental health, and early intervention for children with disabilities, with the federal programs administered by various entities within the U.S. Departments of Education and Health and Human Services. To a large extent, these funding programs are designed to identify and serve young children who are exposed to significant risk factors such as poverty, violence, and family disruption.

Healthcare

Because almost all young children come into contact with the healthcare system to receive immunizations and well-child care, it becomes a primary gateway for identification and entry into services. However, it is estimated that 14% of all children 0–6 years and 20% of low-income young children remain uninsured (Budetti, Berry, Butler, Collins, & Abrams, 2001), thus making identification of emotional and behavior problems through healthcare a difficult path to access for many young children.

Two federal programs, Medicaid and the State Children's Health Insurance Program, increase access to medical care by providing health insurance for low-income children. Medicaid mandates include the Early and Periodic Screening, Diagnostic and Treatment (EPSDT) program of services, which is intended to provide comprehensive preventive healthcare, including behavioral healthcare, to children. The periodic screenings must include a mental health screen, and all medically necessary services identified through the screening must be provided, including a wide array of behavioral health services, whether or not they are part of the state plan (Bazelon Center for Mental Health Law, 1999). However, despite mandates, most young children on Medicaid do not receive regular EPSDT screenings and even fewer receive the mental health screening component (Pires, Stroul, & Armstrong, 2000; U.S. General Accounting Office [USGAO], 2001).

Although the American Academy of Pediatrics (American Academy of Pediatrics Committee on Children with Disabilities, 2001), has developed a policy statement on developmental surveillance, screening and referral of infants and young children, these activities do not always occur within medical practices. Large proportions of behavioral health problems in young children are undetected by pediatricians, although the use of screening tools appears to increase identification rates (Stancin & Palermo, 1997). Even when psychosocial problems are identified, children may not be referred to services, and not all of those who are referred actually receive appropriate interventions (Horowitz, Leaf, Leventhal, Forsyth, & Speechley, 1992). Notable barriers to identification and appropriate referral include physician training variables, time constraints, financial disincentives, reluctance to label young children, and perceived lack of services (Navon, Nelson, Pagano, & Murphy, 2001; Relgado & Halfon, 2002; Stancin & Palermo, 1997).

Early Care and Learning

As large numbers of young children are cared for outside of their family home, early care and learning settings provide a second primary pathway for screening children and referral for further assessment and intervention. However, many children receive care in programs that do not necessarily provide routine developmental screenings. These include relative care, family childcare homes, and private center-based care. The government-funded programs of subsidized childcare, Head Start and Early Head Start,

Title I preschool programs, and state prekindergarten programs vary in their mandates for screening and referring children.

Federally funded Head Start and Early Head Start are designed as comprehensive child development programs for low-income children and their families and include mandates for developmental screening, referral for further assessment and mental health services. Although Head Start's universal screening requirement is an important tool for early identification, there is some evidence that mental health problems are under-identified or misidentified in Head Start children and that some children with emotional and behavioral problems are diagnosed with and receive treatment for speech and language problems instead (Lopez, Tarullo, Forness, & Boyce, 2000). In addition, Head Start programs do not always have access to adequate resources to meet the mental health intervention needs of their children (Lopez et al., 2000).

Funds from Title I of the Elementary and Secondary Education Act, reauthorized in 2002 as the No Child Left Behind Act, may be used by local school districts to establish preschool programs that must adhere to Head Start Performance Standards, including the mandates for screening and mental health services. In 1999–2000, 175 school districts, 17% of those receiving Title I funds, directed money to preschool programs (USGAO, 2000).

Serving the largest number of young children of all the federal early care and learning programs, the Child Care and Development Fund (CCDF) distributes funds to states to subsidize child care for low-income working families. Although the federal legislation contains no requirements for developmental screenings or child/family services other than child care, some states do impose screening requirements in at least some components of their subsidized child care programs (National Child Care Information Center [NCCIC], 2002a). In addition, CCDF earmarks funds for quality improvement that may be used for mental health activities (Administration for Children and Families [ACF], 1999).

Finally, 36 states have established and funded prekindgarten programs and, in 2001, 16 of these states required developmental screenings (Horton & Bowman, 2002).

Early Intervention and Education for Children with Disabilities

An additional significant pathway for identification and entry into services for young children with mental health needs is provided by the Individuals with Disabilities Education Act (IDEA), sections of which are designed to address and fund services for young children with disabilities, including those with social/emotional delays and disabilities. These are entitlement programs, mandated to serve all eligible children. Part C of IDEA, covering children from birth through the third birthday, is meant to create statewide systems of early intervention consisting of outreach, early identification, screening, assessment, referral, case management and services to eligible children and their families that are coordinated with other programs and resources. Section 619 of Part B of IDEA provides funds to states for child find activities and special education services for children aged 3–5 years, typically provided in school-based, classroom settings. Services to children in Part C and Part B are to be based on individual need and driven by the child's Individual Family Service Plan (Part C) or Individual Education Plan (Part B).

Part C and Part B programs serve young children with all types of disabilities and few disaggregated data are available bearing on the effectiveness of these systems in identifying and intervening with children with social and emotional problems. However, findings from the National Early Intervention Longitudinal Study indicate that social and behavioral problems are severely under-addressed by Part C programs (Hebbeler et al., 2001; U.S. Department of Education [USDOE], 2001).

Child Welfare

Young children are heavily represented in child welfare systems and constitute a particularly vulnerable group of children with well-documented mental health needs (Halfon, Mendonca, & Berkowitz, 1995). Each state has its own child welfare system that encompasses protective services, family reunification, foster care, and adoption, but federal programs administered through the Administration for Children and Families provide much of the funding for the state systems. Allowable uses of federal funds include developmental screenings, information and referral for families, home visiting, mental health treatment, and family support services (Cavanaugh, Lippitt, & Moyo, 2000).

However, state child welfare programs, struggling with limited resources, are not able to ensure that young children are screened and identified systematically and receive services at needed levels (Dicker, Gordon, & Knitzer, 2000). Although children in foster care are eligible for Medicaid and use a high proportion of Medicaid mental health services (Halfon, Berkowitz, & Klee, 1992), in most communities there are less-than-optimal linkages and collaboration between child welfare and the healthcare, early intervention, and mental health systems (Dicker et al., 2000).

Mental Health

Historically, few services for young children and their families have been provided through the formal public mental health system (Knitzer, 2000; 2001). Only about $1/2$% of children aged 0–5 years received care in community mental health facilities in 1997 (Pottick & Warner, 2002). The major federal funding for mental health is the Community Mental Health Services Block Grant Program administered through The Center for Mental Health Services, which awards grants to states to support services and the development of systems of community-based care for children with serious emotional disturbance (SED). However, due to the many competing demands on these funds and the SED requirement for children, very little of the money goes to children under 6 years (Cavanaugh et al., 2000). Although Medicaid and state mental health dollars also contribute to funding of public mental health services, some state mental health agencies by policy do not address services for children under 6 years (Knitzer, 2000). Many impediments to paying for mental health services for the 0–6 age group exist in the Medicaid system, including requirements for diagnostic labeling and difficulty reimbursing nontraditional interventions such as consultation and parenting education (Knitzer 2000, 2001). As a further complication, under state Medicaid managed care reforms, few behavioral health services are delivered to young children (Stroul, Pires, & Armstrong, 2001).

Taken together, these pathways present a complex and disconnected structure of multiple entrances into services supported by different funding streams with numerous eligibility criteria. Although a broad net is cast across systems, it is one with many holes in which services are available only to specific sets of eligible children, accessed within isolated service arenas or programs, and rife with missed opportunities for identifying children in need of assessment and intervention. Although these problems may be most conspicuous within the systems of health and child care, which come in contact with large numbers of children, they are a pervasive concern systemwide. In the experience of parents seeking help for their young children, the system is often perceived as fragmented, difficult to navigate, and replete with barriers and restrictive, often conflicting, eligibility requirements (Powell, 2002).

ADDRESSING MENTAL HEALTH CHALLENGES IN YOUNG CHILDREN: EXISTING SERVICES AND SERVICE DELIVERY STRATEGIES

The existing services and service delivery strategies for ensuring healthy social and emotional development for young children can be conceptualized as a tripartite system of (1) universal interventions aimed at all young children, (2) selective preventive interventions for children who are at risk for disrupted social and emotional development, and (3) targeted interventions for children who manifest emotional or behavior problems. The existing array of services is described in this section, including established intervention programs that are widely available, emerging strategies that are gaining wide acceptance, demonstrations of innovative service delivery models, and specific intervention packages and approaches that have demonstrated effectiveness.

Universal Interventions

Programs and services that assist caregivers, both familial and out-of-home, to provide nurturing care that supports emotional and social development can be considered preventive interventions that would benefit all young children. Although the evidence is clear that the quality of child care impacts child behavior and adjustment, due to economic realities, the quality of child care remains highly variable (Shonkoff & Phillips, 2000). Strategies for promoting social and emotional well-being within child care include responsive and relationship-based caregiving for infants and toddlers (Graham, White, Clarke, & Adams, 2001; Honig, 2002) and social skills instruction in preschool classrooms through curriculum infusion, incidental learning strategies, and formal social skills training curricula (Katz & McClellan, 1997).

Developmental and parenting information is widely available in most communities and offered through a variety of settings and formats. An approach for making such information accessible to parents that is being tried in several national initiatives is the incorporation of developmental specialists into pediatric practices to provide materials, answer parents' questions, discuss developmental and behavioral issues, perform developmental screenings and, if necessary, refer for further assessment or services (Eggbeer, Littman, & Jones, 1997; Minkovitz et al., 2001).

Selective Interventions

Selective interventions target particular populations of young children and their families who are considered at risk due to broad factors such as poverty, or specific conditions such as parental substance abuse or domestic violence. Demonstration programs for low-income children and their families that are intensive and comprehensive and combine quality preschool with parenting support have been shown to impact both short- and long-term social outcomes (Shonkoff & Phillips, 2000; Yoshikawa, 1995). However, such programs are costly and are not widely available.

Home visiting programs for parents of infants, toddlers, and preschoolers who are considered at-risk provide health, developmental and parenting information, skills training, and support. These include Healthy Start, Healthy Families America, Early Head Start, the Nurse Partnership, and a variety of small-scale state and local programs. Although evaluation results from these programs are somewhat mixed, there is evidence that such programs can positively impact both immediate social—and emotional indicators and long-term social outcomes (Mathematica Policy Research, 2002; Olds et al., 1998). Home visiting programs have increasingly been recognized as providing opportunities for teaching responsive caregiving to parents, and identifying and addressing parental depression, substance abuse, and domestic violence, all of which are known risk factors for poor social and emotional outcomes for children (Graham et al., 2001).

Early care and learning programs for children at risk present another venue for providing selective preventive interventions. As with universal prevention strategies, these most often take the form of social skills training for children, skill building for teachers, parenting education, or some combination of these three approaches. A growing strategy for delivering such interventions is the use of mental health consultants. Consultants engage in a variety of activities aimed at strengthening programmatic capacity to provide high quality, responsive caregiving, including training teachers to observe and understand behavior, addressing staff stress and emotional health, and conducting support and educational groups for families (Cohen & Kaufmann, 2000).

Packaged intervention programs that combine child social skills training, teacher training, and/or parent training curricula are also available and have demonstrated success in decreasing conduct problems when implemented in classrooms of low-income young children (McMahon, Washburn, Felix, Yakin, & Childrey, 2000; Webster-Stratton, Reid, & Hammond, 2001a).

Adult treatment settings, including domestic violence and homeless shelters, substance abuse and mental health treatment programs, and teen parent programs, have become recognized contexts for reaching young children at high risk (Knitzer, 2000). An array of services may be available to the children of parents receiving services, ranging from screening and referral to relationship-based child care, therapeutic nurseries, psychoeducational groups, and family therapy. Project Before, operating though several community mental health centers serving a region of rural Kansas, is an example of a program delivering both family support and child development services to families with mental health or substance abuse problems. The program combines home visiting, case management, and wraparound strategies using staff who are trained in early childhood development as well as mental illness and substance abuse intervention and employs staff who are themselves in recovery. Program goals center on strengthening parent–child relations and informal family support networks, ensuring access to healthcare and child care, and addressing economic and safety issues (Knitzer, 2000; Simpson, Jivanjee, Koroloff, Doerfler, & Garcia, 2001).

Targeted Interventions

Early childhood programs can also serve as settings for intervening with individual children who are already displaying problematic behaviors and are in need of high-intensity interventions. Again, the use of mental health consultants is a primary strategy for ensuring such children receive appropriate treatment. Consultants may screen and identify children with serious problems, assist parents in obtaining appropriate community services, and may also work with program staff to develop child and family intervention plans. In some cases consultants provide interventions themselves, or they may train teachers to implement interventions with ongoing clinical supervision and monitoring provided by the consultant. Typical strategies include development of individualized classroom-based behavior plans, "pull out" sessions with individual children or groups of children using play therapy or social skills training approaches, crisis intervention, and training and counseling for families (Cohen & Kaufmann, 2000).

Packaged interventions implemented through preschool or kindergarten settings, such as First Steps to Success (Walker et al., 1998) and the Dinosaur/Incredible Years Curriculum (Webster-Stratton, Reid, & Hammond, 2001b), target young children presenting with conduct problems and have shown promising results in evaluations. These packages combine different components including social skills training delivered to individuals or in a small-group format, and training and coaching for teachers and parents (Joseph & Strain, 2003). For example, in the Webster-Stratton program, therapists meet weekly with small groups of children for 6 months for sessions focused on teaching anger management and problem-solving skills, empathy, and play and friendship skills. Teaching tools include videotape modeling, role-play, puppets, stories and games. Parents and teachers are trained to provide support and reinforcement for use of the new skills at home and school.

An approach receiving increasing attention and use with young children with challenging behaviors is Positive Behavior Support (Carr et al., 2002). This model provides individualized, comprehensive, family-centered support to ensure families and other caregivers have the knowledge and resources needed to address child behavior problems and teach new skills (Fox, Dunlap, & Cushing, 2002). It is ecologically based and uses functional assessment, functional communication training and person-centered planning to produce meaningful outcomes for the child and family in home, child care, and other community settings (Dunlap & Fox, 1996; 1999; Fox, Dunlap, & Powell, 2002).

The established continuum of services for children with serious emotional disturbances includes outpatient therapy, therapeutic classrooms, day treatment, inpatient and crisis intervention programs, and wraparound services. Little is known about the extent to which these services are available to young children in local communities, although there is widely held concern that few providers in community mental health centers and in the private mental health sector have training, expertise, or interest in serving young children (Shonkoff & Phillips, 2000; Simpson et al., 2001). Part B Preschool programs often take the form of day treatment or therapeutic classrooms, but there are no data available on the numbers of children with social and emotional disabilities being served in these settings, or on their effectiveness.

The state that appears to have come the furthest in developing its early childhood behavioral health capacity and systematizing services statewide at all of the above three levels is Vermont. The Children's Upstream Services Project (CUPS), utilizing both national and state financing, has relied on regional interagency teams with representatives from child care, health, substance abuse, adult mental health, and domestic violence agencies, to develop and implement strategic plans for early childhood mental health services based on system-of-care principles (Simpson et al., 2001). With emphasis on a continuum of services and integrating mental health into existing child-serving agencies, regional plans have included home visiting for families with newborns, mental health personnel within pediatric practices to provide screenings and developmental information, play groups, parent peer support, mental health consultation to child care programs, and services such as case management, respite, crisis intervention, and intensive home- and child-care-based therapeutic interventions for children with identified problems (Kaufmann & Perry, 2002). To build capacity, a state-level CUPS learning team has developed a set of early childhood mental health core competencies and facilitates regional trainings as well as providing an ongoing support and supervision network.

TOWARD A COMPREHENSIVE SYSTEM OF CARE FOR ENSURING EMOTIONAL AND SOCIAL WELL-BEING OF YOUNG CHILDREN

Although it is clear that a coherent integrated system of early childhood mental health services does not currently exist, there is an emerging consensus on the principles and best practices needed to guide and undergird such a system, as well as the challenges that must be addressed in efforts to build such a system.

Principles and Best Practices

In contrast to traditional mental health approaches that treat children in isolation, emerging approaches are grounded in ecological theory, risk and resilience concepts, and transactional models and thus the focus of intervention becomes relationships and other aspects of the environments in which children function (Simpson et al., 2001). The child is served within the context of family and other caregiving environments by delivering interventions in the settings in which children naturally spend their time such as home, child care, and other community settings, rather than in offices or clinics (Knitzer, 2000).

Such strengths-based approaches recognize families as the most influential and enduring force in their children's lives and embrace a family-professional partnership model in which families actively participate in decision making (Simpson et al., 2001). Services are designed according to family needs, goals, and preferences, and include attention to the family's cultural and ethnic values. This is a capacity-building model in which families are supported in securing the resources and skills that allow them to create nurturing environments, facilitate social competence, and ameliorate challenging behaviors and emotional problems; the role of the professional shifts from that of expert to collaborator and facilitator (Powell, Batsche, Ferro, Fox, & Dunlap, 1997).

Social and emotional problems in young children are determined by multiple influences at multiple levels, necessitating that interventions be broad-based and family-centered, viewing the family as a whole and addressing the varied levels of child, family, and out-of-home care (Knitzer, 2000; Shonkoff & Phillips, 2000). A continuum of supports is provided, individualized to match the content and intensity needs of the child and family. For example, in some cases parental substance abuse or mental health issues will need to be addressed and in others basic conditions such as family economic security and access to health care may need attention.

Systems Issues and Challenges

The ideal early childhood mental health delivery system would provide universal screening for all young children to ensure early identification, timely and seamless referral and access to services, and an array of integrated services using evidence-based practices and grounded in the principles articulated in the previous section. System-building efforts to move the field forward towards this vision will need to address several critical issues.

Funding

Restrictions in the funding streams that support behavioral health services for young children often present barriers to providing effective identification and intervention based on best practices. Requirements for diagnostic labeling can make early childhood programs and others serving young children hesitant to identify children in need of services and also make it difficult to fund selective intervention services for children experiencing multiple risk conditions before they develop clinical disorders (Knitzer, 2000, 2001; Lopez et al., 2000; NCCIC, 2002b). In addition, interventions that are not strictly child focused such as child care program consultation and parent- or relationship-focused services are not always reimbursable (Knitzer, 2001; Simpson et al., 2001). Finally, the lack of a dedicated and secure funding stream for early childhood mental health services means that community agencies and programs wanting to offer such services must engage in the often time-consuming and frustrating endeavor of seeking and pulling together funds from multiple sources, each with its own restrictions, eligibility guidelines, and reporting requirements.

Workforce Development

There is widespread agreement on the need to expand the workforce of professionals with the training and expertise to provide effective prevention and intervention services for young children's emotional and social development, especially for infants and toddlers (Kaufmann & Perry, 2002; Shonkoff & Phillips, 2000). This will necessitate interdisciplinary training that teaches clinical competencies for working with both children and families, as well as skills for working collaboratively with families and other professionals, and delivering nontraditional services in natural settings (Fox et al., 2002; Knitzer 2000).

Collaboration and Coordination

As is clear from the discussion of the multiple pathways through which young children enter and receive mental health services, numerous systems and disciplines are involved. Each discipline has its own philosophy, history, professional culture, and each system has its own funding streams, purposes and priorities, producing formidable challenges for collaboration (Knitzer, 2000). No public entity has a mandated responsibility for early childhood mental health; thus there is no designated or obvious leadership to initiate system building or collaborative efforts at the national, state, or local level. However, at the community level there has been increasing recognition of the need to address these issues, and recent publications have drawn attention to state and local initiatives that incorporate creative blending of funding streams, cross-system approaches, collaborative partnerships, and innovative service delivery strategies; many include the integration of developmental and mental health screening and services into health care, home visiting programs, child care, child welfare, or adult service settings (Dicker et al., 2001; Johnson, Knitzer, & Kaufmann, 2002; Kaufmann & Perry, 2002; Knitzer, 2000, 2001; Simpson et al., 2001).

CONCLUSION

The amount of attention paid to the mental health of young children, and especially infants and toddlers, is just now attaining significant levels. Professionals, advocates and, more gradually, policy makers are noting the clear connection between early social-emotional foundations and social adaptation in later childhood, adolescence, and adulthood. There are currently a number of pathways, including policies and funding streams, that provide the means for identifying and serving young children with, or at risk for, mental health problems; however, these pathways are generally disconnected, underfunded, and inadequately evaluated. For the most part, despite the existence of considerable knowledge regarding effective strategies of prevention on multiple dimensions of practice (Fox, Dunlap, Hemmeter, Joseph, & Strain, 2003), effective mental health services for young children are not available in many communities (Smith & Fox, 2003). Still, this picture of generally discouraging service delivery is mitigated to some extent by the encouraging emergence of heightened awareness and data-based demonstration programs at both the program and systems level. These developments offer reason for optimism as early childhood mental health matures over the coming decades.

REFERENCES

Administration for Children and Families. (1999). *Child Care and Development Fund program instruction*. Retrieved December 6, 2002 from
   http://www.acf.dhhs.gov/programs/ccb/policy1/current/pi9905/pi9905.pdf
American Academy of Pediatrics Committee on Children with Disabilities (2001). Developmental surveillance and screening of infants and young children. *Pediatrics, 108,* 190–196.
Bazelon Center for Mental Health Law. (1999). *Where to turn: Confusion in Medicaid policies on screening children for mental health needs*. Washington, DC: Author.
Budetti, P., Berry, C., Butler, P., Collins, K., & Abrams, M. (2000). *Assuring the healthy development of young children: Opportunities for states*. New York: The Commonwealth Fund.

Campbell, S. B. (1995). Behavior problems in preschool children: A review of recent research. *Journal of Child Psychology and Psychiatry, 36*, 113–149.

Campbell, S. B., Shaw, D. S., & Gilliom, M. (2000). Early externalizing behavior problems: Toddlers and preschoolers at risk for later maladjustment. *Development and Psychopathology, 12*, 467–488.

Carr, E. G., Dunlap, G., Horner, R. H., Koegel, R. L., Turnbull, A. P., Sailor, W. et al. (2002). Positive behavior support: Evolution of an applied science. *Journal of Positive Behavior Interventions, 4*, 4–16.

Cavanaugh, D. A., Lippitt, J., & Moyo, O. (2000). *Resource guide to selected federal policies affecting children's social and emotional development and their readiness for school.* Chapel Hill, NC: University of North Carolina, FPG Child Development Center.

Cohen, E., & Kaufmann, R. (2000). *Early childhood mental health consultation.* Washington, DC: Center for Mental Health Services.

Dicker, S., Gordon, E., & Knitzer, J. (2001). *Improving the odds for the healthy development of young children in foster care.* New York: National Center for Children in Poverty.

Dunlap, G., & Fox, L. (1996). Early intervention and serious problem behaviors: A comprehensive approach. In. L. K. Koegel, R. L. Koegel, & G. Dunlap (Eds.), *Positive behavioral support: Including people with difficult behavior in the community* (pp. 31–50). Baltimore: Brookes.

Dunlap, G., & Fox, L. (1999). A demonstration of behavioral support for young children with autism. *Journal of Positive Behavior Interventions, 1*, 77–87.

Eggbeer, L., Littman, C. L., & Jones, M. (1997, June–July). ZERO TO THREE's Developmental Specialist in Pediatric Practice Project. *Zero to Three, 17*, 1–6.

Fox, L., Dunlap, G., & Cushing, L. (2002). Early intervention, positive behavior support and transition to school. *Journal of Emotional and Behavioral Disorders, 10*, 149–157.

Fox, L., Dunlap, G., Hemmeter, M. L., Joseph, G. E., & Strain, P. S. (2003). The teaching pyramid: A model for supporting social competence and preventing challenging behavior in young children. *Young Children, 58*, 48–52.

Fox, L., Dunlap, G., & Powell, D. (2002). Young children with challenging behavior: Issues and considerations for behavior support. *Journal of Positive Behavior Interventions, 4*, 208–217.

Graham, M., White, B., Clarke, C., & Adams, S. (2001). Infusing infant mental health practices into front-line caregiving. *Infants and Young Children, 14*, 14–23.

Halfon, N., Berkowitz, G., & Klee, L. (1992). Mental health utilization by children in foster care in California. *Pediatrics, 89*, 1238–1244.

Halfon, N. G., Mendonca, A., Berkowitz, G. (1995). Health status of children in foster care: The experience of the Center for the Vulnerable Child. *Archives of Pediatric and Adolescent Medicine, 149*, 386–392.

Hebbeler, K., Wagner, M., Spiker, D., Scarborough, A., Simeonsson, R., & Collier, M. (2001). *A first look at the characteristics of children and families entering early intervention services.* Menlo Park, CA: SRI International.

Honig, A. (2002). *Secure relationships: Nurturing infant/toddler attachment in early care settings.* Washington, DC: National Association for the Education of Young Children.

Horowitz, S. M., Leaf, P. J., Leventhal, J. M., Forsyth, B., & Speechley, K. N. (1992). Identification and management of psychosocial developmental problems in community-based primary care pediatric practices. *Pediatrics, 89*, 480–485.

Horton, C., & Bowman, B. T. (2002). *Child assessment at the preprimary level.* Chicago: Erickson Institute.

Huffman, L. C., Mehlinger, S. L., & Kerivan, A. S. (2000). *Risk factors for academic and behavioral problems at the beginning of school.* Chapel Hill, NC: University of North Carolina, FPG Child Development Center.

Johnson, K., Knitzer, J., & Kaufmann, R. (2002). *Making dollars follow sense: Financing early childhood mental health services to promote healthy social and emotional development in young children.* New York: National Center for Children in Poverty.

Joseph, G. E., & Strain, P. S. (2003). Comprehensive evidence-based social-emotional curricula for young children: An analysis of efficacious adoption potential. *Topics in Early Childhood Special Education, 23*, 65–76.

Katz, L. G., & McClellan, D. S. (1997). *Fostering children's social competence: The teacher's role*. Washington, DC: National Association for the Education of Young Children.

Kaufmann, R., & Perry, D. F. (2002). Promoting social and emotional development in young children: Promising approaches at the national, state and community levels. *Kauffman Early Education Exchange, 1*, 80–96.

Knitzer, J. (2000). Early childhood mental health services: A policy and systems development perspective. In J. P. Shonkoff & S. J. Meisels (Eds.), *Handbook of early childhood intervention* (pp. 416–438). New York: Cambridge University Press.

Knitzer, J. (2001). *Building services and systems to support the healthy emotional development of young children: An action guide for policymakers*. New York: National Center for Children in Poverty.

Lavigne, J. V., Gibbons, R. D., Christoffel, K. K., Rosenbaum, D., Arend, R., Smith, K. et al. (1996). Prevalence rates and correlates of psychiatric disorders among preschool children. *Journal of the American Academy of Child & Adolescent Psychiatry, 35*, 204–214.

Lopez, M. L., Tarullo, L. B., Forness, S. R., & Boyce, C. A. (2000). Early identification and intervention: Head Start's response to mental health challenges. *Early Education and Development, 11*, 266–282.

Mathematica Policy Research (2002). *Making a difference in the lives of infants and toddlers and their families: The impacts of Early Head Start*. Princeton, NJ: Author.

McMahon, S. D., Washburn, J., Felix, E. D., Yakin, J., & Childrey, G. (2000). Violence prevention: Program effects on urban preschool and kindergarten children. *Applied and Preventive Psychology, 9*, 271–281.

Minkovitz, C., Strobino, D., Hughart, N., Scharfstein., D, Guyer, B., & the Healthy Steps Evaluation Team. (2001). Early effects of the Healthy Steps for Young Children Program. *Archives of Pediatric and Adolescent Medicine, 155*, 470–479.

National Child Care Information Center (2002a). *Table of state tiered strategies*. Retrieved April 30, 2003 from http://www.nccic.org/faqs/tieredstrategiestable.pdf

National Child Care Information Center (2002b). Child Care and Mental Health Leadership Forum: Group discussion and recommendations. *Child Care Bulletin, 25*, 4–7.

Navon, M., Nelson, D., Pagano, M., & Murphy, M. (2001). Use of the Pediatric Symptom Checklist in strategies to improve preventive behavioral health care. *Psychiatric Services, 52*, 800–804.

New Freedom Commission on Mental Health. (2003). *Achieving the promise: Transforming mental health care in America. Final Report*. DHHS Pub. No. SMA-03-3832. Rockville, MD: Department of Health and Human Services.

Olds, D., Henderson, C., Cole, R., Eckenrode, J., Kitzman, H., Luckey, D. et al. (1998). Long-term effects of nurse home visitation on children's criminal and anti-social behavior: 15-year follow-up of a randomized trial. *Journal of the American Medical Association, 280*, 1238–1244.

Pires, S. A., Stroul, B., & Armstrong, M. I. (2000). *Health care reform tracking project: Tracking state health care reforms as they affect children and adolescents with behavioral health disorders and their families—1999 impact analysis*. Tampa, FL: University of South Florida.

Pottick, K. J., & Warner, L. A. (2002). More than 115,000 disadvantaged preschoolers receive mental health services. *Update: Latest Findings in Children's Mental Health*. New Brunswick NJ: Institute for Health, Health Care Policy, and Aging Research, Rutgers University.

Powell, D. (2002). *Social and emotional needs of young children and their families in Hillsborough County*. Tampa, FL: Children's Board of Hillsborough County.

Powell, D. S., Batsche, C. J., Ferro, J., Fox, L., & Dunlap, G. (1997). A strength-based approach in support of multi-risk families: Principles and issues. *Topics in Early Childhood Special Education, 17*, 1–26.

Powell, D., Fixsen, D., & Dunlap, G. (2003). *Pathways to service utilization: A synthesis of evidence relevant to young children with challenging behavior*. Tampa, FL: Center for Evidence-Based Practice: Young Children with Challenging Behavior, University of South Florida.

Relgado, M., & Halfon, N. (2002). *Primary care services: Promoting optimal child development from birth to three years.* New York: The Commonwealth Fund.

Sameroff, A. J., & Fiese, B. H. (2000). Transactional regulations: The developmental ecology of early childhood intervention. In J. P. Shonkoff & S. J. Meisels (Eds.), *Handbook of early childhood intervention* (pp. 135–159). Cambridge, UK: Cambridge University Press.

Shonkoff, J. P., & Phillips, D. A. (2000). *From neurons to neighborhoods: The science of early childhood development.* Washington, DC: National Academy Press.

Simpson, J. S., Jivanjee, P., Koroloff, N., Doerfler, A., & Garcia, M. (2001). *Promising practices in early childhood mental health.* Washington, DC: American Institutes for Research, Center for Effective Collaboration and Practice.

Smith, B., & Fox, L. (2003). *Systems of service delivery: A synthesis of evidence relevant to young children at risk of or who have challenging behavior.* Tampa, FL: Center for Evidence-Based Practice: Young Children with Challenging Behavior, University of South Florida.

Stancin, T., & Palermo, T. M. (1997). A review of behavioral screening practices in pediatric settings: Do they pass the test? *Developmental and Behavioral Pediatrics, 18,* 183–194.

Stroul, B. A., Pires, S. A., & Armstrong, M. I. (2001). *Health care reform tracking project: Tracking state health care reforms as they affect children and adolescents with behavioral health disorders and their families.* Tampa, FL: University of South Florida.

Sturm, R., Ringel, J., Bao, C., Stein, B., Kapur, K., Zhang, W. et al. (2000). *National estimates of mental health utilization and expenditures for children in 1998.* Los Angeles: Research Center on Managed Care for Psychiatric Disorders.

U.S. Department of Education (2001). *To assure the free appropriate public education of all children with disabilities: Twenty-third annual report to Congress on the implementation of the Individuals with Disabilities Education Act.* Jessup, MD: Education Publications Center.

U.S. General Accounting Office (2000). *Title I preschool education. More children served, but gauging effect on school readiness difficult.* Washington, DC: Author.

U.S. General Accounting Office. (2001). *Medicaid: Stronger efforts needed to ensure children's access to health screening services.* Washington, DC: Author.

Walker, H. M., Kavanaugh, K., Stiller, B., Golly, A., Severson, H. H., & Feil, E. G. (1998). First steps to success: An early intervention approach for preventing school antisocial behavior. *Journal of Emotional and Behavioral Disorders, 6,* 66–80.

Webster-Stratton, C., & Hammond, M. (1998). Conduct problems and level of social competence in Head Start children: Prevalence, pervasiveness, and associated risk factors. *Clinical Child and Family Psychology Review, 1,* 101–123.

Webster-Stratton, C., Reid, J., & Hammond, M. (2001a). Preventing conduct problems, promoting social competence: A parent and teacher training partnership in Head Start. *Journal of Clinical Child Psychology, 30,* 283–302.

Webster-Stratton, C., Reid, J., & Hammond, M. (2001b). Social skills and problem-solving training for children with early-onset conduct problems: Who benefits? *Journal of Child Psychology and Psychiatry, 42,* 943–952.

Yoshikawa, H. (1995). Long-term effects of early childhood programs on social outcomes and delinquency. *The Future of Children 5,* 51–75.

Yoshikawa, H., & Knitzer, J. (1997). *Lessons from the field: Head Start mental health strategies to meet changing needs.* New York: National Center for Children in Poverty.

3

School Psychology Services

STEVEN W. LEE and T. RENE JAMISON

SCHOOL PSYCHOLOGY SERVICES

American psychology has long recognized the contextual influence of practice in training psychologists. For example, psychologists are trained to work in industry (industrial–organizational psychologists), rehabilitation centers (rehabilitation psychologists), clinical settings (clinical psychologists), medical clinics and hospitals (pediatric and health psychologists), and in the military (military psychologists) to name a few. Like many other settings, schools have their own unique culture, procedures, and organization (Sarason, 1971). School psychologists (SPs) are specially trained to work within the context of school or educational settings. It is this special expertise and orientation to the practice of psychology in schools that is the focus of this chapter.

School psychology is first and foremost a profession and subspecialty of psychology. SPs, trained in the knowledge base of psychology, use their skills to help students, their teachers and parents overcome educational, social, interpersonal, or emotional problems that interfere with the student's progress in school. A unique aspect of school psychology services includes the degree to which the SP works with other adults to help a child in need. Through regular collaboration with teachers, administrators, parents, and paraprofessionals, the SP engages in problem solving with teachers or parents and on various types of multidisciplinary teams. This aspect of their work is frequently referred to as the "paradox of school psychology" (Gutkin & Conoley, 1990), where effective services to children are attained through the psychologist's ability to work with adults.

STEVEN W. LEE and T. RENE JAMISON • School Psychology Program, University of Kansas, Lawrence, Kansas 66045.

Roles and Functions of School Psychologists

Although SPS serve many functions in the schools, their primary roles include providing psychological assessment, individual and group consultation, and counseling/intervention services. SPS are also frequently involved in the planning and implementation of prevention programs as well as serving as a resource for program evaluation efforts in schools.

Within these domains of practice, their training provides special skills unique to the profession. For example, in the assessment arena, SPS are especially trained in tools and instruments that facilitate the diagnosis of specific learning disabilities, and mental retardation along with various emotional and behavioral disorders that negatively influence learning. Highly specific academic tests, well-developed classroom observations tools, and curriculum-related assessment instruments provide an armamentarium of tools unique to the profession.

School psychologists typically work from a developmental and ecological perspective. In this way, psychological assessments attend equally to within-child variables (i.e., development, attitudes, physical) and ecological variables, which include the influence of the classroom and home environments on classroom behavior and academic progress.

SPS primarily served as "gatekeepers" for special education up until the late 1970s (Brown, 1981). There was a decrease in the ratio of SPS to students (Carey & Wilson, 1995), which left more time for SPS to provide services other than assessment (e.g., consultation, counseling, prevention programming). The following sections outline services provided by SPS.

TYPES OF PROBLEMS OR DISORDERS ENCOUNTERED BY SCHOOL PSYCHOLOGISTS

Typical Referrals for School Psychological Services

Although the role of the school psychologist has changed, SPS still spend the most time on assessment-related activities, followed by consultation (Bramlett, Murphy, Johnson, Wallingsford, & Hall, 2002). Referrals for school psychologist services mainly involve academic problems and behavior problems. Of these, Bramlett and colleagues identified academic problems as the most frequent type of referrals, specifically reading problems. With regard to behavior problems, externalizing behavior problems were referred more often than internalizing behavior problems. These referrals suggest SPS spend much of their time addressing academic and externalizing behavior problems.

Diagnostic Taxonomies Used by School Psychologists

Multidisciplinary teams (i.e., including SPS) must identify whether students qualify for special education services based on the presence of a disability. The disability categories that are used in schools (Individuals

Table 1. Principles and Disability Categories of IDEA 1997

Principles of IDEA 1997
  Principle 1: Zero Reject or Free Appropriate Public Education (FAPE)
  Principle 2: Nondiscriminatory Evaluation
  Principle 3: Individualized Education Programs (IEP) or the Individual Family Service Plan
    (IFSP)
  Principle 4: Least Restrictive Environment (LRE)
  Principle 5: Due Process or "Procedural Safeguards"
  Principle #6: Parent Participation

Disability Categories Covered under IDEA 1997 (for children aged 6–21 years)
  Hearing Impairments and Deafness
  Speech and Language Impairments (S-L)
  Visual Impairments and Blindness
  Serious Emotional Disturbance (SED)
  Specific Learning Disabilities (LD)
  Other Health Impaired (OHI)
  Traumatic Brain Injury (TBI)
  Orthopedic Impairments
  Autism
  Developmentally Delayed (DD) — children aged 3–9 years only

---

with Disabilities Education Act [IDEA], 1997) are quite different from the categorical systems often used in clinical settings (i.e., Diagnostic and Statistical Manual—Fourth Edition [DSM-IV]; American Psychiatric Association [APA], 1994).

IDEA 1997

A student is eligible for special education services if that student has a disability (as defined in IDEA) and special education or related services are needed because of that disability (IDEA, 1997). There are 10 categories (see Table 1) that can be used to identify a disability for children aged 6–21 years. An additional category is used for children aged 3–9 years (i.e., Developmentally Delayed) experiencing "developmental delays" in one or more of five areas of development (i.e., physical, cognitive, communication, social or emotional, and adaptive). To determine eligibility for special education services, a comprehensive evaluation must be conducted following parental consent. Additionally, when students are identified with a disability under IDEA, their disability must affect their educational performance to be eligible for services. The evaluation must be nondiscriminatory, conducted by a multidisciplinary team, employ a variety of psychometrically sound instruments, and should be conducted in the child's native language or mode of communication (IDEA, 1997). If the child is eligible for special education services, an Individualized Education Plan (IEP) is written by the multidisciplinary team outlining special education and related services, goals and benchmarks for progress, and evaluation and data collection procedures (Jacob-Timm & Hartshorne, 1998).

Section 504 of the Americans with Disabilities Act (ADA)

In addition to using IDEA (1997) to place students in special education programs, SPS provide services to students with disabilities in the regular education classroom. Specifically, students with a disability (as defined by ADA) who need accommodations in the classroom or school that do not meet IDEA requirements, may be eligible for services under Section 504 of the ADA. Through Section 504, an accommodation plan is written to provide adjustments in the regular education classroom to help the student (Jacob-Timm & Hartshorne, 1998). An evaluation is needed to determine whether the student is eligible for accommodations.

Diagnostic and Statistical Manual of Mental Disorders—Fourth Edition (DSM-IV)

SPS are often trained in using the DSM-IV as a diagnostic tool. Although the DSM-IV is not the diagnostic taxonomy used in most schools, SPS often utilize this system when identifying possible psychological disorders in children. In addition, familiarization with the DSM-IV allows SPS to effectively communicate with other mental health professionals (e.g., clinical psychologists, counseling psychologists, psychiatrists) when collaborating about students. The primary difference between DSM-IV and IDEA is that IDEA identifies global classifications of students and criteria for identification, while the DSM-IV follows a medical model orientation and uses severity specifiers and a polythetic format.

PSYCHOEDUCATIONAL ASSESSMENT

SPS are involved with developmental screenings, psychoeducational evaluations in the schools, and transition planning for adolescents in special education. A variety of instruments are used in the assessment process. These instruments include intelligence tests, academic tests, observation systems, personality and behavior instruments, and adaptive behavior instruments. These, along with other professionals, provide a majority of the psychoeducational assessment data used in decision making for educational placement.

Intellectual Assessment

SPS have been administering intelligence tests (IQ tests) for over 100 years (Fagan & Wise, 2000). IQ tests (Wechsler Intelligence Scale for Children—Third Edition [WISC-III], Stanford-Binet—Fifth Edition [SB-V], Woodcock-Johnson Tests of Cognitive Abilities [WJ-III-Cog.]) are individually administered, standardized, norm-referenced instruments that provide a broad measure of cognitive ability. These instruments provide standard scores and percentile ranks that can be used to make comparisons of students to their peer group and to identify individual cognitive strengths and weaknesses. IQ tests, as part of a battery of tests, provide information used in classifying students into disability categories (e.g., learning disabled, mentally retarded, gifted; see Table 1).

Intelligence tests have been criticized for not providing useful information regarding treatment or instructional planning for students (Gresham & Witt, 1997). Regardless of this criticism, intelligence tests continue to be used in schools when making decisions regarding educational placement and instructional recommendations. In fact, a recent survey of SPS indicated that approximately 22 hours a week are spent on assessment-related activities and that on average, SPS administer about 14 intelligence or ability tests per month (Hosp & Reschly, 2002).

Academic Assessment

Salvia and Ysseldyke (1995) have identified five types of decisions that can be made from academic assessment data, which include referrals for an evaluation, academic screenings, classification, instructional planning, and progress monitoring. Academic assessment is crucial in determining areas of academic strength and weakness, progress monitoring, and to provide information regarding placement in special education. Academic assessment tools can identify broad skill areas or specific skill areas.

Broadband Instruments

Broad-based measures of academic assessment include both norm-referenced (i.e.,Woodcock-Johnson Test of Achievement—Third Edition [WJ-III]) and criterion-referenced tests. Broad criterion-referenced tests also exist to identify proficiency of global academic skills (e.g., Brigance Diagnostic Inventory of Basic Skills). Criterion-referenced tests examine mastery of academic skills, and usually compare the student's performance to a standard of skill acquisition (Shapiro, 1996). These tests can be used in screenings and often contain items that are very similar to what students are asked to learn in schools. Both normative and criterion-referenced tests may be useful in determining the student's current academic skills, but are less useful in monitoring progress or providing direction for instruction interventions.

Narrowband Instruments

Narrowband instruments focus on specific skills within broad areas. Norm-referenced narrowband instruments (e.g., KeyMath; Test of Written Language [TOWL]) are often administered following a broadband instrument. These tools provide more information about the student's specific skills needed to design academic interventions for the student.

Curriculum-based assessment (CBA) methods provide valuable information that can be used to determine instructional strategies. Curriculum-based assessment methods also include curriculum-based evaluation (CBE) and curriculum-based measurement (CBM). These can be used to monitor student progress on specific skills in the local curriculum, compare students using schoolwide or district-generated norms (CBM), and to identify patterns of errors that may be helpful in determining where skill breakdowns occur and which instructional strategies may be beneficial for the student (CBE).

Assessing the Academic Environment

Although one single assessment method may not be appropriate to answer all of the five questions identified by Salvia and Ysseldyke (1995), the combination of academic assessment methods can provide information to make appropriate instructional recommendations and educational placement. In addition to academic testing, an assessment of the academic environment is frequently conducted to identify classroom and instructional variables that influence student learning, and to identify the student's reaction to academic tasks in their natural environment.

Classroom and Behavioral Observations

SPS use classroom observations, along with test data, to generate hypotheses about why a student may be having difficulty in particular areas of school or learning. Behavioral observations that occur within the classroom provide information about academic engagement, interactions with peers and teachers, problem-solving skills, as well as student reactions to the classroom environment. Shapiro (1996) suggests a systematic-direct observation approach as the best practice when collecting observation data. Classroom observations provide an opportunity for the psychologist to observe students in their natural setting, allow for a broader role than the traditional diagnostic approach, and often provide a sense of accountability for both the psychologist (e.g., follow-up with teacher) and for the teacher (e.g., integrity of intervention implementation). SPS use a variety of observation methods, both unstructured (i.e., anecdotal event recording, antecedent, behavior, consequence recording) and structured (i.e., event or frequency recording, duration recording, time-sampling procedures).

Personality and Behavioral Assessment

Personality assessment is the process of collecting data about student behavior, social–emotional functioning, and affective difficulties (Knoff, 1995). SPS use objective techniques (e.g., trait scales) and some projective techniques to collect this data. Trait scales (e.g., State–Trait Anxiety Inventory) examine relatively stable personality traits through self-report measurement, which is used along with other data to develop working hypotheses about the student's social–emotional functioning. SPS also use projective techniques (e.g., Kinetic Family Drawing, Children's Apperception Test, Incomplete Sentences) to help develop working hypotheses about the student.

Behavior rating scales or questionnaires (e.g., Behavior Assessment Scale for Children [BASC], Child Behavior Checklist [CBCL]) may be used to identify global areas of student behavior problems. These global tests are frequently followed by instruments that focus on specific behavior problems or symptoms (Reynolds Adolescent Depression Scale [RADS], Childhood Depression Inventory [CDI]). Although these instruments are widely used, psychometric properties, response bias, and second- or third-party respondent problems should be considered during interpretation.

One behavior assessment method used by SPS is functional behavioral assessment (FBA). FBA identifies environmental conditions and/or variables that support or maintain problem behavior (McComas & Mace, 2000). Systematic manipulation of antecedents and consequences are made to identify the function of the behavior. A mini-experiment method is used to test hypotheses about the function of student behavior and data from the assessment is used to design interventions. The reauthorization of IDEA (1997) required that an FBA be conducted and a behavior intervention plan (BIP) be implemented prior to disciplinary action for children with disabilities. Thus, it is important for SPS as well as other educators, to be familiar with FBA approaches and processes.

Adaptive Behavior Assessment

Adaptive behavior has traditionally been identified as "personal independence and social responsibility, or the skills that are necessary to take care of oneself and get along with others" (AAMR, 1992 as cited in Harrison & Robinson, 1995, p. 753). Today, adaptive behavior encompasses a broader scope of skills, which are developmental, and increase in number and complexity as an individual grows older. More recent definitions of mental retardation require that greater emphasis be put on adaptive behavior. Although adaptive behavior rating scales (e.g., Vineland Adaptive Behavior Rating Scales, Scales of Independent Behavior) provide valuable information about all children, they are usually administered when students are suspected of being mentally retarded.

Infant, Preschool, and Developmental Testing

Although many SPS primarily work with school-aged children, some also provide services to infants, toddlers, and preschoolers. IDEA (1997) mandates that services must be provided for children aged 3–21 years, and recommends that services are provided to children birth to 3 years old. States that provide services for these very young children are eligible for additional funds from the federal government. Because some of the children are not attending schools, states and local communities must locate children to determine if special services are needed. Children are typically referred or identified following a visit to the pediatrician, a community screening (e.g., Child Find), preschool screenings, or kindergarten roundup (Preator & McAllister, 1995). Psychologists may administer developmental screening tests to identify areas of potential developmental delay.

SPS then work with other professionals to provide services to those children prior to attending school and/or when the child is school-aged.

INDIRECT INTERVENTION: CONSULTATION

Consultation is a primary mode of intervention used by SPS to effect therapeutic change for children. Consultation is an indirect service in which the consultant (SP), after receiving a referral (or verbal request for assistance) from a teacher or parent, uses a problem-solving process to generate targeted interventions to be implemented by the classroom teacher and/or parent.

Consultation differs from a medical model orientation that has historically guided the provision of health (including mental health) services. In the medical model orientation, a referral is made to the psychologist who assesses the "ill" child and then reports his/her diagnostic impressions and plan for treatment back to the referral source. The psychologist prescribes a treatment program that is typically implemented through counseling or some other direct method of implementation. This model assumes that the problem (illness) resides within the child and largely ignores the surrounding environment. The process is prescriptive as the psychologist tells the parent/teacher what will be done to "cure" the child. If direct treatment is not successful, little has been done to alleviate the stress surrounding the child's problems. This model features one-way communications and very little serious collaboration.

The consultation model used by most SPS assumes a collaborative and ecological stance toward the assessment-treatment process. Whereas the path to treatment in this model also begins with the referral from the teacher or parent, the psychologist (consultant) broadly assesses not only the child, but also environments and people that are a critical part of the child's life. After the assessment information is collected, collaborative consultation takes place between the psychologist/consultant and the parent or teacher. In this model, treatment is implemented by the teacher or parent and occurs in daily interaction with the child. The focus in this model is on environmental variables and daily interaction and not on the child only. The process is not prescriptive but rather features a collaborative orientation with mutually agreed upon targets for change as well as goals and interventions. Open and ongoing communications are part of the process with continued use of a problem-solving orientation. This approach takes a different posture toward the parent or teacher (consultee). The consultee is assumed to be a competent professional (teacher) that has unique knowledge of the child and their profession, and can meaningfully contribute to the development and implementation of a successful intervention.

Mental Health Consultation

Gerald Caplan (1963) developed the first comprehensive model of mental health consultation during his work in Israel in 1949 with large numbers of immigrant children with a staff far too small to provide traditional services. Caplan emphasized a lack of professional objectivity as the principal barrier preventing the consultee from success in working with the child. When this problem is encountered, the consultant uses verbal and nonverbal approaches called "theme interference reduction techniques" to help the consultee regain an objective view of the problem leading to more effective intervention approaches. Medway and Updyke (1985) completed a meta-analysis on 24 studies that examined mental health consultation and found positive effects for the approach on consultees and to a lesser extent on children.

Behavioral Consultation

Behavioral consultation arose from classical and operant conditioning theories, but it was strongly influenced by social learning theory in late 1960s and 1970s. The notion of the situational specificity of behavior and reciprocal determinism (Bandura, 1978) gave rise to Bergan's (1977) model of behavioral consultation. For Bergan, the consultant's role is to provide psychological information to the consultee in the form of behavioral techniques designed to remediate the problem at hand, and hopefully prevent future occurrences. The behavioral consultant works to develop a collegial relationship with the consultee, while at the same time carefully structuring the verbal exchanges in an effort to influence the consultee to operationally define the problem, and then select and implement an intervention plan based on behavioral principles.

Conjoint behavioral consultation (CBC; Sheridan & Colton, 1994) and ecobehavioral consultation (Gutkin, 1993) are two related consultation models that have evolved from behavioral consultation. In CBC, the consultant includes the child's parents along with the teacher in the consultation process. In this way, improved communication between home and school and more complete information increases the support, ownership, and responsibility for implementation and follow-through on interventions. A related goal of CBC is to prevent future occurrences of the problem by improving the knowledge and skills of the teacher and parents. By involving the home and school in the process, the chance for generalization of the behavior to these two key settings is evident.

Gutkin (1993) argued to expand the concept of behavioral consultation to include more distal environmental variables in the consultation process. In ecobehavioral consultation, the consultant seeks to understand and collect data on the ecological context of the problem that may include both proximal and distal variables. By taking into account the relevant systems of influence (Bronfenbrenner, 1979), interventions developed from this perspective are much more likely to be successful.

In a review of the effectiveness of consultation, Sheridan, Welch, and Orme (1996) found that "behavioral consultation (BC) studies have afforded the most consistently positive results. Specifically, of all BC studies reviewed ($N = 21$), 95% reported at least one positive outcome..." (p. 344). Sheridan, Eagle, Cowan, and Mickelson (2001) found significant effect sizes on the average for the use of CBC with 52 children with learning and/or behavioral problems.

Group Consultation

The various types of multidisciplinary teams that work in schools offer opportunities for SPS to consult with groups that include teachers, parents, and other professional staff. Prior to the initiation of a complete psychoeducational assessment, the school makes proactive efforts to solve the student's problem(s) within the classroom environment. These teams have many names including student assistance teams, teacher assistance teams, pre-referral teams, or intervention assistance teams to name a few.

SPS frequently function as group consultants and facilitate these team meetings. In this role, they assist the team to define the problem, set goals, brainstorm solutions, select and implement trial interventions, and evaluate the effectiveness of the treatment. A review of the effectiveness of these teams suggests that they have not been effectively studied. For example, Welch, Brownell, and Sheridan (1999) found that half of the published studies on school-based problem-solving teams used no methodological design. In most studies, consumer satisfaction with the process was the most frequently cited outcome measure.

Evaluating Outcomes in School Consultation

Consultation services have been evaluated with three different types of measures: (1) outcome measures; (2) process measures and; (3) satisfaction and preference surveys. Outcome measures of consultation include the degree to which the child is ultimately helped as a result of his/her teacher or parent engaging in consultation. To this end, classroom observations of behavior, individual or group achievement tests, curriculum-based measures, behavior rating scales, goal attainment ratings, or measures of effect size are typically used to measure outcome effectiveness.

Process measures are used to assess treatment integrity or to detect the nature and quality of interactions that take place between the consultant and consultee. Measures of this sort include the Consultation Analysis Record (CAR; Bergan & Tombari, 1975; Bergan & Kratochwill, 1990). The CAR has been used in behavioral consultation research to assess the influence of types of verbalizations on the consultee. Satisfaction and preference surveys include instruments that are designed to provide the consultant with feedback on teachers' preferences for consultation approach (e.g., mental health or behavioral consultation), satisfaction with the process and benefits of participating in consultation.

COUNSELING AND OTHER SERVICES

Although counseling is a service provided by SPS, many schools also have counselors and/or social workers that also provide counseling services. As a result, counseling is rated as being of lesser importance as a service (as compared to assessment and consultation) provided by SPS (Rosenfeld, Leung, & Oltman, 2000). Counseling, when provided, is typically short-term in nature and related more to adjustment problems at school or home rather than to severe psychopathology. Severe and chronic mental health problems are generally beyond the competence and scope of services provided by the school psychologist and these cases are typically referred to professionals outside the school. SPS may provide individual or group counseling services (Millman, Schaefer, & Cohen, 1980) for problems such as: (1) social isolation; (2) school refusal; (3) noncompliance; (4) test or generalized anxiety; (5) stealing; (6) cheating; (7) impulsivity/distractibility; (8) low self-esteem and; (9) overdependency. Tharinger and Stafford (1995) suggest a seven-stage model for individual school-based counseling that includes: (1) deciding whether the child is an appropriate referral/candidate for counseling. If appropriate, the counseling plan would be developed and would include: (2) gaining a working alliance with the child; (3) identifying goals; (4) developing a plan for change that may involve teacher consultation; (5) implementation of the counseling plan; (6) assessing progress and planning for termination and; (7) follow-up to evaluate the success of the counseling program.

Other services provided by SPS include organizational consultation, program evaluation, transition services, and developing prevention programs. Consistent with their background in consultation, SPS interested in systems change work to improve conditions in schools, school district, or communities. Whereas organizational change efforts may use a problem-solving approach, a number of system variables such as political, cultural, quality-of-life, and organizational climate must be considered before organizational change can take place (Knoff, 1995).

The development and implementation of new and innovative programs in the schools require an effective program evaluation effort. SPS are frequently called upon to lead a program evaluation effort to assess curricular, social, or discipline innovations.

Through their work with special populations in the schools, SPS are frequently involved in planning transition services for special education students as they begin to reach the end of their school career. With less than 25% of special education students becoming fully employed after high school (Levinson, 1995), the IDEA amendments require transition planning for all students with IEPs by age 16. SPS training in learning and development, psychological assessment, consultation, and intervention makes them vitally important team members when planning for the transition of a student to independent living.

A stronger emphasis of primary and secondary prevention of school problems has resulted from the realization that society does not have adequate resources to provide intervention services to all students in schools that need them (Albee, 1968). From another perspective, the development of skills, or the reduction of risk factors in children that reduce the likelihood of academic problems or psychopathology seems to be within the purview of schools (Adelman & Taylor, 2000). SPS are well suited to work on prevention programs due to their holistic view of children, knowledge of the school climate and culture, and their research and measurement knowledge.

INNOVATIVE MODELS OF SCHOOL PSYCHOLOGY SERVICES DELIVERY

Within the past 10 years, there has been an increase in school-based mental health programs. Perhaps the most well known of these are the Memphis City Schools Mental Health Clinics (MCSMHC; Pfeiffer & Reddy, 1998). The MCSMHC is a state-licensed mental health center that offers a full array of mental health services (e.g., consultation, counseling, crisis intervention, chemical dependency) while maintaining a mission of support to special education staff and students. In addition, the MCSMHC offers unique prevention and health promotion activities. This site provides doctoral internship training in school psychology and was the first to be recognized by the American Psychological Association's first Award of Excellence in School Psychological Services Programs.

Project ACHIEVE (Knoff & Batsche, 1995) is an exemplary, building-wide school reform process that focuses on enhancing teachers' problem-solving and classroom management skills, providing comprehensive services to below average students, and improving parental involvement in education. In Project ACHIEVE, school psychologists play critical roles in training and consulting with staff as well as providing services to children. Project ACHIEVE has shown impressive results in reducing discipline referrals and improving academic achievement.

SUMMARY AND CONCLUSIONS

SPS provide services primarily to students within the school setting through psychoeducational assessment, individual and group consultation, and counseling and intervention. Following the Education of All Handicapped Children Act (PL 94–142) in 1975, the demand for SPS and these services has increased. SPS receive specialized training to work with children and their families to identify variables that may be negatively affect a student's learning. SPS are trained in the use of intellectual assessment, academic assessment, personality and behavioral assessment, and adaptive behavior assessment. SPS use these instruments, along with record review, interviews, and observations, to identify learning disabilities, mental retardation, and behavior problems. More recently, the role of the SP has changed, with the emphasis on consultation and intervention rather than solely on assessment-related activities. SPS have also been involved in many reform and partnership programs designed to best serve the needs of children and their families. SPS provide individual consultation services to teachers and parents, group and individual counseling with students, and are crucial members of educational teams that make decisions about student learning.

Future Directions in School Psychology

Undoubtedly there are many changes ahead for school psychology as a profession. However, there are several future directions for school psychology that will have the most profound impact on the practitioner and researcher. In the assessment arena, an increasing emphasis on evaluative instruments that provide better links to interventions will continue to lead to greater use of functional behavior assessment and curriculum-based assessment tools. This movement seems to be leading to a decreasing emphasis on intelligence tests and the development of shorter instruments. In addition, the SP will need to consider the ecology of the student's environment along with the ability to better assess environmental influences on the student's behavior.

Research on behavioral and group consultation has led to calls for the use of functional behavior assessment in the consultation process. The increased use of functional behavior assessment in consultation will improve the rigor of the process and increase the chances of isolating effective interventions through the use of experimental methods. The aftermath of the recent school shootings has led to improved approaches in crisis consultation and counseling. In this vein, SPS view their role in the development of school crisis plans as quite important (Rosenfeld et al., 2000).

If the recent past provides an indication of the immediate future, then the emphasis on the use of evidence-based interventions (EBI) will continue to grow (Kratochwill & Stoiber, 2002). EBIS are those intervention approaches that have garnered enough scientific evidence through rigorous experimentation and replication to be deemed "evidence-based." The movement toward the use of EBIS in practice will influence researchers, thus improving their research methods in an effort to enhance the practitioner's and consumer's confidence in psychoeducational interventions.

Finally, the limited resources of social service agencies and schools have led to improved partnerships between state and local community groups that seek to serve children and their families. Links between schools, mental health agencies, law enforcement, and other child service organizations are recognized as ways to provide a continuum of care and pool scarce resources. From an ecological and treatment generalization standpoint, it makes good sense for these types of partnerships for children to grow and prosper.

REFERENCES

Adelman, H. S., & Taylor, L. (2000). Moving prevention form the fringes into the fabric of school improvement. *Journal of Educational and Psychological Consultation, 11*, 7–36.

Albee, G. W. (1968). Conceptual models and manpower requirements in psychology. *American Psychologist, 23*, 317–320.

American Psychiatric Association. (1994). *Diagnostic and statistical manual of mental disorders (IV)*. Washington, DC: Author.

Bandura, A. (1978). The self system in reciprocal determinism. *American Psychologist, 33*, 344–358.

Bergan, J. R. (1977). *Behavioral consultation*. Columbus, OH: Merrill.

Bergan, J. R., & Kratochwill, T. R. (1990). *Behavioral consultation and therapy*. New York: Plenum.

Bergan, J. R., & Tombari, M. L. (1975). The analysis of verbal interactions occurring during consultation. *Journal of School Psychology, 13*, 209–226.

Bramlett, R. K., Murphy, J. J., Johnson, J., Wallingsford, L., & Hall, J. D. (2002). Contemporary practices in school psychology: A national survey of roles and referral problems. *Psychology in the Schools, 39*, 327–335.

Bronfenbrenner, U. (1979). *The ecology of human development*. Cambridge, MA: Harvard University Press.

Brown, D. T. (1981). Graduate training in school psychology. *Journal of Learning Disabilities, 14*, 378–379.

Carey, K. T., & Wilson, M. S. (1995). Best practices in training school psychologists. In A. Thomas & J. Grimes (Eds.), *Best practices in school psychology III* (pp. 171–190). Washington, DC: National Association of School Psychologists.

Caplan, G. (1963). Types of mental health consultation. *American Journal of Orthopsychiatry, 33*, 470–481.

Fagan, T. K., & Wise, P. S. (2000). Historical development of school psychology. In *School psychology: Past, present, and future* (2nd ed., pp. 19–60). White Plains, NY: Longman Publishing Group.

Gresham, F. M., & Witt, J. C. (1997). Utility of intelligence tests for treatment planning, classification, and placement decisions: Recent empirical findings and future directions. *School Psychology Quarterly, 12*, 249–267.

Gutkin, T. B. (1993). Moving from behavioral to ecobehavioral consultation: What's in a name? *Journal of Educational and Psychological Consultation, 4*, 95–99.

Gutkin, T. B., & Conoley, J. C. (1990). Reconceptualizing school psychology from a service delivery perspective: Implications for practice, training and research. *Journal of School Psychology, 15*, 203–223.

Harrison, P. L., & Robinson, B. (1995). Assessment of adaptive behavior. In A. Thomas & J. Grimes (Eds.), *Best practices in school psychology III* (pp. 753–762). Washington, DC: National Association of School Psychologists.

Hosp, J. L., & Reschly, D. J. (2002). Regional differences in school psychology practice. *School Psychology Review, 31*, 11–29.

Individuals with Disabilities Education Act of 1997 (PL-105-17), 20 U.S.C. Chapter 33.

Jacob-Timm, S., & Hartshorne, T. S. (1998). Ethical-legal issues in the education of pupils with disabilities under IDEA. In *Ethics and law for school psychologists* (pp. 95–174, 148–167). New York: Wiley.

Knoff, H. M. (1995). Best practices in facilitating school-based organizational change and strategic planning. In A. Thomas & J. Grimes (Eds.), *Best practices in school psychology III* (pp. 849–864). Washington, DC: National Association of School Psychologists.

Knoff, H. M., & Batsche, G. M. (1995). Project ACHIEVE: Analyzing a school reform process for at-risk and underachieving students. *School Psychology Review, 24*, 579–603.

Kratochwill, T. R., & Stoiber, K. C. (2002). Evidence-based interventions in school psychology: Conceptual foundations of the Procedural and Coding Manual of Division 16 and the Society for the Study of School Psychology Task Force. *School Psychology Quarterly, 17*, 341–389.

Levinson, E. M. (1995). Best practices in transition services. In A. Thomas & J. Grimes (Eds.), *Best practices in school psychology III*. Washington, DC: National Association of School Psychologists.

McComas, J. J., & Mace, F. C. (2000). In E. S. Shapiro & T. R. Kratochwill (Eds.), *Behavioral assessment in schools: Theory, research, and clinical foundations* (pp. 78–103). New York: The Guilford Press.

Medway, F. J., & Updyke, J. F. (1985). Meta-analysis of consultation outcome studies. *American* Journal of Community Psychology, 13, 489–505.

Meyers, J., & Nastasi, B. K. (1999). Primary prevention in school settings. In C. R. Reynolds & T. B. Gutkin (Eds.), *The handbook of school psychology* (3rd ed.). New York: Wiley.

Millman, H. L., Schaefer, C. E., & Cohen, J. J. (1980). *Therapies for school behavior problems: A handbook of practical interventions.* San Francisco, CA: Jossey-Bass.

Pfeiffer, S. I., & Reddy, L. A. (1998). School-based mental health programs in the United States: Present status and a blueprint for the future. *School Psychology Review, 27*, 84–96.

Preator, K. K., & McAllister, J. R. (1995). Assessing infants and toddlers. In A. Thomas & J. Grimes (Eds.), *Best Practices in School Psychology III* (pp. 775–788). Washington, DC: National Association of School Psychologists.

Rosenfeld, M., Leung, S. W., & Oltman, P. K. (2000). *A practice analysis of certified school psychologists.* Princeton, NJ: Educational Testing Service.

Salvia, J. A., & Ysseldyke, J. E. (1995). *Assessment in special and remedial education* (6th ed.). Boston: Houghton Mifflin.

Sarason, S. B. (1971). *The culture of the school and the problem of change.* Boston: Allyn & Bacon.

Shapiro, E. S. (1996). *Academic skills problems: Direct assessment and intervention* (2nd ed.). New York: The Guilford Press.

Sheridan, S. M, & Colton, D. L. (1994). Conjoint behavioral consultation: A review and case study. *Journal of Educational and Psychological Consultation, 5*, 211–228.

Sheridan, S. M., Eagle, J. W., Cowan, R. J., & Mickelson, W. (2001). The effects of conjoint behavioral consultation: Result of a 4-year investigation. *Journal of School Psychology, 39*, 361–385.

Sheridan, S. M., Welch, M., & Orme, S. F. (1996). Is consultation effective? A review of outcome research. *Remedial and Special Education, 17*, 341–354.

Tharinger, D., & Stafford, M. (1995). Best practices in individual counseling of elementary-age students. In A. Thomas & J. Grimes (Eds.), *Best practices in school psychology III* (pp. 893–908). Washington, DC: National Association of School Psychologists.

Welch, M., Brownell, K., & Sheridan, S. M. (1999). What's the score and game plan on teaming in schools: A review of the literature on team teaching and school-based problem-solving teams. *Remedial and Special Education, 20*, 36–49.

4

Providing Services within a School-Based Intensive Mental Health Program

ANNE K. JACOBS, CAMILLE RANDALL, ERIC M. VERNBERG, MICHAEL C. ROBERTS, and JOSEPH E. NYRE

As outlined in the Individuals with Disabilities Education Act (IDEA, 1990, 1997), emotional disturbance (ED) is designated by a multidisciplinary team, including the parents, when a child shows a number of difficulties in functioning. Within the group labeled ED, impairments in functioning range from relatively mild difficulties that can typically be managed in regular educational settings (with additional supports) to moderate or severe disturbances in multiple domains (Hodges, 2004). It is this more severely disturbed spectrum of children with serious emotional disturbance (SED) that is most in need of the intensive mental health service model described here. Children with severe SED struggle to function day by day, despite efforts of family members, school personnel, and mental health professionals. Within the classroom, they may withdraw and refuse to participate in learning exercises or may become disruptive, interfering with other students' learning. Coexisting learning disabilities often hinder educational progress, and compound the interference produced by difficulties in mood and behavior. All of these factors contribute to long-term academic failure and low rates of graduation from high school (Duchnowski, 1994; Rubin, Daniels-Beirness, & Bream, 1984; U.S. Department of Education, 1991).

ANNE K. JACOBS, CAMILLE RANDALL, ERIC M. VERNBERG, and MICHAEL C. ROBERTS • Clinical Child Psychology Program, University of Kansas, Lawrence, Kansas 66045. JOSEPH E. NYRE • Department of Child and Adolescent, Psychiatry, University of Chicago, Chicago, Illinois 60637; and Department of Pediatrics, Southern Illinois University Medical School, Springfield, Illinois.

Children with SED may also show a variety of bizarre and dangerous behaviors that result in restrictive, out-of-home placement (e.g., residential treatment center, juvenile detention facility, or psychiatric hospitalization). In many instances, a cycle develops wherein the extreme behaviors of children with SED are countered with negative, controlling adult behaviors both at home and at school (Long, 1995; Shores, Gunter, & Jack, 1993).

Over time, mental health professionals have used diverse treatments in an effort to help children with SED. Inpatient hospitalization, residential programs, and day treatment have historically been used to treat children showing severe impairments in functioning. The challenges faced by these services include ensuring the generalization and maintenance of treatment effects after discharge (Weisz, Donenberg, Han, & Weiss, 1995; Weisz, Weiss, & Donenberg, 1992), and difficulties in decreasing the behavior problems of children presenting with multiple psychiatric diagnoses (Jacobs, 2002). Research suggests a pattern in which children with severe impairments who are removed from their typical environments for treatment showed difficulties in functioning once they are returned to their typical settings (Ringeisen & Hoagwood, 2002). Alternatively, systems-of-care approaches relying heavily on community mental health centers (CMHC) offer the possibilities of providing a variety of services on an outpatient basis while children remain at home and in school. Obstacles faced in these systems of care include limited implementation of empirically supported treatments and difficulties in securing resources for sustaining the intensive, coordinated services that children with SED require. Ultimately, it is the schools that are responsible for maintaining the children's behaviors and providing appropriate education for much of the day. Self-contained behavioral disorder (BD) programs are frequently called on to manage the behaviors of children with SED for part or all of the school day. Unfortunately, severely impaired children served through self-contained BD programs alone, or in conjunction with the diverse services available from community mental health centers or private practice mental health professionals, often continue to show poor outcomes overall (Greenbaum et al., 1996; Osher, Osher, & Smith, 1994). Families, researchers, and clinical practitioners continue to search for effective models for working with children with SED.

CHARACTERISTICS OF THE INTENSIVE MENTAL HEALTH PROGRAM

The Intensive Mental Health Program (IMHP) is a school-based therapeutic classroom designed to address the needs of children with moderate-to-severe SED through diverse, comprehensive services (Vernberg, Roberts, & Nyre, 2002). One unique characteristic of the IMHP is to require children's continued enrollment in their original, neighborhood school for half of their school day to facilitate the goal of an eventual full-time transition back to the neighborhood school. The neighborhood schools, then, are committed to maintaining educational ownership for IMHP students and creating solutions (often in consultation with IMHP staff) for demanding behaviors with extant resources for the portion of the day the IMHP students attend. Although the IMHP is school-based, each child's individualized behavior program follows him or her throughout the day at the neighborhood school, home, and any extracurricular activities. The IMHP strives for a consistent behavioral program to be in effect for the child for all hours he or she is awake. If nocturnal enuresis is a presenting problem, the behavioral program may even extend into sleeping hours.

The IMHP is also characterized by its provision of an array of evidence-based psychosocial and biomedical treatments. Modalities include individual therapy, group therapy, evaluations of medication trials, social skills training, anger management, relaxation, and instruction of other coping skills. Services for medically fragile children are also coordinated and implemented as needed in specific cases. The IMHP staff provides consistent consultation on the children's behavior across settings, therapeutic needs, and academic progress with parents, guardians, and other service providers in an effort to synthesize therapeutic modalities. The IMHP organizes service coordination with all other service providers so as to prevent the piecemeal services between agencies and to encourage the generalization of treatment effects once the child transitions out of the IMHP. Finally, the program is characterized by its rigorous collection and evaluation of data from empirically valid measures. Information is constantly gathered on children's functioning in a variety of settings from a variety of informants. These data are evaluated weekly in team and supervision meetings to inform clinical decisions. This informational database has also been analyzed to add to the growing body of literature on the effective treatment of children with SED (e.g., Greenbaum et al., 1996; Hoagwood & Cunningham, 1992; Osher et al., 1994). Taken together, these characteristics address the significant emotional, behavioral, and academic needs of children with SED and endeavor to produce more positive outcomes for this high-risk population.

CREATION AND COST OF THE IMHP

The IMHP was created in 1996 to address the challenges of serving children with SED in the schools and is a joint venture between the Lawrence Public Schools and the Clinical Child Psychology Program at the University of Kansas. It began with one half-day classroom and expanded to four classrooms within 5 years. The IMHP can now serve 24 children in a district with 5,500 elementary school children. Faculty and postdoctoral fellows from the Clinical Child Psychology Program serve as clinical supervisors for master's level psychologists, who are students enrolled in the doctoral program at KU. The classroom therapists are employed directly by the school district. Participating special education teachers, paraprofessional teachers, principals, school psychologists, and social workers are all employees of the Lawrence Public Schools. The annual cost for providing these intensive services, including salaries for the core classroom staff, currently averages $9,300 per child. After federal and state reimbursement for special education services, the average cost to the school district is reduced to under $6,000 per child. Compared to alternative settings such as juvenile detention centers, residential treatment centers, and inpatient hospitalization, the IMHP costs significantly less (Nyre, Vernberg, & Roberts, 2003). The strong investment of money and space made by the school district helps ensure the ownership and stability of high-quality services through the IMHP.

STAFF REQUIREMENTS OF THE IMHP

Due to the extreme behaviors demonstrated by the children admitted to the IMHP and the intensity of services provided, a ratio of three staff for six children is maintained in each classroom. The core classroom staff includes (a) a special education teacher, who serves as the lead teacher; (b) a paraprofessional teacher, who assists both in academic and behavioral interventions; and (c) two master's level therapists, who alternate days in the classroom, provide individual and group therapy, coordinate and monitor the implementation of the service plan, and conduct home visits. Outside of the classroom are doctoral-level psychologists who provide supervision and consultation for the behavioral and therapeutic interventions implemented in the classroom, neighborhood schools, and in-home interventions. A school social worker is assigned to each classroom and aids the implementation of the service plan with the neighborhood school and outside service providers. A school psychologist provides consultation regarding the Individualized Education Plan (IEP) service plan implementation, school policies and procedures, and state and federal educational regulations. Each classroom has a treatment, outcome, and process consultant (TOP), who collects, analyzes, and presents data to inform clinical decision making and for research purposes. A child psychiatrist may also serve as part of the team to consult regarding medication management.

Nine guiding principles were central in the development of the IMHP as a program to obtain better outcomes for children with SED who were not succeeding in public schools despite receiving numerous services (Vernberg et al., 2002). The children requiring placement in the IMHP typically present with more than one psychiatric diagnosis, have numerous service providers, and have homes characterized by stress, and sometimes chaos. The nine guiding principles were influenced by the research on empirically supported treatments for children (e.g., American Academy of Child and Adolescent Psychiatry, 1997; Lonigan & Elbert, 1998) and the Child and Adolescent Service System Program (CASSP) principles (Day & Roberts, 1991). The IMHP principles are: (a) maintain placement in the child's home and neighborhood school, (b) emphasize an empirical approach to guide interventions, (c) focus on cognitive and behavioral skill development, (d) attend to cross-setting linkages and events, (e) emphasize generalization and maintenance of treatment outcomes, (f) collaborate with family members and other service providers involved with the child, (g) view assessment and diagnosis as an ongoing process, (h) maintain a developmental focus, and (i) cultivate an authoritative parenting style for adults involved with the child. These nine guiding principles are central to the service delivery features and the treatment features of the IMHP.

SERVICE DELIVERY FEATURES

Service delivery features are held constant across all children in the IMHP and are organized into six areas of service: therapeutic classroom, neighborhood school, home, collaboration, transition, and supervision.

Therapeutic Classroom

Children are expected to attend the classroom 3 hours a day, 5 days a week. They receive at least 30 minutes of individual therapy twice a week and 40 minutes of group therapy (social skills group) 4 days each week. Group check-in, where children share thoughts, feelings, and goals, occurs for 15 minutes each day (i.e., processing group). The intensity of services necessitates a child-to-staff ratio that is relatively smaller than typical special education services. No more than six children are in a classroom with three staff members. The IMHP develops and follows an individualized behavior plan that utilizes a modified token economy. Classroom staff rate children's attainment of individual target behaviors on individualized point sheets and complete daily symptom rating forms every day. Children who earn a specified percentage of their points are allowed to participate in daily free time and special activities each week. Those who do not earn the needed percentage of points use the free time to do academic work. Gotcha tickets ("Gotcha being good"), part of the modified token economy, are earned by the children every day. Children can turn in their tickets for small toys during Gotcha ticket shopping, which is held once a week for older children and twice a week for the younger group. Whereas the point sheet feature is a type of response-cost system, the Gotcha system primarily utilizes positive reinforcement. It also allows staff to monitor how frequently each child receives praise and positive feedback.

Neighborhood Schools

Children are expected to attend their neighborhood schools for 3 hours each school day. Similar to the therapeutic classroom, the teachers in the neighborhood school rate students' target behaviors on their point sheets and utilize consistent behavioral strategies during the portion of the day that they attend. Gotcha tickets are also used to reward desired behaviors in the neighborhood school. Especially as children approach transitioning back to their neighborhood schools full time, the Gotcha system is faded or schools are encouraged to set up their own reward systems.

Home

Home service features include ongoing collaboration with their parents or caregivers, with the goal of maintaining children in a family setting whenever possible. Parents and guardians are trained in behavioral strategies, taught how to rate target behaviors on the point sheet, and are encouraged to hand out Gotcha tickets each day. Parents also agree to participate in home visits by the IMHP staff at least twice a month. The content of these visits reflects the family's need and may include family therapy, monitoring cleanliness and safety, providing help with basic needs, consultation on specific problem behaviors, or simply checking up on family progress toward goals for their children.

Collaboration

While children are in the IMHP, several collaboration features are offered. The masters-level therapists take the lead on the behavioral and therapeutic interventions without disrupting helpful service provision already in place. The IMHP staff coordinates services and thus draws from expertise already present in the children's lives. This activity is no small feat because many enrollees received numerous services prior to their admission to the IMHP; as an extreme example, one child had over 20 independent service providers. Unfortunately, for children referred to the IMHP, such services have often been accessed in a piecemeal fashion, with no overall treatment plan or complete assessment of the various factors at play in the children's lives.

The IMHP staff developed a number of documents and procedures in an effort to provide better service coordination. IMHP staff distributes a *collaborative contacts form*, listing contact information for all service providers, to everyone involved with the child within the child's first month in the program. During this first month, the IMHP therapists also develop and distribute a *comprehensive service plan* to all service providers listing specific goals and objectives in multiple settings and domains of functioning (Vernberg et al., 2002). The IMHP staff collaborates with neighborhood school staff weekly regarding the children's behavior and the use of the behavior management system. Core Team meetings involving the parents or guardians, neighborhood school staff, and all involved service providers are organized by IMHP staff every 4–6 weeks for each child. If the children are receiving psychotropic medications, as many do, the IMHP staff meets with the medication prescriber and provides a summary of target behaviors and daily symptom ratings at least once a month.

Transitions

As children begin to function at a level where they can successfully transition to their neighborhood school full time, as evidenced by the various data collected, the IMHP staff holds a transition meeting with the neighborhood school and service providers. A written agreement detailing the timeline for the transition and any services to be provided following the transition is developed and signed by all involved parties. The implementation of this transition plan is reviewed with the child's team 2 and 4 weeks after the transition to ensure that the plan is going smoothly or to problem-solve around any difficulties that arise. Although each transition plan is individually tailored to the child's needs, a gradual increase in time spent in the neighborhood school, supported by consultation and careful monitoring by IMHP staff, are hallmarks of the transition process. IMHP personnel also contact the family and neighborhood school staff 3 and 6 months after the transition is completed to provide additional consultation and support as needed.

Supervision

Clinical supervision features occur throughout the child's treatment in the IMHP. Therapists complete a comprehensive evaluation form for each child. This evaluation includes developmental and behavioral history and assessment of current functioning across several domains. It is completed within each child's first month in the program and is updated at least once a month. Therapists discuss each child's case with a doctoral-level psychologist during clinical supervision at least once a week. Social skills and emotion management groups are planned during supervision and care is taken to ensure that didactic and experiential material addresses each child's level of comprehension or functioning. Supervision is also available during nonscheduled times as crises emerge. The entire IMHP classroom staff meets together once a week for at least 40 minutes to review classroom procedures and discuss each child's progress.

PSYCHOLOGICAL TREATMENT FEATURES

The treatment features are child-specific, based upon the information gathered by the IMHP team regarding each child's strengths and emotional, behavioral, and academic concerns. These features are the "active ingredients" of each child's treatment and are delivered by way of the service delivery features. The service plan developed under IDEA regulations and procedures provides a brief summary of the treatment features for each child and is organized by the following domains: home, therapy, medical, academic, and service coordination. Plans are distributed to the child's family and all involved service providers and are modified in consultation with everyone involved in the child's care. Treatment features are further categorized into case conceptualization, treatment selection, and treatment implementation.

The therapists develop a comprehensive case conceptualization for each child within 1 month of admission. A thorough case history is gathered along with an evaluation of current functioning that includes information from empirically supported, psychometrically sound, age-appropriate measures. The IMHP team gathers information from multiple informants including the children, parents or guardians, neighborhood school staff, other service providers, and direct observation of the children in a variety of settings. Based on the presenting concerns, therapists incorporate information from available practice parameters for assessment and case conceptualization (e.g., American Academy of Child and Adolescent Psychiatry, 1997). Therapists create the case formulation by considering numerous paradigms (e.g., biological, behavioral, cognitive, cognitive-behavioral, family systems, attachment, and cultural and socioeconomic factors). This case conceptualization is reviewed and modified as additional information becomes available.

The course of treatment closely follows the initial case conceptualization. When selecting appropriate treatments, the IMHP staff first works with the child's parents and neighborhood school staff to agree upon treatment goals or measurable targets for change. These treatment goals fall into a variety of areas including biological regulation, overt behavior, social cognitions, and relations with family members, peers, and teachers. Additional environmental factors that may cause or maintain undesirable behavior also become a focus of the treatment goals. Therapists select interventions that are appropriate to the case conceptualization and treatment goals and that have been determined to be efficacious or probably efficacious (Lonigan & Elbert, 1998).

Treatment implementation is fine tuned through clinical supervision each week. During these supervision times, Research consultants present graphs of behavioral data from the Daily Point Sheets and Daily Symptom Rating scales. Therapists and supervisors rely on these data as objective behavioral indicators of child functioning. The progress of treatment implementation in the IMHP, neighborhood school, and the child's home is reviewed, as well as the child's progress in individual and group therapy. Supervisors provide guidance on difficulties that arise in individual or group therapy or in working with the family, neighborhood school, and other service providers. Supervisors use relevant research to guide therapists through treatment decisions. A semistructured supervisory format maintains a solution-focused atmosphere and ensures that previously assigned therapeutic tasks are attempted or achieved.

ADMISSION TO THE IMHP

Children are referred to the IMHP by the multidisciplinary team in their neighborhood school when a critical need for services has been identified. This need becomes evident when these children continue to function poorly despite receiving numerous services in their neighborhood schools, including placement in Behavior Disorders classrooms, and, often, services from outside service providers. Children may be referred to the IMHP following inpatient hospitalization or a serious attempt to harm themselves or someone else. Once the referral has been made, the IMHP staff conducts an evaluation of the child's functioning. Information is gathered from the family and other adults involved in the child's life. Therapists also glean information from standardized behavioral scales and observations in the neighborhood school. If the IMHP Admissions Team deems the referral appropriate, the IMHP sends representatives to the child's IEP meeting to discuss the evaluation and recommendation for admission to the IMHP. The decision to place a child in the IMHP is made by the multidisciplinary team, including the child's parents, at the neighborhood school. If the family and team agree to admission, the services provided by the IMHP are documented in the child's IEP. The neighborhood school staff maintains responsibility for the child's IEP.

DIAGNOSES AND BACKGROUND OF CHILDREN IN THE IMHP

All children admitted to the IMHP have demonstrated dangerous, disorganized, or severely disruptive behaviors. They have received at least one Diagnostic and Statistical Manual—Fourth Edition [DSM-IV] diagnosis, though most have more than one diagnosis on record. A majority of IMHP students are diagnosed with a disruptive behavior disorder. Many also display symptoms of anxiety and mood disorders. Approximately one third of the children enrolled in the first 5 years displayed psychotic features at some point during treatment (Vernberg, Jacobs, Nyre, Puddy, & Roberts, 2004), and a significant proportion of the children meet the criteria for Posttraumatic Stress Disorder. In addition to emotional and behavioral difficulties, many of the children also have learning difficulties. Otherwise well-functioning families may have difficulty addressing the index child's extreme behaviors. However, 70% of the families have a history characterized by notable family dysfunction such as domestic violence, child abuse or neglect, out-of-home placement for the child, or parental psychiatric or substance abuse problems (Vernberg et al., 2004). These families have often been involved with child protection, juvenile corrections, and community mental health services. At the time of admission, 20% of the children were living out of the home in foster care, therapeutic group homes, the juvenile detention center, or other residential settings (Vernberg et al., 2004).

PROVIDING THE NECESSARY PHYSICAL STRUCTURE WITHIN THE SCHOOLS

Several elements of the IMHP physical environment have been found to be helpful in providing the service delivery and treatment features. Classrooms that are large enough to provide space for group therapy separate from the academic space help children distinguish between school work and the types of activities associated with psychotherapy. If a child becomes overly disruptive during group therapy or academics, the separate spaces in the classroom allow the child or the rest of the class to be moved to stop possible social reinforcement or modeling of inappropriate behavior. Having a seclusionary time-out room inside the IMHP classroom has been extremely advantageous. Close proximity allows children to be moved quickly to time-out, which prevents or reduces time in physical restraint and reduces the risk to others. Staff observing the child in time-out can easily signal other staff if they need to be relieved or require additional help keeping the child safe. Occasionally, children become so disruptive in time-out that it becomes necessary to have the rest of the class temporarily relocate (to the library, for instance). IMHP staff supervises all seclusion-ary time-outs closely. Behaviors displayed before and during time-outs are carefully documented and are reviewed and signed by at least two staff members. Parents receive a copy of the time-out log.

For the modified token economy, having a closet or cabinet space available for housing the Gotcha ticket store helps keep the items organized and separate from personal belongings or classroom materials. It also allows the store items to be secured out of the children's view during nonshopping times, thereby avoiding distractions during academic and therapy time. Finally, having toys and games that encourage social skills practice during earned free time is important to the overall classroom climate and for the generalization of learned skills.

PROVIDING THERAPY WITHIN THE SCHOOLS

Some school principals have been able to provide a consistent, private location for individual therapy when a classroom has been placed in their school building. In other cases, therapists balance needs for confidentiality and avoid disrupting the routines of other students as they search for a suitable space for therapy. Some spaces offered by schools for individual therapy, despite being private and nondisruptive to other students, are not deemed appropriate for use. More humorous examples from our history include staff bathrooms and chemical-laden cleaning closets. Using classrooms during off-periods or the offices of half-day staff can be good compromises. It has been important to review rules to encourage children to respect the classrooms and offices of others. Though it is preferable to have individual therapy in a standard location each session, this has not always possible. In these cases, both the child and therapist remain flexible, moving themselves and needed therapeutic materials to different locations. The lack of a consistent individual therapy room may have limited the use of certain therapeutic tools such as sand trays or large dollhouses. Typically, arrangements that are satisfactory to both the therapist and other school staff have been negotiated with a little effort.

MEASURING EFFECTIVENESS

Daily Measures

The IMHP received a 3-year grant in 2001 from the U.S. Department of Education for the purpose of evaluating outcomes. This grant allowed the hiring of research assistants (TOP consultants), who are not school system employees, for each of the four classrooms. The TOP consultants collect various outcome measures that help inform therapists' treatment decisions as well as contribute to the overall evaluation of the IMHP. The Daily Point Sheet and Daily Symptom Ratings are two important sources of information on child behavior. The Daily Point Sheet serves three functions: (a) as a tool for changing child behavior, (b) as a source of communication between adults in all the children's settings, and (c) as data for use in evaluating outcomes. When marking the point sheet, school staff provide a data point for every 5 minutes of the child's school day. Parents and guardians provide qualitative ratings of child behavior after school, around bedtime, and during the family's morning routine. IMHP staff completes the Daily Symptom Ratings after the children leave the classroom each day. Symptoms are rated on a 9-point scale, providing a useful gauge of child behavior as well as medication effects ratings. TOP consultants graph information from the Daily Point Sheets and the Daily Symptom Ratings weekly for use in group supervision, team meetings, and Core Team meetings with parents and other service providers. These continuous records of functioning help staff examine patterns of child behavior, possible intervention effects, and maintain an accurate clinical picture of each child. This is especially helpful in cases where those involved with the child encounter a series of crises and may lose sight of the overall course of treatment and long-term gains relative to baseline functioning.

Outcome Measures

A number of additional assessment measures also are used throughout each child's involvement with the IMHP. Measures and frequencies are: (a) Child and Adolescent Functioning Assessment Scale (CAFAS; Hodges, 2000; Hodges, Wong, & Latessa, 1998) completed three times a year; (b) Behavioral Assessment System for Children (BASC; Reynolds & Kamphuis, 1992) completed twice a year by parents, IMHP teachers, and neighborhood school teachers; (c) Diagnostic Interview for Children and Adolescents (DICA: Welner, Reich, Herjanic, Jung, & Amado, 1987) at intake; (d) Parenting Stress Index (PSI: Abidin, 1995) once a year; (e) Hope Scales (Snyder et al., 1996, 1997) for adults and children once a year; and (f) HOME Scale (Caldwell & Bradley, 1994) twice a year. As the study continues, efforts are made to collect the CAFAS and BASC at 6 months and 1 year following discharge.

INITIAL OUTCOMES

Child Functioning

The funded project to evaluate the effectiveness of the IMHP is still in progress at the time of this writing. However, initial outcomes were explored in a study by Vernberg et al. (2004) using CAFAS ratings completed from information in the children's files. A significant majority of the 50 children

(84%) included in this study showed clinically significant improvement in their overall functioning as measured by the total CAFAS score. An examination of the individual CAFAS scales found that the children improved significantly in their behaviors at school and home, behaviors toward others, expression of moods and emotions, self-harm, and problems in thinking. Significant improvement was not found in their behaviors in the community, though levels of impairment on this scale were relatively low at admission. Significant changes were also not seen on the two caregiver scales that rate the family's ability to meet the material needs of the child and the family's ability to provide social support. In some cases, caregiver impairment was rated as becoming worse over time. This finding may reflect a more thorough observation of the child-rearing environment by the therapist over the course of treatment. Overall, changes in functioning were positive over time and the majority of the children in the program successfully transitioned back into their neighborhood schools full time.

Factors Related to Outcomes

Factors related to IMHP children with good outcomes versus poorer outcomes have been examined (Nyre, Roberts, Jacobs, Puddy, & Vernberg, 2002). Results highlight the complexity of the children's cases, as well as the importance of the IMHP's emphasis on service coordination. Better agreement and coordination among the IMHP staff, family members, neighborhood school personnel, and outside service providers were linked to better outcomes for children in the IMHP. Better outcomes were found for children who showed greater participation in individual and group cognitive-behavioral therapy and the individualized behavior management system. Particular strengths of the IMHP appear to be found in the therapeutic interventions addressing difficulties in depressed or anxious mood and self-harm. Children who did not respond as well to IMHP interventions tended to be older, received less support from service providers, and had been diagnosed with more DSM-IV diagnoses. Low responding children remained in the IMHP almost twice as long as other children before transitioning full time back to their neighborhood schools. This finding may reflect more entrenched habits, more severe or complex presenting concerns, or more variable approaches among concurrent environments and systems.

Family Involvement

Given the apparent importance of family participation (Nyre et al., 2002), investigators examined levels of family involvement in treatment and child functioning (Richards, Bowers, Lazicki-Puddy, Krall, & Jacobs, 2002). Family involvement was measured by (a) parents' completion of the Daily Point Sheet ratings, (b) written notes to IMHP staff in the comments section of the point sheet, (c) attendance at Core Team and other treatment meetings, and (d) facilitating home visits by therapists. Parents who wrote more notes to IMHP staff on the Daily Point Sheet had children who engaged in less self-harmful behaviors and demonstrated greater improvements in overall functioning at discharge. Parents who had greater attendance at IMHP Core Team meetings also demonstrated a greater ability to provide a safe and supportive home environment for their children. Finally, in families where the caregivers were less able to meet their children's material needs, it was found that IMHP therapists made more frequent home visits to try to help enhance their resources.

FUTURE DIRECTIONS

Initial studies of the effectiveness of the IMHP for treating children with SED show promising results. The completion of the grant project will permit more comprehensive outcome studies, integrating information from all the measures administered to children, their families, and school staff. Outcomes for children receiving services in the IMHP will be evaluated against outcomes for comparison groups of children who received services from a local community mental health center or who received special educational services for at least half their school day each week. The evaluation of the IMHP and comparison groups will include behavioral and financial data.

The rich level of data collected in the IMHP evaluation will allow interesting examinations of processes and outcomes. Individual factors that predict varying child outcomes can be explored. Similarly, examinations of the functioning of systems in which children live can be conducted. Current projects address aspects of service coordination in the IMHP and satisfaction with the IMHP by various stakeholders (e.g., children, parents or guardians, neighborhood school staff). Children with SED present clinically with a diverse number of symptoms and experiences. Treatment response for subgroups of children, such as children exposed to single traumas versus children who endured a series of traumatic events, can be explored.

Children with severe SED can pose challenges to service delivery, but positive gains can be made with the type of service organization and delivery provided through the IMHP. One possible way to replicate the IMHP model, in part, would be to examine the effects of the critical treatment components (e.g., enhanced behavior management, consultation, service coordination, family involvement, individual therapy, group therapy, and process groups) when applied to a typical, self-contained BD program. Additional replications could involve integrating clinical child psychologists to address the diverse needs of children with severe SED within a school.

One of the strengths of the IMHP is its linkage to a university. This aspect provides a large number of qualified therapeutic staff, a strong empirical foundation, and program evaluation expertise or staff. School districts without nearby universities could establish linkages with local professional psychologists and other mental health providers possessing expertise in treatment of severe childhood disorders. When integrating outside professionals, it is important to clearly delineate roles so as to avoid turf issues between outside psychologists and psychologists already within the school. Creating an environment of mutual respect between diverse professionals, collaborating as a team, and turning to the scientific literature to solve differences of opinion are ways in which turf problems have been minimized through the IMHP (Roberts, Jacobs, Puddy, Nyre, & Vernberg, 2003). The model of IMHP service delivery not only shows promise in outcomes for children with severe SED, but it also provides a favorable example of child-focused, professional collaboration.

REFERENCES

Abidin, R. (1995). *Parenting Stress Index professional manual* (3rd ed.). Odessa, FL: Psychological Assessment Resources, Inc.

American Academy of Child and Adolescent Psychiatry. (1997). Practice parameters for the assessment and treatment of children and adolescents with conduct disorder. *Journal of the American Academy of Child and Adolescent Psychiatry, 36*(10 Supplement), 122S–139S.

Caldwell, B. M., & Bradley, R. H. (1994). Environmental issues in developmental follow-up research. In S. L. Friedman & H. C. Haywood (Eds.), *Developmental follow-up* (pp. 235–256). San Diego: Academic.

Day, C., & Roberts, M. C. (1991). Activities of the Child and Adolescent Service System Program from improving mental health services for children and families. *Journal of Clinical Child Psychology, 20*, 340–350.

Duchnowski, A. J. (1994). Innovative service models: Education. *Journal of Clinical Child Psychology, 23*(Suppl.), 13–18.

Greenbaum, P. E., Dedrick, R. F., Friedman, R. M., Kutash, K., Brown, E. C., Lardieri, S. P. et al. (1996). National Adolescent and Child Treatment Study (NACTS): Outcomes for children with serious emotional and behavioral disturbance. *Journal of Emotional and Behavioral Disorders, 4*, 130–146.

Hoagwood, K., & Cunningham, M. (1992). Outcomes of children with emotional disturbance in residential treatment for educational purposes. *Journal of Child and Family Studies, 1*, 129–140.

Hodges, K. (2000). *Child and Adolescent Functional Assessment Scale* (3rd ed.). Ypsilanti, MI: Eastern Michigan University.

Hodges, K. (2004). Child and Adolescent Functional Assessment Scale (CAFAS). In M. E. Maruish (Ed.), *The use of psychological testing for treatment planning and outcome assessment* (3rd ed., pp. 405–442). Hillsdale, NJ: Lawrence Erlbaum.

Hodges, K., Wong, M. M., & Latessa, M. (1998). Use of the Child and Adolescent Functional Assessment Scale (CAFAS) as an outcome measure in clinical settings. *Journal of Behavioral Health Services & Research, 25*, 325–336.

Individuals with Disabilities Education Act. (1990). Pub. L. No. 101-476; 20 U. S. C. Chapter 33.

Individuals with Disabilities Education Act, Amendments. (1997). Pub. L. No. 105-17.

Jacobs, N. J. (2002). A program evaluation assessing outcomes of youth admitted to a psychiaric community facility: A study of the impact of policy change over time (Doctoral dissertation, University of Kansas, 2002). *Dissertation Abstracts International, 63*, 2587.

Long, N. J. (1995). Why adults strike back: Learned behavior or genetic code? *Journal of Emotional and Behavioral Problems, 4*, 11–15.

Lonigan, C., & Elbert, J. (Eds.). (1998). Special issue on empirically supported psychosocial interventions for children. *Journal of Clinical Child Psychology, 27*, 138–226.

Marsh, D. T., & Fristad, M. A. (Eds.). (2002). *Handbook of serious emotional disturbances in children and adolescents*. New York: Wiley.

Nyre, J. E., Roberts, M. C., Jacobs, A. K., Puddy, R. W., & Vernberg, E. M. (2002, August). Treating SED in an intensive school-based mental health program. In E. M. Vernberg (Chair), *EBT and children who are impulsive, aggressive, psychotic, and failing.* Symposium conducted at the annual convention of the American Psychological Association, Chicago.

Nyre, J., Vernberg, E. M., & Roberts, M. C. (2003). Serving the most severe of serious emotionally disturbed students in school settings. In M. D. Weist, S. W. Evans, & N. A. Lever (Eds.), *Handbook of school mental health: Advancing practice and research* (pp. 203–222). New York: Kluwer.

Osher, D., Osher, T., & Smith, C. (1994). Toward a national perspective in emotional and behavioral disorders. *Beyond Behavior, 6,* 6–17.

Reynolds, C. R., & Kamphuis, R. W. (1992). *Behavior Assessment System for Children: Manual.* Circle Pines, MN: American Guidance Association.

Richards, M. M., Bowers, M. J., Lazicki-Puddy, T., Krall, D., & Jacobs, A. K. (2002, October). *The influence of family involvement on changes in child functioning within a school-based intensive mental health program.* Poster presented at the Kansas Conference in Clinical Child and Adolescent Psychology, Lawrence, Kansas.

Ringeisen, H., & Hoagwood, K. (2002). Clinical and research directions for the treatment and delivery of children's mental health services. In D. T. Marsh & M. A. Fristad (Eds.), *Handbook of serious emotional disturbance in children and adolescents* (pp. 33–55). New York: Wiley.

Roberts, M. C., Jacobs, A. K., Puddy, R. W., Nyre, J. E., & Vernberg, E. M. (2003). Treating children with serious emotional disturbances in schools and the community: The Intensive Mental Health Program. *Professional Psychology: Research and Practice, 34,* 519–526.

Rubin, K. H., Daniels-Beirness, T., & Bream, L. (1984). Social isolation and social problem solving: A longitudinal study. *Journal of Consulting and Clinical Psychology, 52,* 17–25.

Shores, R. E., Gunter, P. L., & Jack, S. L. (1993). Classroom management strategies: Are they setting events for coercion? *Behavioral Disorders, 18,* 92–102.

Snyder, C. R., Hoza, B., Pelham, W. E., Rapoff, M., Ware, L., Danovsky, M. et al. (1997). The development and validation of the Children's Hope Scale. *Journal of Pediatric Psychology, 22,* 399–421.

Snyder, C. R., Sympson, S. C., Ybasco, F. C., Borders, T. F., Babyak, M. A., & Higgins, R. L. (1996). Development and validation of the State Hope Scale. *Journal of Personality and Social Psychology, 2,* 321–335.

U.S. Department of Education. (1991). *To assure the free appropriate public education of all children with disabilities: Annual report to Congress on the implementation of the Individuals with Disabilities Act* (13th ed.), Washington, DC: Author.

Vernberg, E. M., Jacobs, A. K., Nyre, J. E., Puddy, R. W., & Roberts, M. C. (2004). Innovative treatment for children with serious emotional disturbance: Preliminary outcomes for a school-based intensive mental health program. *Journal of Clinical Child and Adolescent Psychology, 33,* 359–365.

Vernberg, E. M., Roberts, M. C., & Nyre, J. (2002). School-based intensive mental health treatment. In D. T. Marsh & M. A. Fristad (Eds.), *Handbook of serious emotional disturbances in children and adolescents* (pp. 412–427). New York: Wiley.

Weisz, J. R., Donenberg, G. R., Han, S. S., & Weiss, B. (1995). Bridging the gap between lab and clinic in child and adolescent psychotherapy. *Journal of Consulting and Clinical Psychology, 63,* 688–701.

Weisz, J. R., Weiss, B., & Donenberg, G. R. (1992). The lab versus the clinic: Effects of child and adolescent psychotherapy. *American Psychologist, 47,* 1578–1585.

Welner, Z., Riech, W., Herjanic, B., Jung, K. G., & Amado, H. (1987). Reliability, validity, and parent–child agreement studies of the Diagnostic Interview for Children and Adolescents (DICA). *Journal of the American Academy of Child and Adolescent Psychiatry, 26,* 649–653.

5

Inpatient Pediatric Consultation–Liaison

Applied Child Health Psychology

BRYAN D. CARTER and RENEE T. VON WEISS

As the scope of this book illustrates, there are many forms and modalities of mental health services for children and their families. One such venue is that of Pediatric Consultation–Liaison (Peds C/L). Within this modality, a specialized child mental health consultant (typically a pediatric psychologist or child psychiatrist) advises the physician or provides direct services to medically hospitalized children regarding behavioral, emotional, or familial aspects of the child's symptoms and illness (Drotar, Spirito & Stancin, 2003; Kazak, 2002). As a subspecialty practice, Peds C/L represents perhaps the most active collaboration between pediatricians and child psychologists and psychiatrists (Olson, Mullins, Chaney, & Gillman, 1994; Walker, 1988).

PREVIOUS RESEARCH ON PEDIATRIC CONSULTATION–LIAISON SERVICES

Despite a long history of Peds C/L services (Fritz, 1990; Lewis, 1994; Lewis & King, 1994; Roberts, Mitchell, & McNeal, 2003; Routh, 1985; Stabler, 1988), there is a relative dearth of studies characterizing the array of services provided by Peds C/L services despite their centrality to hospital-based pediatric psychology and child psychiatry. In one of the first studies of referral problems to a Peds C/L service, Drotar (1995)

BRYAN D. CARTER • Kosair Children's Hospital, University of Louisville School of Medicine, Louisville, Kentucky 40202.   **RENEE T. VON WEISS** • Children's Hospital of Minneapolis, Minneapolis, Minnesota 55404.

surveyed 528 children and adolescents who were pediatric inpatients. The most frequently reported referral questions included evaluation of developmental delay, adaptation and adjustment to chronic illness or physical disability, concerns regarding the psychological factors in physical symptom presentation, behavior problems, and managing psychological crises (Drotar et al., 2003).

Olson et al. (1988) at the University of Oklahoma Health Sciences Center (where the first formal training program in pediatric psychology was established) conducted a retrospective review of the records of 749 inpatient referrals seen by their pediatric psychology service at Oklahoma Children's Hospital over a 5-year period. Referrals seen, in order of greatest frequency, were depression or suicide attempt, adjustment problems to chronic illness, and behavior problems. General Pediatrics requested consultations most frequently, followed by Surgery and Adolescent Medicine. Almost a third of the children seen for in-hospital consultation were subsequently seen for outpatient follow-up. Health care professionals making referrals were generally very satisfied with the services of the Peds C/L team and expressed a high likelihood of making future referrals for consultation.

In a similar study, Rodrigue and colleagues (1995) conducted an archival review of 1,467 records of in-hospital ($n = 448$) and outpatient ($n = 1,019$) referrals to a health sciences center-based pediatric psychology service at the University of Florida Health Sciences Center from 1990 to 1993. General Pediatrics (40%), Pediatric Hematology or Oncology (31%), Adolescent Psychiatry (15%), Pediatric Intensive Care (5%), and the Burn Unit (4%) accounted for most of the inpatient referrals. The most common reason for referral (inpatient and outpatient) was assessment of cognitive or neuropsychological functioning (reflecting the strong psychological assessment orientation of this particular Peds C/L service) followed by externalizing behavior problems, comprehensive psychological evaluation, presurgery or transplant evaluation, and adjustment problems to chronic illness. A retrospective survey of 143 referring health professionals indicated generally high overall satisfaction with service quality.

In the Knapp and Harris 10-year review of clinical reports (1998a) and treatment outcome (1998b) studies on pediatric consultation–liaison child psychiatry, the authors surveyed both the categorical (illness-specific) and noncategorical investigations into the psychiatric care of medically ill children. They concluded that pediatric consultation–liaison services are increasingly playing a role in meeting the emotional and behavioral needs of pediatric inpatients via facilitation of individual and family adaptation to the stressors associated with chronic illness.

Carter et al. (2003) at the University of Louisville School of Medicine conducted a prospective case-controlled study of pediatric inpatients referred for consultation at Kosair Children's Hospital. One hundred and four referrals were matched with nonreferred controls for age, gender, and illness type or severity and completed parent- and self-report behavioral rating scales to assess for adjustment or functioning. Nurses completed in-hospital ratings of behavioral or adjustment difficulties. Goal attainment and satisfaction ratings were obtained from the referring physicians, parents or guardians, and the consultant. Results from this, the only case-controlled study of Peds C/L services, indicated that referrals exhibited more behavior, adjustment or coping difficulties than nonreferrals by parent-, nurse- and self-report. Some of the most frequently employed interventions included coping strategies interventions, cognitive and behavioral therapies, and case management. Referring physician and consultant ratings of goal attainment were high, as were physician ratings of satisfaction and parent or guardian ratings of overall helpfulness of the Peds C/L service.

THE CHILDREN'S HOSPITAL ENVIRONMENT

Setting Characteristics

As a consultant, the Peds C/L professional must constantly be cognizant of the fact that they are seeing the pediatric patient "by invitation" of the attending physician and their medical team, and may be one of many consultants asked to provide input to the case (Drotar, 1995; Fritz, 1993a). Thus, for the consultant as an "outsider," there are certain expectations and rules of etiquette that are critical to follow, which requires a sophisticated understanding of the structure and hierarchy of the medical system in general, and the consultant's specific health care setting. The consultant role is thus one of collaboration with the system of medical care, not resistance to it. This knowledge and awareness are critical to the success of the consultation process, and maximizes the development of recommendations and interventions that can be implemented with the support and participation of the health care team.

As Fritz (1993a) has indicated, one component of understanding the medical system is developing a working knowledge of children's hospital systems in general, as well as the unique aspects of the hospital environment in which the consultant is operating. In general, there are three basic types of hospitals, each with their own unique mission and values: the university-based or affiliated hospital, the public hospital, and the private hospital. University-based or affiliated hospitals, in which most Peds C/L services tend to be established, emphasize training and the furthering of medical knowledge as well as competent comprehensive care of the medically ill child. As such, numerous members of the medical team, who may rotate on various services, often have multiple contacts with each patient. Therefore, during an extended hospital stay, a patient is likely to have multiple health care providers involved in one's care, increasing the complexity of the communication process.

In contrast, public hospitals, typically consisting of city and county hospitals, have a mission to care for all patients regardless of ability to pay. Budgetary issues and problems with continuity of care and patient follow-through following discharge, are often of primary concern. As a result of these constraints, there is often a "minimalist" approach to the care of patients (Fritz, 1993a) due to the many complicating factors that may impinge upon more comprehensive care of the patient.

The private hospital is typically serviced by community pediatricians, most of who are in solo or group private practice settings (Fritz, 1993a). In contrast to the university hospital, where attendees and trainees frequently rotate services, pediatricians in the community often have long-term relationships with their patients. Therefore, it is extremely important to be in close communication with the primary pediatrician and to discuss recommendations with them before presentation to the patient and family, nursing staff, and health care team. One consideration somewhat unique to the private hospital setting relates to payment for services provided, such as who charges for the service, how the services is paid for, and what the insurance company is willing to reimburse (Drotar, 1995).

Increasingly, to survive in the competitive health care marketplace, medical schools and hospitals have had to be flexible in their structure and organization, leading to a less clear delineation of academic and nonacademic hospitals. For example, large for-profit hospital corporations have contractually run some university hospitals, and many private hospitals have become affiliated with university medical center settings, with resident training and research collaborations. The Peds C/L consultant will need to be cognizant of the impact of these various structural arrangements on their practice in each setting.

Personnel Characteristics: The Hierarchy

In addition to having an understanding of the hospital system, it is also important for the consultant to develop a "who's who" knowledge base of the component members of the medical team and hospital system. Within the hospital hierarchy, the *attending pediatrician or attending pediatric specialist* has the ultimate responsibility for both the patient and the medical trainees. In a training-hospital setting, the *pediatric residents and fellows* (specialists in training) are an integral part of the hospital staffing. Pediatric residents are at different levels in their training and are still learning many of the basic procedures in the practice of their clinical skills. Furthermore, they are continually rotating through different services in the hospital. *Medical students* also are very involved on the unit. Because they are in their first years of training, they do not have significant experience, but are often involved in charting and write-ups and may even be more thorough in their descriptions than the other members of the team. For the Peds C/L consultant, familiarity with the roles and responsibilities of the *nursing staff*, as well as a strong collaborative connection, are critical (Drotar, 1995). Nurses typically have the most contact with the patients or families and make up the largest proportion of clinical staff in the inpatient setting. Because nurses are in the most advantageous position for observing patient and family behaviors in the hospital, they often are the first to alert the attending and house staff physicians to concerns that lead to referral of cases to the Peds C/L service. If the consultant neglects nursing staff perceptions and concerns, the effectiveness of the consultation can be seriously hindered.

Hospital *social workers* are another important component of the hospital staff, with the specific roles of the social worker varying from hospital to hospital. It is critical that the consultant have a working relationship with the social services staff and understand what resources they provide to prevent role confusion, redundancy, and lack of coordination (Drotar, 1995; Fritz, 1993a). Many times the social workers have extensive knowledge of specific community resources, and serve as the liaison between the hospital and local child protective and other social services. Similarly, it is important to understand the role of the *child life specialists* (Fritz, 1993a), whose main role it is to facilitate the child's adjustment in the hospital environment, trying to make their experience as "normal" and comfortable as possible, so that the child and parents can function despite the stresses of being hospitalized. Finally, the *ward or unit secretary* can be an invaluable resource in helping the consultant and team via coordinating the patients' schedules, organizing paperwork, among other things.

Procedurally, the Peds C/L consultant is faced with multiple challenges and obstacles even before beginning the consultation proper. In the era of managed care and utilization review, children's hospital stays have gotten progressively shorter. On average, children in the United States are admitted to hospitals for 3–4 days from admission to discharge (Drotar, 1995). Thus, the consultant today may typically face a rather narrow window of time in which to complete the consultation. Under frequent utilization review, there are often pressures on the attending physician to get patients out of the hospital as quickly as is medically possible, particularly when the hospital census is high and there are children waiting for hospital beds. To complicate matters, physicians may inadvertently delay the decision to request a Peds C/L consultation while they are awaiting the findings of various medical tests. The consultant is then faced with walking into the patient's hospital room, with the patient "packed up" and ready to go, balloons tied securely to the Radio Flyer wagon. The patient and family perception is often that the consultant is keeping the child in the hospital at the very time they are excitedly anticipating going home. These health care environment factors have resulted in Peds C/L professionals having to perform their services ever more efficiently and expediently (Drotar et al., 2003). Often, faced with multiple referrals, the consultant needs to triage cases for their more or less emergent status to avoid the undesirable experience of showing up on the ward to evaluate the referral, only to learn that the patient has been discharged home (Fritz & Spirito, 1993c).

THE PROCESS OF CONSULTATION

The Referral Process

Requests for inpatient pediatric consultations are made for a wide array of presenting problems and referral questions. Many of the referrals are made to address the following concerns: the differential diagnosis of organic versus psychogenic contributors to symptom presentation;

adherence problems to medications and treatments; coping and adjustment to chronic illness and trauma; pain management; decision making for organ transplantation; behavior problems that present management difficulties in the hospital; assessment and disposition of suicidal ideation or attempt; end-of-life issues; difficulties with parents or family members that impact on the child's care and adjustment; and arranging for post-hospitalization follow-up (Carter et al., 2003; Fritz, 1993b; Kremer & Wasserman, 1994; Lewandowski & Baranoski, 1994; Olson et al., 1994). On many Peds C/L services, patients and their families are seen for protocol consultation, where the consultant is typically requested to meet and evaluate all new patients on a particular service as a matter of routine to screen for psychosocial needs. This is particularly true of services that care for patients with serious chronic and life-threatening illness such as diabetes, cystic fibrosis, renal diseases, and childhood malignancies and hematologic disorders. Many times the Peds C/L consultant working with these specialty services will have involvement at the outpatient clinics to provide continuity of care and opportunity for collaborative planning and intervention.

The referral process may range considerably from service to service and from case to case. The call to request a consultation may be made by the unit secretary on the nursing unit where the patient is hospitalized, a medical student, pediatric resident or subspecialty fellow, the patient's nurse or clinical nurse specialist, hospital social worker, or even the attending physician. In teaching hospital settings, the attending physician often delegates such responsibility to the resident or medical student. Thus, there is room for considerable distortion of information about the specific referral problem(s) in the busy daily schedule of the medical team.

The broad variety of problems referred for consultation, and the ever-pressing time constraints of inpatient work, demand that the consultant give careful consideration to the screening and management of referrals in their system (Carter et al., 2003; Drotar, 1995). Also, in many seemingly straightforward case consultation referrals, there may be intricate systems-related issues that will influence both staff perceptions of the problem definition and, in turn, the management strategies employed (Mullins, Gillman, & Harbeck, 1992).

Perhaps the most desirable mechanism for getting a referral, that is, for accuracy of problem definition, is via a direct face-to-face contact between the consultant and the referring physician. Though it may seem obvious, it cannot be overstated that the success of any consultation is highly dependent on the consultant and consultee coming to a consensus as to the specific definitions of the referral problem(s) and desired outcome(s) from the consultation. Without such agreement, it is increasingly likely that the consultee will be dissatisfied with the process and outcome of the consultation. From a systems perspective, it is most important to inquire about the nature of the referring professional's interactions with the patient and their family members, the expectations they have of the consultation, and their beliefs about the type of assistance they (the referring professional or team) should receive (Kazak, 2002). This model assumes a shared responsibility for problem solution involving a collaborative alliance of the patient, their family members, physicians and hospital staff, and the consultant.

Setting the Goals for the Consultation

After establishing the general nature of the consultation request with the referring physician or medical team member, the consultant must establish contact with the parent or guardian and, depending on age and developmental status, the pediatric patient. Often, when an inpatient consultation is requested by the attending physician, the patient, or their parent or guardian have limited input to the process and may even have objections to being evaluated by a psychologist or psychiatrist. Thus, it is important to encourage the referring physician to discuss their reasons for requesting the consultation with the family and patient before the consultant comes to meet with them. It is seldom helpful or effective for the referring physician to suggest that the patient needs psychological or psychiatric help, even in those consultations where the referring physician suspects that the patient's symptoms have a primarily functional basis, for example, conversion or somatization disorders. Rather, the referring professional might be advised to reframe the recommendation for Peds C/L involvement as a frequently employed and natural mechanism for helping all parties better understand the patient's or family's problems and to come up with a solution in which all members can play a role, and that will facilitate patient or family functioning in the midst of the medical stressors.

Ideally, when the consultant initiates contact with the patient and their family, all concerned will have at least a general agreement as to one or more problem areas that need to be addressed in the consultation. Once the consultant has met with the patient and parent(s) or guardian(s), mutually agreed upon and achievable goals for the assessment and disposition can be delineated. Goals should be fairly specific, problem-focused, and within achievable time frames. As Carter and colleagues (2003) found in their case-controlled study, clear delineation of consultation goals at the outset of the process was associated with consistently high referring professional ratings of consultation goal attainment as well as professional and patient or family satisfaction with the service.

Pre-assessment Communication with Hospital Staff

It is critical for the consultant to review the patient's clinical presentation with the referring physician, house staff, and nursing unit staff. Often there is some degree of discrepancy between various team members' perception of the actual need for a consultation, and a failure on the part of the consultant to address this factor may contribute to some "splitting," or even overt sabotage, of intervention efforts by the disagreeing team member(s) (Robertson, Robison, & Carter, 1996). For example, the authors have had experiences where nursing staff on another shift have actively undermined behavioral protocols when they felt that their input was not solicited or valued on the case, or they identified with some characteristic of the child or family that made them want to be "protective" of the child from the ill-advised efforts of the psychologist or psychiatrist. Such events need to be handled tactfully by the consultant to build the trust and confidence of the medical team and the patient or family.

Assessment

Consultations for hospitalized children typically follow a medical model whereby the consultant conducts an assessment of the referred pediatric patient and advises the referring physician and medical team about the findings and management of psychosocial aspects of the patient's care (Drotar et al., 2003). Even this more traditional model entails a complex process involving multiple interviews with child, family, and staff, repeated behavioral observations, perhaps formal psychological assessment, communication of findings to the hospital staff via written, telephone, and face-to-face contacts, and implementation of intervention procedures often under tight time constraints of competing medical procedures and insurance limitations (Drotar, 1995).

Parent- or Guardian-Based Information

Multisituational assessment methods have distinct advantages for the Peds C/L consultant, although time and logistical constraints often demand a highly streamlined process, heavily reliant upon clinical interviewing, history taking, and behavioral observation. Various parent-report measures of child behavioral problem, such as the Child Behavior Checklist (CBCL; Achenbach, 1991) and Behavioral Assessment System for Children-Parent Report Form (BASC-PRF; Reynolds & Kamphaus, 1998), may assist the consultant in obtaining normatively referenced data regarding more pervasive difficulties in adjustment that may contribute to the child's presentation in the hospital. In their case-controlled study of Peds C/L referrals, Carter et al. (2003) found that referred patients had significantly more externalizing and internalizing behavioral problems on the CBCL than their nonreferred hospitalized peers, suggesting that pre-hospitalization behavioral difficulties are likely to assist in predicting the need for referral.

Patient-Based Information

Self-report and direct psychological assessment (e.g., developmental and cognitive tests) measures may be more difficult to obtain with in-hospital consultation referrals due to a number of factors including the pediatric patient's physical condition, nonavailability due to absence from their room for diagnostic tests and treatments, uncooperative behaviors, and the distressing aspects of being in the hospital environment that make it difficult for the patient to concentrate; for example, pain, emotional upset, frequent interruptions, and so on. Nonetheless, such instruments may provide efficiency in assessing referrals when such questions as the child's cognitive ability to understand illness- and treatment-related information and procedures is in question, or concerns about the level of psychological distress and adjustment are of paramount importance. In the Carter et al. (2003) study, referrals had significantly higher scores on the self-report version of the BASC and on the Children's Depression Inventory (CDI; Kovacs, 1992) than children and adolescents who were not referred to the Peds C/L service, suggesting the potential usefulness of self-report measures.

Nursing-Based Observations

Input of the nursing staff is extremely helpful, if not critical, in assessing a referred patient. In addition to a thorough review of the patient's medical history and current treatment plans, nursing notes and gathering observational information from the nursing staff, who have frequent contact with the child and their family, can often be quite revealing as to the actual meaning behind the medical record notes (Drotar, 1995). Kronenberger, Carter, and Thomas (1997) developed a 47-item nurse-completed measure of a child's behavior during medical hospitalization titled the Pediatric Inpatient Behavior Scale (PIBS). The PIBS has 10 factor-analytically derived subscales covering a variety of internalizing and externalizing behaviors that may directly impact the child's ability to function in the hospital setting. The PIBS has acceptable interrater reliability, high internal Causey, & Carter, 2001). Kronenberger, Carter, and Lombird (1999) found that 7 of the 10 PIBS subscales (Oppositional-Noncompliant, Positive-Sociable, Withdrawal, Conduct Problems, Distress, Anxiety, Overactive) had very strong internal consistency reliability and discriminant validity, leading to the recommendation that the three remaining PIBS subscales be used with caution. The PIBS represents much-needed efforts to expand the array of tools available to assess coping and adjustment in the medically hospitalized child and adolescent.

Assessing Family and Systems Factors

As Kazak (2002) observed, there has been an increasing emphasis on family-centered perspectives in conceptualizing and treating chronic illness in children. This has been objectively reflected over the past decade in a doubling of the number of empirical studies published in the *Journal of Pediatric Psychology* that include data from multiple members of the family. However, this aspect has been more characteristic of the explicative research literature (e.g., Spirito & Stark, 1994), whereas being slower to develop in the clinical intervention literature and often involving integration of individual and family-based treatment procedures (e.g., Kazak, Penati, Brophy, & Himelstein, 1998; Wysocki et al., 2000). Systems-based perspectives go beyond focusing on the family system, positing that the reciprocal interaction with the health care and other systems requires a broad-based collaborative approach (McDaniel, Hepworth, & Doherty, 1992).

Communication of Findings and Recommendations

There are multiple ways in which the consultant communicates their findings and recommendations to the referring physician, health care team, and the parents and child. Communications to the hospital staff are routinely provided via a consultation report or progress note entry in the patient's medical chart. In the senior author's (BC) hospital setting, there is a separate "Consults" tabbed section to the chart. However, it is our practice to place our initial consultation report in the "Progress Notes" tabbed section, as this is the place in the chart typically reviewed first by the treatment team when they pick up the chart. The unit secretary typically will move the report to the "Consults" tabbed section if the patient is in the hospital over an extended period of time. Consultation reports are typically fairly brief, specific and problem-focused, with brief descriptions of the presenting problem(s), a developmental and medical history, a review of current treatments and medications, a summary of the consultant's evaluation of the referral problem, and specific recommendations for intervention and disposition. Additional entries of ongoing interventions provided by the consultant are documented in the "Progress Notes" section of the chart. Our team has developed a two-page Pediatric Consultation Form that organizes these data in a format that ensures the key areas are covered in the report. More detailed reports are often needed for complex referral questions involving formal psychological testing, complex child protective issues (e.g., factitious-disorder-by-proxy), and others. Finally, hospitals are increasingly moving toward electronic records systems, which may provide more creative (and sometimes cumbersome) ways to communicate with the health care team.

Ideally, the Peds C/L consultant also provides the referring physician and members of the health care team feedback via telephonic or, even better, face-to-face communication. The increased interpersonal communication of face-to-face discussion with a colleague can maximize the usefulness of the consultation, clarify roles in arranging a disposition for the referral, and even provide opportunities for informal teaching (Drotar, 1995).

Finally, the patient and their parents will often request information about the findings and recommendations of the consultation evaluation. This can be an important part of the trust-building phase of a therapeutic relationship, if the consultant is going to be involved in providing such services while the patient is in the hospital, or via outpatient follow-up in the clinic or the consultant's office. Many families are initially quite defensive about the prospect of being evaluated by a psychologist or psychiatrist, particularly if the request is to evaluate possible psychogenic factors contributing to their symptom presentation. Such clinical challenges call for considerable empathy, skill, and tact on the part of the Peds C/L consultant.

Additionally, with increasingly shorter hospital stays in recent years, the Peds C/L consultant is often required to arrange for follow-up services for referred cases. Extensive knowledge of community and regional resources is required to insure maximal efficacy and continuity of care beyond the hospital setting.

PRACTICE ARENAS OF PEDIATRIC CONSULTATION

Arenas of Intervention: The Five C's of Pediatric Consultation

One way of characterizing the activities of the Peds C/L team is according to the arenas of practice or intervention into which most case referrals can be categorized. A convenient alliterative pneumonic device might be called the "Five C's of Consultation: Crisis, Coping, Compliance (Adherence), Communication and Collaboration." These are overlapping arenas, for example, assisting a patient and their family with coping with their illness and treatment procedures is also likely to improve adherence with treatment and involve improving communication between patient or family and their treatment team.

Crisis

Patients and families referred for Peds C/L service involvement are often in an initial state of shock and disbelief about the seriousness of the child's illness or injury and the bewildering details and decisions of medical evaluation and treatment (Drotar & Zagorski, 2001). As such, they often are in need of very focused interventions to give them some sense of basic understanding and control. The consultant must be capable of empathically engaging in active listening so as to determine the patient's or family's view of the situation and to create a working relationship. Additional skills include crisis intervention, needs assessment, providing direction, mobilization of social supports, finding areas for parental or child control and interpreting and reframing child or family reactions to staff. Pollin (1994, 1995) has developed a medical crisis counseling model that has the following components: the primary focus is on the medical condition; interventions target normalizing the emotional distress experienced; the consultant helps the patient and family identify concrete actions that can be taken to cope successfully. These procedures are particularly relevant to children and families in crisis in a pediatric trauma setting.

Coping

One of the areas in which pediatric psychology and C/L child psychiatry have made the greatest contribution is in understanding how children cope with and adapt to medical stressors (Harbeck-Weber, Fisher, & Dittner, 2003). During the course of medical evaluation to establish a diagnosis, and in the process of medical treatment, the child may be exposed to a multitude of stressors. These include acute stressors such as venipunctures, injections, minor surgeries, and more lengthy procedures such as hospitalizations, major surgeries, repeated painful dressing changes, chemotherapy, among others. In the case of chronic illnesses such as diabetes, cystic fibrosis, various childhood cancers, chronic renal disease, hemophilia, sickle cell disease, and others, the child and family may face months, years, or even a lifetime of stressful and hassling procedures and lifestyle modifications, often with an uncertain course and outcome.

Both developmental and individual factors play a major role in determining the child's adaptation to the stressors of illness or injury and treatment. Younger children are generally more vulnerable due to their limited linguistic and cognitive abilities, because the child's knowledge and understanding of health concepts, their ability to employ internal coping resources and to access external supports are more limited than that of older children and adolescents (Harbeck-Weber & Peterson, 1993). Various perspectives have been employed in conceptualizing children's preferred coping styles, as well as the applicability of various coping strategies to the demands of different stressful situations (Peterson, Oliver, & Saldana, 1997). In anticipation of a stressful experience, some children may attempt to gather information and familiarize themselves with the procedures (sensitizers), whereas others may avoid conversation about the stressors and refuse to look at or distract themselves from the specific stressful stimuli (repressors). These different coping styles have been shown to be associated with the child's adaptation to surgery and hospitalization, lower rates of salivary cortisol production (a physiological indicator of stress response), and child cooperation pre- and postsurgery (Harbeck-Weber et al., 2003).

Rothbaum, Weisz, and Snyder (1982) have conceptualized children's coping somewhat differently, along the dimensions of the extent to which the child modifies their objective situation (primary control) versus focusing on modifying their own emotional and behavioral reactions to the stressor (secondary control). There is some evidence suggesting that primary control strategies are most effective when employed to cope with stressors over which the child has control, whereas secondary control strategies are most effective with uncontrollable stressors (Compas, Malcarne, & Banez, 1992).

Interventions in facilitating child and family coping often begin with providing basic information and education about their illness and treatment procedures. This educational component might be facilitated by the use of videotaped or in vivo models that demonstrate the use of positive coping strategies and teach mastery skills. Additional coping interventions might involve cognitive-behavioral and strength-building interventions, coping strategies intervention, the use of operant reward programs, integrating parent participation, evaluating and mobilizing family and social supports, assisting patient and family in understanding and navigating the complex medical system, directive and expressive medical play therapy, pain and anxiety management skills training (relaxation, distraction, imagery, emotive imagery, hypnosis), sensitizing medical staff to individual child needs and perceptions, and psychopharmacologic medications to decrease anxiety and improve mood.

Finally, it cannot be overly emphasized that systems factors, both family and health care system related, play a crucial role in children's coping with both short-term and chronic health concerns. These aspects of the pediatric patient's "social ecology" (Thompson & Gustafson, 1996; Wallander, Varni, Babani, Banis, & Wilcox, 1989) may influence coping and adjustment more than illness-related or demographic factors. Such family environment variables as parental freedom from serious psychopathology, family adaptability, cohesion, encouraging emotional expression, communication and conflict resolution skills have been shown to impact on the child's coping with their illness and treatment (Wallander & Thompson, 1995). Indeed, family-based interventions with such health conditions as diabetes (Wysocki et al., 2000), recurrent abdominal pain (Sanders, Shepherd, Cleghorn, & Woolford, 1994), and sickle cell disease (Kell, Kliewer, Erickson, & Ohene-Frempong, 1998), have been demonstrated to improve child adjustment and decrease behavioral problems.

Compliance (Adherence)

The authors have employed the term "compliance" for this section to be consistent with our alliterative teaching device. However, the term "adherence" is preferable (and used here as a synonym) as it implies the cooperative and collaborative participation of the patient with the health care team in maximizing the patient's or family's approximation of the recommended medical care regimen.

Adherence to medical treatment regimens is a major pediatric health concern (La Greca & Bearman, 2003), with estimates on nonadherence as high as 50% in some studies, and even higher for patients with chronic illnesses necessitating long-term behavior changes in the child and caretakers (Rapoff, 1999). Unlike most adult patients, children's adherence to their medical regimens is more heavily influenced by developmental and family factors. The very complexity of the medical management of many chronic and serious pediatric illness, for example, severe asthma, insulin-dependent diabetes, cystic fibrosis, and others, often necessitate stressful role relationship changes within the family that require considerable reorganization and redistribution of time and responsibilities, and possibly impact on such factors as marital satisfaction and parent adjustment (Quittner, Espelage, Opipari, Carter, & Eigen, 1998). Thus, the failure to adhere to prescribed medical regimens may be due to a variety of factors including lack of education and training (information and skills) in the regimen, difficulty in understanding the procedures (cognitive and learning ability skills), fearfulness and anxiety (emotional issues), interference of the treatment with normal activities and functioning (developmental and lifestyle change issues), and parent or child dynamics (family factors), among others.

The very process of monitoring adherence presents methodological challenges for the patient, family, and health care team. Multiple methods might be employed including direct observations of the patient's behavior; assays of blood, urine, or saliva; self-report via diaries or 24-hour recall, health care provider ratings, counting remaining medications, and a variety of monitoring devices, for example, blood glucose meters (La Greca & Bearman, 2003). Each of these methods has inherent limitations such as labor intensity, unreliability, expense, susceptibility to deception, and others. Even within the more closely controlled confines of the inpatient setting, pediatric patients and their families may fail to administer medications on schedule or in the appropriate doses, refuse to follow dietary guidelines, fail to follow physical activity guidelines, or be uncooperative with medical procedures that involve pain and discomfort. Interventions likely to be employed to facilitate patient and family adherence in the inpatient pediatric setting include the following: information and education; teaching mastery skills (role play, reversal, rehearsal); behavioral management contracting; removing barriers to compliance; monitoring and charting performance of medical treatment components; altering family or health care system dynamics; normalizing or reframing the patient's condition; altering patient or family lifestyle behaviors; altering expectations of family or health care providers to coincide with realistic developmental needs; negotiation and compromise. Since a comprehensive review of the pediatric adherence intervention literature is beyond the scope of this chapter, the reader is advised to see the excellent review by La Greca and Bearman (2003).

Communication

The Peds C/L consultant to inpatient pediatric units often must confront situations where staff have initiated the referral due to encountering behavioral difficulties with the child or their family that are proving disruptive to the functioning of the hospital unit. The patient and family, at times unaware of the referral, are often at the point of significant frustration and defensiveness as the consultant steps into a potentially volatile situation. Such conditions require strong skills in communication and diplomacy, and great sensitivity to patient, family, and medical team issues (Brown & Macias, 2001). This situation is greatly facilitated by the Peds C/L consultant arranging and coordinating staffings on complex cases, maintaining a regular presence at service rounds and team meetings, engaging in ongoing collaborative relationships with hospital staff, assisting with increasing cultural sensitivity, and respectively reframing patient or family and staff behaviors to facilitate understanding. Effective consultant involvement with such multidisciplinary teams is maximized when roles are clearly delineated, relationships are well established and ongoing, and there are realistic expectations of just what the consultant can provide (Brown & Macias, 2001).

Collaboration

Although this area is listed as the last of the five C's, it is perhaps the most pervasive in that it underlies, to a great extent, the potential successfulness of practice in the other four arenas. Indeed, so important is the collaborative relationship to the conduct of pediatric consultations that Drotar (1995) titled the opening chapter of his book *Consulting with Pediatricians: Psychological Perspectives*, "Evolution of collaboration among psychologists and pediatricians: A brief history." Drotar provided historical documentation of the struggles in the evolution of this relationship in service, teaching, and research. We have found that some of our best professional service collaborations with our pediatric colleagues have often evolved out of collaborations in research. Perhaps the communication skills developed in establishing research goals and procedures facilitate understanding and communication about clinical issues with patients and their families.

FINANCIAL AND INSURANCE ISSUES

One of the greatest administrative challenges to Peds C/L services is the lack of adequate funding, particularly in the current fiscal environment of managed care (Drotar & Zagorski, 2001), mental health carve-outs, state and federal budget deficits, reductions in Medicaid benefits, and so on. With the advent of managed care, and particularly behavioral health carve-out plans, adequate reimbursement for services has become a struggle for many Peds C/L services, particularly broad-based services that do not have substantial financial backing from specialty services, for example, hematology–oncology, endocrinology, and others. Typically, managed care plans require preauthorization for services, which can be difficult to obtain prior to initiating the consultation process in the busy and rushed hospital setting. Many times the consultation needs to be completed before the authorization has been formally obtained, placing the financial risk on the Peds C/L service. Even when authorized, many insurance companies deny payment for a variety of reasons, which may have to be appealed for reimbursement.

Because most pediatric hospitals in the United States maintain policies of admitting all patients, regardless of ability to pay, they are particularly vulnerable to economic factors. Additionally, these hospitals also are likely to admit patients who are initially designated as "self-pay," that is, they have no insurance or Medicaid coverage. Such hospitals are heavily dependent on local, regional, and state assistance to cover the expenses of caring for these patients. This dependence also makes these facilities particularly vulnerable to economic downturns when these funds are in short supply, or unavailable. Furthermore, in many states, Medicaid plans will not reimburse for the services of a psychologist or psychology and psychiatry trainees on the Peds C/L service.

Most insurance plans are geared toward more traditional service delivery mechanisms, such as outpatient mental health, inpatient psychiatric, or psychiatric day treatment. For example, the daily in-hospital contacts needed to assess, execute, and manage behavioral interventions for treatment adherence and coping in a child with a serious illness often do not fit the template employed for review of claims by the mental health care-outs of most insurance plans. These factors contribute to often chronic problems in funding Peds C/L services, despite the fact that referring physicians and health care workers see them as often essential to the management of the child's medical illness and overall welfare (Carter et al., 2003). Consequently, by necessity Peds C/L services often need to seek additional sources of funding, such as grant and contract support. Many hospitals and specialty services underwrite a significant portion of Peds C/L services to offset the unacceptable losses that would otherwise be incurred.

Recently, a new set of CPT codes (Current Procedural Terminology) has been developed specifically for services in health psychology, established in collaboration between the American Medical Association and the American Psychological Association. Whereas these Health and Behavior Codes are most appropriate for a broad array of Peds C/L services, their use has been problematic for a number of reasons. For one, services provided using Health and Behavior Codes are to be billed to the patient's medical (not mental health) benefits, using the ICD-9 diagnostic code for their physical condition (not a DSM-IV or ICD-9 mental health diagnostic code). Whereas Medicare recognizes these services provided by a psychologist, many Medicaid, managed care, and other insurance plans have been reticent to recognize these codes. The bills are frequently forwarded by the physical health benefits plan to the carved-out mental health component, where they are not readily recognized and where no preauthorization has been obtained or documented. The request for payment is then denied, because the service was billed under the medical diagnosis, instead of the psychiatric diagnosis. Hopefully, these codes will eventually receive recognition and acceptance in the health care and insurance industries, minimizing the difficulties experienced during this transition.

TRAINING ISSUES

Changes in health care have been accompanied by corresponding changes in pediatric psychology. Currently, there is not a standardized approach to training in Peds C/L (Spirito et al., 2003). With the expansion of pediatric psychology programs, there has been growing emphasis on the need to identify standards of training in specific areas of pediatric psychology, such as Peds C/L. In 1999, the Society of Pediatric Psychology commissioned a task force to recommend how current pediatric psychology training should be done at the predoctoral, intern, and postdoctoral levels (Spirito et al., 2003). One of the core recommendations of this report was that trainees should have experiences in interdisciplinary settings (e.g., health centers and hospitals), as well as experience working with a variety of health care providers (e.g., physicians, nurses, physical therapists, etc.) in multidisciplinary activities, such as interdisciplinary and teaching rounds. Moreover, the committee explicitly recommended training in Peds C/L. Although the committee expanded Peds C/L to include consultation in general, the main points are applicable to Peds C/L.

Specifically, the members of the task force recommended that trainees be versed in the various models of consultation and have the ability to complete focused and brief consultations with patients and family members, as well as with the medical staff (Spirito et al., 2003). It was also recommended that pediatric psychologists have experience in consulting with nonmedical professionals concerning the psychosocial aspects of pediatric medical conditions. The committee also commented that pediatric psychologists often act as a liaison between members of the medical staff or between medical staff and families.

To achieve these competencies in consultation–liaison, the committee recommended that trainees have both didactic and experiential learning experiences, including readings and seminars related to the models of consultation, communication between physicians (medical staff) and patients, and issues of professional stress and burnout. Furthermore, it was recommended that training include observation of supervisors conducting consultations and presentations by faculty to medical staff and physicians. It also was recommended that students have opportunities to conduct consultations, relay feedback to the referring physicians, and participate in all aspects of writing in the medical chart notes.

Results from a survey of pediatric psychology predoctoral internships suggest that consultation–liaison is increasingly being incorporated into training programs (Mackner, Swift, Heidgerken, Stalets, & Linscheid, 2003). All of the survey respondents (i.e., 35 of 52 programs) reported their programs provided opportunities in Peds C/L. On average, departments received 362 consults per year, with a range between 10 and 1,430. Among the subspecialties, trainees most often had consultation experiences in hematology or oncology, neurology, gastroenterology, adolescent medicine, and pulmonary medicine. The most frequent disease group reported was diabetes, followed by developmental disabilities, traumatic brain injury, and cystic fibrosis. Results indicated that pain management was the most frequently used intervention. Feeding interventions, as well as coping and support with rehabilitation and bone marrow transplants, were also commonly employed.

The training program within the University of Louisville School of Medicine in the Division of Child & Adolescent Psychiatry is similar to many of the programs described in Mackner et al.'s (2003) study, and follows many of the task force's recommended guidelines (see Spirito et al., 2003). Trainees in our program are involved in multiple areas of Peds C/L. The team comprises a faculty pediatric psychologist (service director), a predoctoral intern, one to two postdoctoral fellows, a child psychiatry fellow, and a graduate student from the health psychology track of a local doctoral program in clinical psychology. A second faculty pediatric psychologist (who works half time in a rehabilitation setting) and part time child psychiatrist, are also part of the team. As the trainees gain more expertise over the course of their rotation, they take on additional responsibility and autonomy. For example, at the beginning of their 4-month rotation, the psychology predoctoral intern usually observes the faculty member conducting a consultation, followed by the intern assisting the faculty member with the consultation. With time, the intern becomes more independent, such that at the completion of the rotation, the psychology intern is able to conduct the majority of the consult by him or herself with only minimal supervision from the faculty member. Child psychiatry fellows rotate on the service every 6 months, whereas the pediatric psychology postdoctoral fellows are on the service the full year of their training. Increasingly, the postdoctoral fellows are able to take on supervisory functions with the predoctoral intern and leadership positions in providing coverage for services where our Peds C/L team has greater involvement, for example, hematology–oncology. As the trainees progress through the rotation, they take on increasingly greater responsibility and autonomy in the consultation process. Peds C/L service rounds conducted three mornings per week and provide an avenue to discuss issues related to consultation, such as effective communication with physicians.

FUTURE NEEDS

Roberts, Brown, and Puddy (2002) urged that increased efforts be made toward the development of evidence-based interventions in clinical practice to improve service delivery within medical systems. For progress to be toward this goal, future research into Peds C/L services needs to verify the disturbances in adaptation experienced by hospitalized children and their families by applying standardized instruments that measure adjustment and psychological functioning in prospective samples of inpatient pediatric referrals, via multiple informants, to avoid the limitations found in measurement by other investigators of Peds C/L services (Harris, Canning, & Kelleher, 1996). In particular, there is a need for information as to whether or not pediatricians and pediatric specialists are sensitive and appropriate in their referrals of specific cases for consultation, identification of the types of psychiatric diagnoses represented among referred pediatric inpatients, and further identification of the clinical issues and needs of these children. Furthermore, more specific information is needed about the efficacy of Peds C/L services in attaining the goals set in the consultation contract between the referring physician and the consultant, as well as general satisfaction with the services from the perspective of the referring physician and the pediatric inpatient's parent or guardian. Finally, the efficacy of our training methods in Peds C/L need to be exposed to empirical investigation as the field moves toward further expanding the roles psychologists and psychiatrists play in inpatient pediatric settings.

REFERENCES

Achenbach, T. M. (1991). *Manual for the child behavior checklist/4–18 and 1991 profile.* Burlington, Vermont: Department of Psychiatry.
Brown, R. T., & Macias, M. (2001). Chronically ill children and adolescents. In J. N. Hughes, A. M. La Greca, & J. C. Conoley (Eds.), *Handbook of psychological services for children and adolescents* (pp. 353–372). New York: Oxford.

Carter, B. D., Kronenberger, W. G., Baker, J., Grimes, L. M., Crabtree, V. M. & Smith, C. (2003). Inpatient pediatric consultation–liaison: A case-controlled study. *Journal of Pediatric Psychology, 28*, 425–432.

Compas, B., Malcarne, V., & Banez, G. (1992). Coping with psychological stress: a developmental perspective. In B. Carpenter (Ed.), *Personal coping: Theory, research and application* (pp. 47–64). Westport, CT: Praeger.

Drotar, D. (1995). *Consulting with pediatricians: Psychological perspectives.* New York: Plenum.

Drotar, D., Spirito, A., & Stancin, T. (2003). Professional roles and practice patterns. In M. C. Roberts (Ed.), *Handbook of pediatric psychology* (3rd ed., pp. 50–66). New York: Guilford.

Drotar, D., & Zagorski, L. (2001). Providing psychological services in pediatric settings in an era of managed care. In J. N. Hughes, A. M. La Greca, & J. C. Conoley (Eds.), *Handbook of psychological services for children and adolescents* (pp. 89–104). New York: Oxford.

Fritz, G. K. (1990). Consultation–liaison in child psychiatry and the evolution of pediatric psychiatry. *The American Academy of Psychosomatic Medicine, 31*, 85–90.

Fritz, G. K. (1993a). The hospital: An approach to consultation. In G. K. Fritz, B. Mattison, D. Nurcombe, & A. Spirito (Eds.), *Child and adolescent mental health consultation in hospitals, schools, and courts* (pp. 7–24). Washington, DC: American Psychiatric Press.

Fritz, G. K. (1993b). Common clinical problems in pediatric consultation. In G. K. Fritz, B. Mattison, D. Nurcombe, & A. Spirito (Eds.), *Child and adolescent mental health consultation in hospitals, schools, and courts* (pp. 47–65). Washington, DC: American Psychiatric Press.

Fritz, G. K., & Spirito, A. (1993c). The process of consultation on a pediatric unit. In G. K. Fritz, B. Mattison, D. Nurcombe, & A. Spirito (Eds.), *Child and adolescent mental health consultation in hospitals, schools, and courts* (pp. 25–46). Washington, DC: American Psychiatric Press.

Harbeck-Weber, C., Fisher, J. L., & Dittner, C. A. (2003). Promoting coping and enhancing adaptation to illness. In M. C. Roberts (Ed.), *Handbook of pediatric psychology* (3rd ed., pp. 99–118). New York: Guilford.

Harbeck-Weber, C., & Peterson, L. (1993). Children's conception of illness and pain. In R. Vasta (Ed.), *Annals of child development* (pp. 133–163). Bristol, PA: Jessica Kingsley.

Harris, E. S., Canning, R. D., & Kelleher, K. J. (1996). The utility of measures of psychopathology, adjustment and impairment in children with chronic illness. *Journal of the American Academy of Child and Adolescent Psychiatry, 35*, 1025–1032.

Kazak, A. E. (2002). Family systems practice in pediatric psychology. *Journal of Pediatric Psychology, 27*, 133–143.

Kazak, A. E., Penati, B., Brophy, P., & Himelstein, B. (1998). Pharmacologic and psychologic interventions for procedural pain. *Pediatrics, 102*, 59–66.

Kell, R., Kliewer, W., Erickson, M., & Ohene-Frempong, M. (1998). Psychological adjustment of adolescents with sickle cell disease: Relations with demographic, medical, and family competence variables. *Journal of Pediatric Psychology, 23*, 301–312.

Knapp, P. K., & Harris, E. S. (1998a). Consultation–liaison in child psychiatry: A review of the past 10 years: Part I: Clinical findings. *Journal of the American Academy of Child and Adolescent Psychiatry, 37*, 17–25.

Knapp, P. K., & Harris, E. S. (1998b). Consultation–liaison in child psychiatry: A review of the past 10 years: Part II: Research on treatment approaches and outcomes. *Journal of the American Academy of Child and Adolescent Psychiatry, 37*, 139–146.

Kovacs, M. (1992). *Children's depression inventory (CDI) manual.* North Tonawanda, NY: Multi-Health Systems.

Kremer, P. K. G., & Wasserman, A. L. (1994). Diagnostic dilemmas in pediatric consultation. *Child and Adolescent Psychiatric Clinics of North America, 3*, 485–512.

Kronenberger, W. G., Carter, B. D., & Lombird, T. (1999). *Correspondence of the Pediatric Inpatient Behavior Scale (PIBS) scores with DSM diagnosis and problem severity ratings in a referred pediatric sample.* Poster presented at the Florida Conference on Child Health Psychology, Gainesville, FL.

Kronenberger, W. G., Carter, B. D., & Thomas. D. (1997). Assessment of behavior problems in pediatric inpatient settings: Development of the Pediatric Inpatient Behavior Scale. *Children's Health Care, 26*, 211–232.

Kronenberger, W. G., Causey, D., & Carter, B. D. (2001). Validity of the Pediatric Inpatient Behavior Scale in an inpatient psychiatric setting. *Journal of Clinical Psychology, 57*, 1421–1434.

La Greca, A. M., & Bearman, K. J. (2003). Adherence to pediatric treatment regimens. In M. C. Roberts (Ed.), *Handbook of pediatric psychology* (3rd ed., pp. 99–118). New York: Guilford.

Lewandowski, L. A., & Baranoski, M. V. (1994). Psychological aspects of acute trauma. *Child and Adolescent Psychiatry Clinics of North America, 3*, 513–529.

Lewis, M. (1994). Consultation process in child and adolescent psychiatric consultation–liaison in pediatrics. *Child and Adolescent Psychiatric Clinics of North America, 31*, 439–448.

Lewis, M., & King, R. A. (1994). Preface. *Child and Adolescent Psychiatric Clinics of North America, 3*, xi–xii.

Mackner, L. M., Swift, E. E., Heidgerken, A. D., Stalets, M. M., & Linscheid, T. M. (2003). Training in pediatric psychology: A survey of predoctoral internship programs. *Journal of Pediatric Psychology, 28*, 433–441.

McDaniel, S., Hepworth, J., & Doherty, W. (1992). *Medical family therapy: A biopsychosocial approach to families with health problems.* New York: Basic Books.

Mullins, L. D., Gillman, J., & Harbeck, C. (1992). Multiple-level interventions in pediatric psychology settings: A behavioral systems perspective. In A. M. LaGreca, L. J. Siegel, J. L. Wallander, & C. E. Walker (Eds.), *Stress and coping in child health* (pp. 371–399). New York: Guilford.

Olson, R. A., Holden, E. W., Friedman, A., Faust, J., Kenning, M., & Mason, P. (1988). Psychological consultation in a children's hospital: An evaluation of services. *Journal of Pediatric Psychology, 13*, 479–492.

Olson, R., Mullins, L., Chaney, J. M., & Gillman, J. B. (1994). The role of the pediatric psychologist in a consultation–liaison service, In R. A. Olson, L. L. Mullins, J. B. Gillman, & J. M. Chaney (Eds.), *The sourcebook of pediatric psychology* (pp. 1–8), Needham Heights, MA.: Allyn and Bacon.

Peterson, L., Oliver, K., & Saldana, L. (1997). Children's coping with stressful medical procedures. In S. Wolchik & L. Sandler (Eds.), *Handbook of children's coping: Linking theory and intervention* (pp. 333–360). New York: Plenum.

Pollin, I. (1994). *Taking charge: Overcoming the challenges of long-term illness.* New York: Times Books.

Pollin, I. (1995). *Medical crisis counseling: Short-term therapy for long-term illness.* New York: Norton.

Quittner, A. L., Espelage, D. L., Opipari, L. C., Carter, B. D., & Eigen, H. (1998). Role strain in couples with and without a child with a chronic illness: Associations with marital satisfaction, intimacy, and daily mood. *Journal of Health Psychology, 17*, 112–124.

Rapoff, M. A. (1999). *Adherence to pediatric medical regimens.* New York: Kluwer/Academic.

Reynolds, C. R., & Kamphaus, R. W. (1998). *Behavior assessment system for children: Manual.* Circle Pines, MN: American Guidance Services.

Roberts, M. C., Brown, K. J., & Puddy, R. W. (2002). Service delivery issues and program evaluation in pediatric psychology. *Journal of Clinical Psychology in Medical Settings, 9*, 3–13.

Roberts, M., Mitchell, M., & McNeal, R. (2003). The evolving field of pediatric psychology: Critical issues and future challenges. In M. C. Roberts (Ed.), *Handbook of pediatric psychology* (3rd ed., pp. 3–18). New York: Guilford.

Robertson, J. M., Robison, B. D., & Carter, B. D. (1996). Splitting on a pediatric consult liaison service. *International Journal of Psychiatry in Medicine, 26*, 93–104.

Rodrigue, J. R., Hoffman, R. G., Rayfield, A., Lescano, C., Kubar, W., & Streisand, R. (1995). Evaluating pediatric psychology consultation services in a medical setting: An example. *Journal of Clinical Psychology in Medical Settings, 2*, 89–107.

Rothbaum, F., Weisz, J. R., & Snyder, S. S. (1982). Changing the world and changing the self: A two-process model of perceived control. *Journal of Personality and Social Psychology, 42*, 5–37.

Routh, D. K. (1985). Psychology, child health, and human development. In A. R. Zeiner, D. Bendell, & C. E. Walker (Eds.), *Health psychology: Treatment and research issues* (pp. 99–111). New York: Plenum.

Sanders, M., Shepherd, R., Cleghorn, G., & Woolford, H. (1994). The treatment of recurrent abdominal pain in children: A controlled comparison of cognitive-behavioral family interventions and standard pediatric care. *Journal of Consulting and Clinical Psychology, 62,* 306–314.

Spirito, A., Brown, R. T., D'Angelo, E. J., Delamater, A. M., Rodrigue, J. R., & Siegel, L. J. (2003). Training pediatric psychologists in the 20th century. In M. C. Roberts (Ed.), *Handbook of pediatric psychology* (3rd ed. pp. 99–118). New York: Guilford.

Spirito, A., & Stark, L. J. (1994). Stressors and coping strategies described during hospitalization by chronically ill children. *Journal of Clinical Child Psychology, 24,* 314–322.

Stabler, B. (1988). Pediatric consultation–liaison. In D. K. Routh (Ed.), *Handbook of pediatric psychology* (pp. 538–566). New York: Guilford.

Thompson, R. J., & Gustafson, K. (1996). *Adaptation to chronic childhood illness.* Washington, DC: American Psychological Association

Walker, C. E. (1988). The future of pediatric psychology. *Journal of Pediatric Psychology, 13,* 465–478.

Wallander, J., Varni, J., Babani, L., Banis, H., & Wilcox, K. (1989). Family resources as resistant factors for psychological maladjustment in chronically ill and handicapped children. *Journal of Pediatric Psychology, 14,* 23–42.

Wallander, J., & Thompson, R. J. (1995). Psychosocial adjustment of children with chronic physical conditions. In M. C. Roberts (Ed.), *Handbook of pediatric psychology* (2nd ed., pp. 124–141). New York: Guilford.

Wysocki, T., Harris, M., Greco, P., Bubb, J., Danda, C., & Harvey, L. (2000). Randomized, controlled trial of behavior therapy for families of adolescents with insulin dependent diabetes. *Journal of Pediatric Psychology, 25,* 23–33.

6

Mental Health Services for Children in Pediatric Primary Care Settings

TERRY STANCIN

Psychologists,[1] and pediatricians have been collaborating to care for children's health and mental health care needs since at least the latter half of the 20th century. However, most of the collaboration between pediatric psychologists and pediatricians has taken place in hospital settings and has focused on children with physical conditions. Recently, there has been interest in expanding opportunities for mental health services in outpatient medical settings, where the majority of children obtain primary and acute medical care. *Primary care* refers to a broad range of health care services delivered in outpatient (ambulatory) medical settings that focus on prevention of illness, promotion of health and wellness, and amelioration of consequences of chronic health conditions. Primary care can be contrasted with acute and urgent care health services that are directed toward sick or injured children. In the United States, primary care providers (PCPs) of children are usually pediatricians and family medicine physicians, with some care also delivered by nurse practitioners, nurse clinicians, or physician assistants.

This chapter describes the basis for this service trend, presents models of service delivery, describes common problems and skills needed to address them in the primary care setting, outlines opportunities for the future, and summarizes available outcome data.

TERRY STANCIN • Department of Pediatrics, MetroHealth Medical Center, Case Western Reserve University School of Medicine, Cleveland, Ohio 44109.

[1]"Psychologist" is used throughout this chapter to refer to doctoral level mental health professionals with advanced training in pediatric psychology. However, many of the activities could be adapted for provision by non-doctoral level mental health clinicians including social workers and nurse specialists.

PEDIATRIC FACTORS

There has been growing interest in psychosocial issues in pediatrics since the late 1960s (e.g., Haggerty, 1986; Starfield & Borkowf, 1969; Task Force on Pediatric Education, 1978), much of which has raised awareness of pediatricians regarding their responsibilities to identify and address mental health needs of children. In a series of studies beginning in the late 1970s, Elizabeth Costello and others (e.g., Costello, 1986; Costello et al., 1988; Goldberg, Regier, McInerny, Pless, & Roghmann, 1979) established that significant behavior problems are present in 11–20% of school age children in primary care. The prevalence rate is even higher for preschool-age children and children from economically disadvantaged families (Lavigne et al., 1993). Moreover, up to 50% of parents express concerns about their child's behavior during routine pediatric appointments (Costello & Shurgart, 1992; Horwitz, Leaf, Leventhal, Forsyth, & Speechley, 1992; Sharp, Pantell, Murphy, & Lewis, 1992; Starfield & Borkowf, 1969). Although the prevalence of childhood behavioral problems in primary care is well documented, PCPs have been shown to identify less than half of the children who might need services (Sharp et al., 1992). Moreover, most patients referred for mental health services by their PCP never make it to their initial appointment. Therefore, although child behavior problems are common in primary care settings, they are clearly underidentified and undertreated (Perrin & Stancin, 2002).

Pediatric leaders have expressed the importance of responding to the mental health needs of children seeking pediatric attention (e.g., Haggerty, 1986; Perrin, 1999). Although pediatricians do receive some training in behavioral and developmental pediatrics, this training is usually minimal and most do not have the skills to adequately address complex psychosocial needs (Perrin, 1999). Even if they had the skills, PCPs probably do not have enough time to adequately care for child mental health needs. Routine well-child care now involves many time-consuming tasks including prevention and early detection of diseases, prevention of unintentional trauma, assessment of family health and safety, immunizations, and comprehensive care of children with chronic health and developmental conditions (Green, 1994). PCPs are expected to address so many issues during routine care that they cannot be expected to be competent or have sufficient time to address the spectrum of mental health issues as well (Perrin & Stancin, 2002).

PEDIATRIC PSYCHOLOGY INFLUENCES

The idea for providing behavioral health services in primary care settings has been advocated by psychologists for many years (e.g., Christophersen, 1982; Drotar, 1993; Roberts & Wright, 1982; Routh, Schroeder, & Koocher 1983). The earliest descriptions of psychological services in primary care (e.g., Smith, Rome, & Freidman, 1967) indicated that they were consultative in nature and primarily involved colocating activities (i.e., behavioral and primary care services provided in the same place).

Carolyn Schroeder's pioneering work with the Chapel Hill Pediatric Psychology Practice raised awareness of the potential scope and impact of a primary care psychology practice (Schroeder, 1979, 1999, 2004; Schroeder, Goolsby, & Stangler, 1974). Dr. Schroeder's visionary practice included clinical, teaching, research, community advocacy, and public health components that continues to serve as a model today. Initially, clinical programs were offered free of charge in exchange for training opportunities for psychology and other mental health trainees. A "call-in hour" gave parents an opportunity to inquire about development and behaviors. Weekly evening parent groups focused on normal development topics. Half-hour "come-in" sessions allowed parents to discuss developmental and behavioral concerns. A developmental screening program identified children at risk for developmental problems. These services were so well received by families and pediatricians that clinical activities were greatly expanded into an integrated, collaborative private practice. Prevention activities included the development of a parent resource library and a series of parent handouts on common behavioral concerns (e.g., toilet training). Direct clinical services for a variety of problems (e.g., negative behaviors, anxiety, attention deficit hyperactivity disorder [ADHD], adjustment issues) were provided. Schroeder (2004) noted that the "treatment" activities she and her group provided were often in the role of consultant to pediatricians or parents who carried out the actual intervention with a child. Interventions focused on brief, problem-focused treatments. The practice emphasized the use of protocols for common problems (e.g., enuresis, sleep problems, negative behaviors) and parent or child groups, which proved to be both cost effective and efficient treatment modalities. Not only were the psychologists "therapists" (providing direct treatment to child, parents, and family), but also they were often educators (of physicians, parents, and teachers), advocates (in court, schools, and community), and case managers (coordinating services among various medical, school and community providers). The practice placed a high value on training of health care providers (medical and mental health) and conducting clinical outcome research.

Interest in primary care is growing in pediatric psychology. Dennis Drotar (1995) featured descriptions of collaborative outpatient pediatric practices in his important text, *Consulting with Pediatricians* (e.g., Hurley, 1995). A special issue of the *Journal of Pediatric Psychology* was devoted to Pediatric Mental Health Services in Primary Care Settings in 1999 (Stancin, 1999). In her Society for Pediatric Psychology Presidential Address, Maureen Black (2002) advocated for pediatric psychologists to develop and evaluate health promotion programs for use in primary care. Recently, Spirito et al. (2003) and others (e.g., Drotar, Spirito, & Stancin, 2003; Perrin, 1999; Stancin, 1999; Wildman & Stancin, 2004) have recommended expansions of pediatric primary care service models, training activities, and research efforts.

Why the increased interest? One explanation is the change in practice patterns and roles for pediatric psychologists in recent years (Drotar et al., 2003). Pediatric psychologists specialize in the evaluation and treatment of psychosocial concerns of children seen in medical settings.

Because children are spending less time in the hospital than in years past, most medical care is now delivered in pediatric ambulatory settings. Pediatric psychologists, who were accustomed to seeing children with medical conditions while they were in the hospital, are now seeing those children in the outpatient clinic instead. Moreover, as noted previously, pediatricians are seeking broader assistance in addressing psychosocial concerns of children in the primary care setting. Thus, opportunities for outpatient collaboration are growing rapidly.

TRADITIONAL VERSUS PRIMARY MENTAL HEALTH CARE

Within traditional primary care settings, mental health services are considered to be separate specialty care. If a PCP recognizes that a child may have a behavioral or emotional problem, then he or she might refer the family to a psychologist in the same way that a referral might be made to a neurologist or gastroenterologist. In most settings, the psychologist is located in a different office, and communication between the medical and mental health provider may be limited to a courtesy call or perhaps a brief letter or report summarizing the specialist's assessment and treatment results. Table 1 outlines some of the differences between traditional child mental health services and primary care mental health services.

There are several problems with this traditional model of mental health service for PCPs and families. First, most children do not receive mental health services from behavioral specialists. Rather, families seek and

Table 1. Comparisons between Traditional and Primary Care Mental Health Service Models

	Traditional model	Primary care model
No. of patients	Few patients	Many patients
Time	50-minute sessions	Flexible time limits (sometimes 15–30-minute sessions)
Patient problem severity	Severe	Mild to moderate
Prevention and early intervention opportunities	Few	Many
Treatment focus	Multiple problems	Targeted, specific problems
Treatment course	Long-term, many sessions	Brief, short term
Treatment period	Termination of case after treatment is completed	Continuity of care: contact occurs as needed throughout childhood
Mental health provider role with family	Single role as therapist	Multiple roles (therapist, teacher, advocate, case manager)
Accessibility to child's PCP	Difficult to access directly	Visible and accessible
Communication with child's PCP	Little or no communication	Prompt, frequent feedback and case discussion

obtain services from PCPs even for problems that are clearly "psychological" (e.g., depression, anxiety, ADHD) (Strosahl, 1998). For example, Cunningham and Freiman (1996) estimated that 44% of all child mental health care in the United States is delivered solely by PCPs. Another problem with the traditional model is that it is often difficult to link families with mental health services after they leave the PCP office. Most families enjoy an ongoing relationship with their PCP, yet that individual may not be involved in ongoing care once an outside psychologist is involved. Moreover, many problems (sometimes referred to as "biopsychosocial conditions") are not presented to PCPs by families as either medical or psychological, but as both (e.g., abdominal pain associated with school avoidance). Families may view traditional mental health services for biopsychosocial conditions as confusing at best, and often as inadequate.

COLOCATION, COLLABORATION, AND INTEGRATION

Three key variables define the service delivery of mental health services in primary care (Strosahl, 1998):

Colocation

Colocation is considered to be a necessary, but not sufficient, condition for primary care mental health services. That is, although it is crucial that behavioral services be located in close proximity to medical services, colocation does not guarantee that practices will be integrated. Moreover, behavioral and medical services need to have overlapping office hours so that providers can have easy access to one another for consultation (Strosahl, 1998).

Collaboration

Collaboration refers to the practice of providers with separate sets of expertise bringing their work together so as to coordinate treatments between the two. Collaboration may occur without colocation, but it always includes a rich exchange of communication between providers (Blount, 1998; Drotar, 1995).

Integration

Integration implies that mental health services are a component of primary care, rather than a specialty service (Blount, 1998). Integrated practices offer behavioral health services to children with and without mental health diagnoses.

Services may vary in primary care settings from being colocated to fully integrated. At one end of the continuum, pediatric and mental health practices may have separate offices, staff, waiting space, and records, but are conveniently located next to one another. Referral is facilitated by location, but interaction between medical and mental health staff may be minimal.

A mid-continuum collaborative practice includes specialty mental health care that is delivered in a primary care setting. In this practice, a psychologist may be part of the primary care team, with shared offices, staff, and possibly records. However, the psychologist sees patients for mental health services determined by screening procedures or PCP referral, and is not necessarily part of routine primary care. The psychologist in this setting may have frequent contact with the medical providers and may follow what has been termed a *collaborative care model* (McDaniel, Campbell, & Seaburn, 1995). Psychologists using a collaborative care model may assume a variety of responsibilities in the primary care practice including organizing and administering developmental and behavioral screening programs, running psychoeducational or therapeutic groups for children and for parents (e.g., related to divorce, ADHD), providing individual counseling, coordinating services for children with chronic health conditions, and communicating with schools and community agencies (Perrin, 1999; Perrin & Stancin, 2002).

At the most fully integrated end of the practice continuum are those that follow a *primary mental health care model*, described as one in which behavioral specialists provide consultative, time-limited services within a primary care setting (Strosahl, 1998). The goal is to provide consultative support to PCPs rather than to take over responsibility for providing all mental health services to the primary care population. Strosahl distinguished between specialty mental health care (behavioral services delivered in a primary care setting) and primary care behavioral health (fully integrated mental health services delivered in primary care settings). A fully integrated care practice focuses on behavioral health issues and the behavioral health provider is considered to be an integral member of the general health care team. Integrated services may be "horizontal" (for an entire population, e.g., behavioral screening) or "vertical" (targeted to a group of patients, e.g., those with ADHD) (Strosahl, 1998).

Strohsahl predicted that the next era of managed health care will involve integrated services as well as development of cost- and quality-oriented delivery systems. A model of integrated service delivery, he argued, is necessary to reduce redundant administrative and infrastructure costs, to address consumer demands for simpler "one-stop shopping" service delivery venues, and to contain utilization and costs because so much of medical treatment hinges on psychological and psychosocial issues (Strosahl, 1998). In a fully integrated practice, patients may be just as likely to be seen by a psychologist or PCP (or both). Which provider sees that child or parent may depend on the setting, the needs of the child and family, interest and skills of the provider, time availability, or economic factors (Schroeder, 2004).

COMMON CHILD MENTAL HEALTH PROBLEMS IN PRIMARY CARE SETTINGS

Although children of all ages are seen in primary care settings, the majority of patients are infants and very young children. This is because infants need to be seen for about a dozen well-child visits during the first

2 years of life for immunizations and other preventive interventions, but only once yearly after the age of 2 years until adulthood (Green, 1994). The relatively large infant and toddler population in primary care settings offers important opportunities for prevention and early intervention services such as developmental monitoring, screening for developmental delay, promotion of healthy parent–child interactions, and detection of parental mental health problems (Drotar et al., 2003; Roberts & Brown, 2004).

Referrals for psychological services from primary care settings may differ considerably from inpatient pediatric psychology referrals. Studies describing the nature of referral problems of children seen for primary care behavioral services have shown that the most frequently referred problems are negative behavior such as tantrums, oppositional behavior, defiance, noncompliance, and aggression (Charlop, Parrish, Fenton, & Cataldo, 1987; Finney, Riley, & Cataldo, 1991; Schroeder, 2004; Sobel, Roberts, Rayfield, Barnard, & Rapoff, 2001). For example, Finney et al. (1991) reported that 56% of children referred in their primary care psychology clinic had behavioral problems such as aggression, sleep and mealtime struggles. Toileting (e.g., enuresis) and somatic (e.g., recurrent abdominal pain) problems were also common reasons for referral. Similarly, Sobel et al. (2001) reported that the 100 children seen for psychological services at two primary care settings were referred for externalizing problems (i.e, disruptive, negative behaviors) (45%), internalizing problems (e.g, depression, anxiety) (23%), school-related problems (e.g., attention, learning) (15%), adjustment problems (7%), diagnosis for medical or psychological problem (4%), habit disorders (4%), and medical problems (3%). The majority of diagnoses made by psychologists were oppositional defiant disorder (22%), ADHD (22%), and adjustment disorder (14.4%).

HOW ARE SERVICES PROVIDED?

There is a broad range of behavioral service options in a primary care setting including consultation, direct clinical services (assessment and treatment), case management, forensics, and community agency involvement (Drotar et al., 2004; Schroeder, 2004). The type and scope of services offered will depend largely upon the philosophy and interests of the providers within the practice. In practices that are more integrated there are larger opportunities for comanagement of patients, with and without mental health diagnoses.

Psychologists in primary care settings need to be cognizant about several issues. First, PCPs may need assistance in identifying children in need of behavioral attention and in linking them to services (Riekert, Stancin, Palermo, & Drotar, 1999). Moreover, they may be most likely to miss the problems in children in earlier or milder stages of development when they are most amenable to early intervention. Results from a recent study by Lochrie and Roberts (2003) using clinical vignettes indicated that PCPs were likely to identify and refer problems that were severe (e.g., severe depression), but were more likely to misidentify the presenting problems when they were mild. Lochrie and Roberts suggest that onsite primary care psychologist providers may be of assistance in teaching PCPs about how behavior problems develop over time so that early intervention could take place.

Screening

Having onsite mental health collaborators helps to facilitate referrals and removes many of the inherent barriers to care for children. However, colocation may not be sufficient to insure that children who would benefit from mental health services will receive them. It is often useful for psychologists in primary care settings to design and implement developmental and behavioral screening protocols and procedures that fit an office practice (Perrin & Stancin, 2002; Stancin & Aylward, 2003; Stancin & Palermo, 1997).

Screening for disease (e.g., lead poisoning) is a concept that is quite familiar to physicians, so it is not surprising that PCPs would be interested in ideas for efficient and accurate ways to identify children in need of developmental or mental health services. By definition, "screening" refers to a process for identifying a child in need of further evaluation and possible treatment, but does not provide a diagnosis. Screening procedures appear to be a cost-effective way to increase the identification of children who might benefit from mental health services, although data on comparative effectiveness of techniques are lacking (Stancin & Palermo, 1997).

In primary care settings, it is sometimes useful to use a two-step screening procedure for child developmental and behavior problems (Simonian, Tarnowski, Stancin, Friman, & Atkins, 1991; Stancin & Aylward, 2003; Stancin & Palermo, 1997). For example, a "first stage" screening measure may be administered to all children in a setting, such as the PCPs' waiting room or in the exam room. First-stage procedures often use parent or caretaker responses on a questionnaire or a short, structured interview that can be completed and scored in less than 10 minutes. For children whose scores exceed a set criterion, a longer, "second-stage" screening procedure may follow to provide more detailed information about the nature and severity of concerns. Second-stage screening instruments tend to be multidimensional in focus and have normative standards by which to evaluate severity of problems (Stancin & Aylward, 2003). In the absence of formal screening procedures, a child's problem is recognized because a parent raises a concern with the PCP during the office visit (Barlow, Wildman, & Stancin, 2002). Ideally, the PCP and parent would then discuss how the family would like to pursue help for the problem.

What Happens When a Behavior Problem Is Identified?

Depending on the skill and interests, the PCP may feel comfortable providing counseling for milder concerns (e.g., sleeping through the night, temper tantrums, picky eating). Other concerns may be referred to the psychologist (e.g., school refusal, depressed mood, learning problems). If a referral is being made, it is important that the family have an opportunity to discuss the referral with the PCP. The family will want to know why they are being referred and what to expect from the psychologist (Drotar, 1995).

PCPs and primary care psychologists should agree on referral procedures and questions. A conversation between the PCP and psychologist prior to the mental health appointment can be useful in clarifying concerns. Moreover, because the PCP usually knows the family well, he or she is often in a position to convey valuable insights about the child and family. During the initial mental health appointment, it is useful to discuss the family's understanding about the reasons for the referral (Drotar, 1995). Some parents express confusion or misunderstanding, especially if the child is viewed to have a medical, not psychological problem. For example, parents may wonder why a child whose problems appear to them to be physical (e.g., abdominal pain, headaches, fatigue) would need to be seen by a psychologist. Indeed, it is sometimes not clear to the psychologist! If the PCP has explained to the family that stress or other psychological factors may be contributing to physical problems, then the psychologist and family can begin to look for sources of stress and develop interventions to reduce symptom severity.

Primary care mental health services differ from traditional services in the level of communication between PCP and psychologist. PCPs expect prompt feedback from the psychologist about their patients (Drotar, 1995), done formally (via letter or chart notes) or informally (in person or by phone). Most PCPs are interested in hearing from psychologists and many participate directly in the implementation of behavioral treatment plans. Most PCPs value psychologist insights and are appreciative of practical, relevant suggestions about how they might also assist the family with behavioral concerns. Communication between psychologist and PCP should not be misconstrued as "casual," in that confidentiality matters must be carefully considered. Therefore, it is important that a family has the opportunity to discuss with the psychologist how and what information can be shared with others, including the PCP.

Intervention Strategies in Primary Care

As was aptly described by Schroeder (2004), mental health interventions in primary care settings may be traditional treatments delivered in nontraditional ways. For example, time constraints are usually more flexible and variable. In primary care settings, the mental health professional often cannot adhere to a 50-minute session but may have only 10 or 15 minutes with a patient. It is not unusual for a patient to have brief, frequent visits and approximate appointment times (Blount, 1998). Treatments tend to be more focused, goal oriented, and didactic (Blount, 1998). Therefore, psychologists tend to be use cognitive-behavioral, solution-focused or family systems treatment approaches. In the referred children described by Sobel et al. (2001), 79% were treated with behavioral techniques (e.g., bibliotherapy, parent training, behavior management), 10.5% with cognitive-behavioral methods (e.g., relaxation, social skills training, problem solving), 8% with supportive counseling, and 2.5% with physical techniques (e.g., diet, exercise). Behavioral treatments in primary care settings also tend to be brief. Sobel et al. (2001) reported that the majority of patients saw a psychologist between one and five times (81%), and that the modal number of sessions was one.

PREVENTION AND PUBLIC HEALTH MODELS

Because children are seen by PCPs longitudinally from infancy, psychologists in primary care settings may have an important role in developing and promoting public health agendas that include prevention and early intervention (Drotar et al., 2003; Roberts & Brown, 2004). It would be especially helpful to implement prevention services targeted at the most frequently occurring issues including negative behaviors and other common problems. Psychologists in primary care have the opportunity to develop and evaluate prevention strategies, and to emphasize training in effective prevention methods (Roberts & Brown, 2004).

Drotar et al. (2003) suggest that psychologists in primary care need to move beyond services for individuals to more broad-based community initiatives. A prevention-based model of primary care mental health services developed in Australia appears to have potential for applicability and effectiveness in the United States (Tynan, 2004). The "Triple P" (Positive Parenting Program) model developed by Matt Sanders, Ph.D., is a comprehensive, integrated system of mental health care that includes both primary care and specialty mental health providers (Sanders, 1999). The Triple P model is based on empirically supported interventions and includes five levels. Level 1 involves education and universal prevention (e.g., television promotional series on common child behavior problems). Level 2 emphasizes brief, problem-specific sessions conducted by PCPs on common, normal behavior challenges. Level 3 focuses on structured individual parent training sessions conducted by PCPs for mild behavioral concerns. Level 4 includes parent group sessions for more severe problems conducted by a mental health specialist (or PCP with additional training). Finally, Level 5 provides for intensive group or individual interventions by a mental health professional. One of the interesting aspects of the Triple P model is that it emphasizes training PCPs to provide basic empirically supported behavioral interventions. Tynan (2004) argued that if PCPs were effective in providing prevention and early intervention services in primary care settings, then psychologists could focus more on program development, evaluation, training and interventions with more severe cases. Clinical trials are currently underway in the United States to study whether the Triple P model can be transported to the United States (Matt Sanders, Ph.D., personal communication, January 17, 2003).

PRACTICE ISSUES

There are several practical considerations when establishing a primary care practice. As in any business arrangement, it is critical that the medical and mental health providers adhere to similar philosophical ideas about their service delivery model. The practice will need to use a common model and language that makes sense to all providers. Setting up a practice requires an investigation of financial matters including a delineation of payers for services, scheduling, and space issues. Prior to implementing any integrated service, Blount (1998) recommends involving not only physicians and office managers, but nursing staff and the entire clinical team in the planning process. Moreover, it is usually important for medical and behavioral providers to have regular structured meetings to discuss cases and practice issues (Blount, 1998).

Confidentiality issues are complex in the primary care setting. Practices need to decide how much of the medical and mental health data needs to be shared and how to document information. As all health care practitioners prepare for federal regulations regarding privacy (i.e., Health Insurance Portability and Accountability Act of 1996 [HIPAA]), they must determine whether to keep a single/joint record or to maintain separate medical and mental health records. Practices that share a single medical record will need to decide how much confidential information is recorded and who will be able to access the records. Families should be clearly informed about how confidentiality will be maintained in an integrated practice.

What Are the Skills Needed to Succeed in a Primary Care Mental Health Service Setting?

Formal, supervised training is important for those who choose to practice in primary care settings, although few mental health professionals have the opportunity. Schroeder (2004) incorporated psychology trainees at all levels in the Chapel Hill practice, as well as social work, medical students, and residents, but this is unusual. The primary care setting may require an attitude shift and a willingness to be accessible, flexible, and creative; not all psychologists have the temperament necessary to succeed in the primary care setting.

In addition to broad clinical child and pediatric psychology training, the successful psychologist in a primary care setting must have a firm grasp of normal child development and behavioral concerns from infancy through late adolescence. Knowledge and facility with behavioral and developmental screening and assessment techniques are essential. The primary care psychologist should be competent to deliver brief, solution-focused, and family systems treatments, often by applying behavioral and cognitive behavioral approaches, to children from birth through adolescents and their parents. The primary care psychologist must possess psychoeducational skills, especially related to parenting behavioral and discipline topics. Often, group therapy skills are important for offering to parent and child groups on a variety of common issues (e.g., ADHD, divorce, social skills). The pediatric primary care psychologist should be comfortable serving as a liaison to schools and other agencies that serve children.

The primary care psychologist must also be familiar with general pediatric medical issues, including anatomy, physiology, disease processes,

pharmacology, and preventive medicine (Blount, 1998). Knowledge about
the evaluation and treatment of psychosocial aspects of child and adolescent chronic and acute medical conditions is essential. The primary
care psychologist must be comfortable discussing a patient's need for
psychopharmacology, although not as a replacement for a psychiatrist
(Blount, 1998). This is a particularly important issue because Sobel et al.
(2001) reported that 44% of the children that received psychological services in their primary care setting were taking medication related to their
psychological diagnoses.

Opportunities in Academic Primary Care Settings

Academic primary care settings offer several additional opportunities
beyond clinical services, where psychologists may be integral to training
a variety of health care professionals and to research activities (Drotar,
1995). Because national accreditation standards and training guidelines
require structured educational experiences in behavior and development
during pediatric residencies (Coury, Berger, Stancin, & Tanner, 1999), pediatric psychologists have often assumed a central or leadership role in
teaching pediatric residents about child mental health needs. Psychologists
in academic primary care settings are ideally situated to provide clinical
supervision ("precepting") for pediatric residents regarding child development and behavioral issues that arise during primary care pediatric office
visits.

Economic Constraints

The medical cost-savings involved when mental health care is integrated into primary practice is compelling, although there are few data
available with pediatric populations than with adult populations. For example, Cummings, Dorken, Pallack and Henke (1990, cited by Blount,
1998) found that focused mental health services targeted toward the highest utilizers of medical care reduced medical costs by as much as 38%
even with the cost of mental health treatment included. Several other cost
benefits derive from higher rates of patient satisfaction, lower provider
turnover, and ultimately increased productivity in the general workforce
(Blount, 1998).

Despite the growing recognition of the importance of delivering mental
health care in pediatric outpatient settings, providers have faced difficult
challenges when trying to obtain reimbursement for services. Coding and
billing are complex issues in any mental health setting, but are particularly
troublesome in primary care. Insurance reimbursement is driven by codes
for diagnosis and procedures, and mental health services in primary care
settings do not always fit neatly into recognizable codes. Many insurance
companies and other third-party payers are unfamiliar with the range of
mental health services in primary care practices and may be reluctant to
agree to payment. For example, brief interventions services may be offered
for behavioral problems when they are in the early problem stage; that is,

parent training in behavior management for parents with a preschool child with oppositional behavior. In this case, reimbursement may be denied because services are provided for mental health conditions that do not meet diagnostic criteria for a mental disorder.

The Diagnostic and Statistical Manual for Primary Care (DSM-PC), Child and Adolescent Version (Wolraich, Felice, & Drotar, 1996), is a coding system developed as a way to describe the kinds of child mental health problems most often treated in primary care settings. This system allows not only child symptoms to be coded (e.g., anxiety), but also incorporates the child's environmental stresses (e.g., divorce). One of the intentions for developing the DSM-PC was the expectation that with an increased number of diagnostic classifications for children, it would be easier to identify children, thus leading to more requests for reimbursement. Although information about the DSM-PC has been disseminated to pediatricians and some psychologists, it has not been adopted by most pediatric practices (Drotar, 1999). Moreover, there are many unanswered questions regarding training and implementation as well as how insurance payers view the DSM-PC codes (Black, 2002; Drotar, Sturner, & Nobile, 2004).

Another reimbursement challenge sometimes occurs with managed care organizations (Drotar & Zagoski, 2001). It is not unusual for medical care to be covered under one payer with mental health care "carved out" and managed by another. In a primary care practice, it is important that care does not become fragmented because of reimbursement issues.

EVALUATION OF BEHAVIORAL HEALTH SERVICES IN PRIMARY CARE SETTINGS

Although research in primary care settings poses difficult obstacles (Drotar & Lemanek, 2001), it is critical that psychologists demonstrate the need for and effectiveness of their services. At a practical level, many PCPs will expect some proof of effectiveness before they will accept nonphysicians as colleagues. Moreover, insurance payers will need to be convinced that interventions are needed before they will be willing to reimburse them. Research evaluating patient and provider satisfaction and effectiveness of mental health services in primary care has been supportive of interventions (Charlop et al., 1987; Finney et al., 1991; Kanoy & Schroeder, 1985; Sobel et al., 2001; Tynan, Schuman, & Lampert, 1999). However, studies have been primarily descriptive in nature and randomized controlled trials that would empirically evaluate the efficacy of primary care interventions compared with other service systems have not been reported (Drotar et al., 2003).

Well-integrated primary behavioral health care services should focus on controlling medical costs while optimizing health care outcomes (Strosahl, 1998). Finney et al. (1991) addressed the question of whether brief targeted therapy for common behavioral problems in a pediatric outpatient clinic would reduce the level of pediatric health care utilization. In this study, not only were treatments effective in decreasing behavior problems, but also there was a decrease in the number of medical visits in the behaviorally treated group that did not occur in a matched comparison group of children from the practice that did not receive behavioral treatment. Similarly, Finney, Lemanek, Cataldo, Katz and Fugua (1989) demonstrated a decrease in medical utilization as well as improvement of pain symptoms among children with recurrent abdominal pain following multicomponent, targeted behavioral therapy.

CONCLUDING REMARKS

Outpatient pediatric clinics and primary care practices are gaining attention from pediatricians and psychologists as important settings for child mental health services. Whereas in the past, much of the collaboration between pediatric psychologists and pediatricians focused on children in hospitals who were physically ill, there are many opportunities to extend work to community practices and academic primary care settings. Pediatricians note that there is a great unmet need for services and pediatric psychologists are eager to respond to those needs.

Although several models have been described, the empirical basis of psychological services in pediatric primary care settings is at an early stage. In many respects, issues overlap with practices in other public and private mental health arenas. Quality of care, access to services, availability of empirically supported interventions, managed care, and reimbursement constraints (to name a few) are as important in primary care as they are in other treatment settings. Pediatric psychologists need to develop and test models that incorporate these broad mental health considerations within the primary care setting and also take advantage of the rich opportunities available for innovation with prevention, intervention, and public health initiatives.

There are many opportunities for psychologists to impact the mental health status of children by providing services in primary care settings, yet integrated models of care in family medicine and internal medicine practices seem to have evolved more rapidly than pediatric models. Why more child mental health professionals have not established such practices as yet is unclear. Possible reasons may include lack of training opportunities necessary to obtain requisite skills, reimbursement patterns that favor services for the most seriously disordered children over early intervention and prevention activities, and perhaps a reluctance of mental health providers to partner with physicians out of concern for being delegated to a secondary status. However, it has been my experience and that of others (e.g., Drotar, 1995; Schroeder, 2004) that pediatricians highly value the contributions psychologists make in service, teaching and research in primary care, and that many welcome us as partners and colleagues. Similarly, many of us psychologists who work in primary care settings cannot imagine working with children without a pediatrician colleague close by with whom to collaborate on the health and mental health care of our patients.

REFERENCES

Barlow, M., Wildman, B., & Stancin, T. (2002, September). *Mother's help-seeking for pediatric psychosocial problems*. Paper presented at the annual meeting of the Society for Developmental and Behavioral Pediatrics, Seattle, WA.

Black, M. M. (2002). Society of Pediatric Psychology Presidential Address: Opportunities for health promotion in primary care. *Journal of Pediatric Psychology, 27*, 637–646.

Blount, A. (1998). Introduction to integrated primary care. In A. Blount (Ed.), *Integrated primary care: The future of medical and mental health collaboration* (pp. 1–43). New York: W.W. Norton.

Charlop, M. H., Parrish, J. M., Fenton, L. R., & Cataldo, M. J. (1987). Evaluation of hospital-based pediatric psychology services. *Journal of Pediatric Psychology, 12*, 485–503.

Christophersen, E. R. (1982). Incorporating behavioral pediatrics into primary care. *Pediatric Clinics of North America, 29*, 261–296.

Costello, E. J. (1986). Primary care pediatrics and child psychopathology: A review of diagnostic, treatment, and referral practices. *Pediatrics, 78*, 1044–1051.

Costello, E. J., Burns, B. J., Costello, A. J., Edelbrock, C., Dulcan, M., & Brent, D. (1988). Service utilization and psychiatric diagnosis in pediatric primary care: The role of the gatekeeper. *Pediatrics, 82*, 435–441.

Costello, E. J., & Shugart, M. A. (1992). Above and below the threshold: Severity of psychiatric symptoms and functional impairment in a pediatric sample. *Pediatrics, 90*, 359–368.

Coury, D., Berger, S., Stancin, T., & Tanner, L. (1999). Curricular guidelines for residency training in developmental and behavioral pediatrics. *Journal of Developmental and Behavioral Pediatrics, 20*, S1–S38.

Cummings, N. A., Dorken, H., Pallack, M. A., & Henke, C. (1990). *The impact of psychological intervention on healthcare utilization and costs*. South San Francisco: The Biodyne Institute.

Cunningham, P. J., & Freiman, M. P. (1996). Determinants of ambulatory mental health services use for school-age children and adolescents. *Health Services Research, 31*, 409–427.

Drotar, D. (1993). Influences on collaborative activities among psychologists and physicians: Implications for practice, research, and training. *Journal of Pediatric Psychology, 18*, 159–172.

Drotar, D. (1995). *Consulting with pediatricians: Psychological perspectives for research and practice*. New York: Plenum Press.

Drotar, D. (1999). The Diagnostic and Statistical Manual for Primary Care (DSM-PC), child and adolescent version: What pediatric psychologists need to know. *Journal of Pediatric Psychology, 24*, 369–380.

Drotar, D., & Lemanek, K. (2001). Steps toward a clinically relevant science of interventions in pediatric settings: Introduction to the special issue. *Journal of Pediatric Psychology, 26*, 385–394.

Drotar, D., Spirito, A., & Stancin, T. (2003). Professional roles and practice patterns. In M. C. Roberts (Ed.), *Handbook of pediatric psychology* (3rd ed., pp. 50–66). New York: Guilford.

Drotar, D., Sturner, R., & Nobile, C. (2003). Diagnosing and managing behavioral and developmental problems in primary care: Current applications of the DSM-PC. In B. W. Wildman & T. Stancin (Eds.), *New directions for research and treatment of pediatric psychosocial problems in primary care*. Westport, CT: Greenwood Publishing.

Drotar, D., & Zagorski, L. (2001). Providing psychological services in pediatric settings in an era of managed care: Challenges and opportunities. In J. N. Hughes, A. La Greca, & J. C. Conoley (Eds.), *Handbook of psychological services to children and adolescents* (pp. 89–107). New York: Oxford University Press.

Finney, J. W., Lemanek, K. L., Cataldo, M. F., Katz, H. P., & Fuqua, R. W. (1989). Pediatric psychology in primary health care: Brief target therapy for recurrent abdominal pain. *Behavior Therapy, 29*, 283–291.

Finney, J. W., Riley, A. W., & Cataldo, M. F. (1991). Psychology in primary care: Effects of brief targeted therapy on children's medical care utilization. *Journal of Pediatric Psychology, 16,* 447–461.

Goldberg, I. D., Regier, D. A., McInerny, T. K., Pless, I. B., & Roghmann, K. J. (1979). The role of the pediatrician in the delivery of mental health services to children. *Pediatrics, 63,* 898–909.

Green, M. (Ed.). (1994). *Bright futures: Guidelines for health supervision of infants, children and adolescents.* Arlington, VA: National Center for Education in Maternal and Child Health.

Haggerty, R. J. (1986). The changing nature of pediatrics. In N. A. Krasnegor, J. D. Arasteh, & M. F. Cataldo (Eds.), *Child health behavior: A behavioral pediatrics perspective* (pp. 9–16). New York: Wiley.

Horwitz, S. M., Leaf, P. J., Leventhal, J. M., Forsyth, B., & Speechley, K. N. (1992). Identification and management of psychosocial and developmental problems in community-based, primary care pediatric practices. *Pediatrics, 89,* 480–485.

Hurley, L. K. (1995). Developing a collaborative pediatric psychology practice in a pediatric primary care setting. In D. Drotar (Ed.), *Consulting with pediatricians: Psychological perspectives* (pp. 159–184). New York: Plenum.

Kannoy, K. W., & Schroeder, C. S. (1985). Suggestions to parents about common behavior problems in a pediatric primary care office: Five years of follow-up. *Journal of Pediatric Psychology, 10,* 15–30.

Lavigne, J. V., Binns, H. J., Christoffel, K. K., Rosenbaum, D., Arend, R., Smith, K. Hayford, J. R., & McGuire, P. A. (1993). Behavioral and emotional problems among preschool children in pediatric primary care: Prevalence and pediatricians' recognition. *Pediatrics, 91,* 649–655.

Lochrie, A. S., & Roberts, M. C. (2003). Pediatricians and family physicians' identification and management of psychosocial problems in primary care, Unpublished manuscript.

McDaniel, S. H., Campbell, T. L., & Seaburn, D. B. (1995). Principles for collaboration between health and mental health providers in primary care. *Family System Medicine, 13,* 283–298.

Perrin, E. C. (1999). The promise of collaborative care. *Journal of Developmental and Behavioral Pediatrics, 20,* 57–62.

Perrin, E. C., & Stancin, T. (2002). A continuing dilemma: Whether and how and to screen for concerns about children's behavior in primary care settings. *Pediatrics in Review, 23,* 264–275.

Riekert, K. A., Stancin, T., Palermo, T. M., & Drotar, D. (1999). A psychological behavioral screening service: Use, feasibility, and impact in a primary care setting. *Journal of Pediatric Psychology, 24,* 405–414.

Roberts, M. C., & Brown, K. J. (2004). Primary care, prevention and pediatric psychology: Challenges and opportunities. In B. W. Wildman & T. Stancin (Eds.), *New directions for research and treatment of pediatric psychosocial problems in primary care.* (pp. 35–60). Greenwich, CT: Information Age Publishing.

Roberts, M. C., & Wright, L. (1982). The role of the pediatric psychologist as consultants to pediatricians. In J. M. Tuma (Ed.), *Handbook for the practice of pediatric psychology* (pp. 251–289). New York: Wiley.

Routh, D. K., Schroeder, C. S., & Koocher, G. P. (1983). Psychology and primary care for children. *American Psychologist, 38,* 95–98.

Sanders, M. R. (1999). The Triple P positive parenting program: Towards an empirically validated multilevel parenting and family support strategy for the prevention of behavior and emotional problems in children. *Clinical Child and Family Psychology Review, 2,* 71–90.

Schroeder, C. S. (1979). Psychologists in a private pediatric practice. *Journal of Pediatric Psychology, 4,* 5–18.

Schroeder, C. S. (1999). Commentary: A view from the past and a look to the future. *Journal of Pediatric Psychology, 24,* 447–452.

Schroeder, C. S. (2004). Reaching beyond the guild. In B. W. Wildman & T. Stancin (Eds.), *New directions for research and treatment of pediatric psychosocial problems in primary care.* Westport, CT: Greenwood Publishing.

Schroeder, C. S., Goolsby, E., & Stangler, S. (1974). Preventive services in a private pediatric practice. *Journal of Clinical Child Psychology, 4,* 32–33.

Sharp, L., Pantell, R. H., Murphy, L. O., & Lewis, C. C. (1992). Psychosocial problems during child health supervision visits: Eliciting, then what? *Pediatrics, 89,* 619–623.

Simonian, S. J., Tarnowski, K. J., Stancin, T., Friman, P. C., & Atkins, M. S. (1991). Disadvantaged children and families in pediatric primary care settings: II. Screening for behavior disturbance. *Journal of Clinical Child Psychology, 20,* 360–371.

Smith, E. G., Rome, L. P., & Freedman, D. K. (1967). The clinical psychologist in the pediatric office. *Journal of Pediatric Psychology, 71,* 48–51.

Sobel, A. B., Roberts, M. C., Rayfield, A. D., Barnard, M. U., & Rapoff, M. D. (2001). Evaluating outpatient pediatric psychology services in a primary care setting. *Journal of Pediatric Psychology, 26,* 395–405.

Spirito, A., Brown, R. T., D'Angelo, E., Delamater, A., Rodrique, J., & Siegel, L. (2003). Society of Pediatric Psychology Task Force Report: Recommendations for the training of pediatric psychologists. *Journal of Pediatric Psychology, 28,* 85–98.

Stancin, T. (1999). Introduction to the special issue on Pediatric Mental Health Services in Primary Care Settings. *Journal of Pediatric Psychology, 24,* 367–368.

Stancin, T., & Aylward, G. P. (2003). Screening instruments: behavioral and developmental. In C. Schroeder & T. Ollendick (Eds.), *Encyclopedia of pediatric and clinical child psychology* pp. 574–577. New York: Kluwer.

Stancin, T., & Palermo, T. M. (1997). A review of behavioral screening practices in pediatric settings: Do they pass the test? *Journal of Developmental Behavioral Pediatrics, 18,* 183–194.

Starfield, B., & Borkowf, S. (1969). Physicians' recognition of complaints made by parents about their children's health. *Pediatrics, 43,* 168–172.

Strosahl, K. (1998). Integrating behavioral health and primary care services: The primary mental health care model. In A. Blount (Ed.), *Integrated primary care, the future of medical and mental health collaboration* (pp. 139–166). New York: W.W. Norton.

Task Force on Pediatric Education. (1978). *The future of pediatric education.* Evanston, IL: American Academy of Pediatrics.

Tynan, W. D. (2004). Interventions in primary care: Psychology privileges for pediatricians. In B. W. Wildman & T. Stancin (Eds.), *New directions for research and treatment of pediatric psychosocial problems in primary care.* Westport, CT: Greenwood Publishing.

Tynan, W. D., Schuman, W., & Lampert, N. (1999). Concurrent parent and child therapy groups for externalizing disorders: From the laboratory to the world of managed care. *Cognitive & Behavioral Practice, 6,* 3–9.

Wildman, B. W., & Stancin, T. (Eds.). (2004). *New directions for research and treatment of pediatric psychosocial problems in primary care.* Westport, CT: Greenwood Publishing.

Wolraich, M. L., Felice, M. E., & Drotar, D. (Eds.). (1996). *The classification of child and adolescent mental diagnoses in primary care: Diagnostic & Statistical Manual for Primary Care (DSM-PC), Child and Adolescent Version.* Elk Grove, IL: American Academy of Pediatrics.

7

Providing a Range of Services to Fit the Needs of Youth in Community Mental Health Centers

JULIANNE M. SMITH-BOYDSTON

Community mental health centers (CMHCS) share a rich history in the United States, which dates back to the period immediately following World War II. Before this time, mental health issues were stigmatized and many people with mental illness remained without effective treatment or were institutionalized (Grob, 1991). After the war, at least three factors converged to improve mental health care. First, rather than simply confining people with mental illness, mental health professionals, and the communities that they served began to value the treatment of patients in less restrictive environments. Second, the advent of psychotropic medications made it increasingly possible for patients to be appropriately discharged from institutions while having their mental health needs met (Grob, 1991). Third, federal funding in the 1960s assisted communities in developing CMHCS to treat a range of disorders. In concert with this funding, federal mandates outlined specific areas that would be targeted by the CMHCS, including outpatient, inpatient, day treatment, emergency services, and educational guidance to the community (Mechanic, 1998). CMHCS were also encouraged to pursue diagnostic and rehabilitation services, training, research, and evaluation. Presently, CMHCS around the country provide a range of services individualized to their own communities and are less bound by clients' abilities to pay than many other service delivery institutions.

Although they serve their specific community needs, CMHCS continue to provide primary services to their individual clients. Services are usually

JULIANNE M. SMITH-BOYDSTON • Bert Nash Center, Lawrence, Kansas 66044.

divided into adult and child services, with treatment ranging from mild difficulties to severe or chronic mental illness. Treatment teams may comprise master's and Ph.D. level psychologists, bachelor's and master's level social workers, counselors, psychiatrists, and nurses. The professionals work together with the goal of providing the most effective resources for the youth and family. An initial intake helps to identify the potential needs of the youth and family that then guides the resulting treatment plan and process as well as potential referral to other resources. During the initial intake, the youth may be identified as severely emotionally disturbed (SED), which indicates that (1) the youth has a diagnosable disorder as defined by the *Diagnostic and Statistical Manual-IV-TR* (*DSM-IV-TR*, American Psychiatric Association [APA], 2000) and (2) this condition affects their functioning in at least one area such as within the family, at school, or in the community. The average percentage of youth identified as SED within the community ranges from 5% to 8% (Friedman, Katz-Leavy, Manderscheid, & Sondheimer, 1996).

Due to the overwhelming needs of youth identified with SED, guidelines have been developed through a systems-of-care to facilitate and govern treatment services (Stroul & Friedman, 1986). This philosophy represents a way to provide comprehensive care to youth and families that may differ in its expression across communities. Core components to a system-of-care include services that are child centered and family focused, and in which the needs of the family are primarily represented. In addition, services should be community-based to ensure that youth are treated in the least restrictive environment. Finally, individuals who provide services in these systems should be culturally competent and be responsive to the differences across families. A primary theme in this philosophy is the difficult task of coordinating services across different public sectors that may be serving youth.

Considering the overlap of mental health services with other public sectors in service of youth with SED, there has been increased focus on the characteristics of youth across sectors and interconnections across settings or systems of care (Garland et al., 2001). Primary sectors of care that have been identified for children include alcohol and drug services, child welfare, juvenile justice, mental health services, and public schools. Garland et al. (2001) found that across sectors, 54% of youth were diagnosed with at least one disorder, with disruptive behavior disorders being diagnosed more often (50%) than anxiety (10%) or mood disorders (7%). In addition, youths with substance abuse difficulties are found in all public sectors, particularly juvenile justice and mental health settings (Aarons, Brown, Hough, Garland, & Wood, 2001). This fact suggests that youth who are behaviorally acting out in aggression or antisocial behavior may be identified in a system with higher frequency, either referred by parents or teachers or because they have broken the law. It also supports using more intensive treatments in these sectors for particular behavior disorders.

Services for youths in CMHCs can be categorized into outpatient and community-based alternatives. Outpatient services encompass more traditional services including individual, family, and group treatment. In addition, medication services are provided on an outpatient basis. Community-based alternatives have been guided by system-of-care principles and are being increasingly used by professionals, particularly for youth identified as SED. Examples of these community-based services include case management, Wraparound Care, Family Preservation, and Multisystemic Treatment (MST). Individual centers may differ in how they carry out these services, but general ideologies are similar across communities.

OUTPATIENT SERVICES

Outpatient services typically make up the largest percentage of consumers at a CMHC. During the initial intake with a client, the therapist gathers information on referral behavior, background history, past assessments and interventions, and present requests to help guide recommendations for particular services that meet the needs of the client. After the intake, service recommendations are then based on the extent of difficulties and family input. If the youth is seen as non-SED or SED with mild symptoms, it is likely they will participate in less intensive individual, family, or group treatment.

Outpatient services are traditionally delivered at the CMHC; however, few studies have evaluated the overall effectiveness of services delivered at CMHCS. Positive treatment changes on externalizing and internalizing Child Behavior Checklist (CBCL) scores have been found between treatment and control groups for school-aged children (Dalton et al., 2000). In addition, although cognitive treatment has been associated with increased treatment success, support has also been found for parent and youth's abilities to use treatment strategies rather than particular treatment methods (Shapiro, Welker, & Jacobson, 1997). Unfortunately, these studies have shown some weaknesses in design in that they often lack experimental control over conditions, and frequently rely on retrospective reviews of client information or therapist report of progress (e.g., Dalton et al., 2000).

Because of the need to provide comprehensive outpatient services in a CMHC, medication prescription and monitoring is fairly routine. Children may be referred to a psychiatrist at a CMHC by outside agencies, such as pediatricians or schools. In addition, ongoing outpatient therapists may refer children to psychiatric services. There are several factors that may prompt a referral to the psychiatrist. These factors include symptom patterns that may be ameliorated with medication intervention such as inattention, hyperactivity, or depression, degree of corresponding comorbid problems, intensity of symptoms that have not changed following outpatient interventions, or parental preference for medication management. When evaluating a new client, psychiatrists gather background history of the family, which also focuses on medical issues of the child and family, referral symptoms, and past interventions used to treat symptoms. During the evaluation, if medication is deemed appropriate, psychiatrists prescribe medication that fits the symptom picture. After a designated time of use, the client and family report to the psychiatrist the perceived effectiveness of the medication and prescriptions are modified as needed.

Some studies have documented the changing patterns of medication use in CMHCs over time (Safer, 1997; Storch, 1998). Storch (1998) compared use in the CMHC to inpatient treatment and found differences in diagnoses, types of medication used, and differences in age at prescription. He reported that 82% of patients in a CMHC received more than one diagnosis, and most common medications prescribed included antidepressants, stimulants, and mood stabilizers. Safer (1997) documented trends across four separate mental health centers from 1988 to 1994, including an increase in medication use overall, increase in polypharmy or the use of more than one medication, and increase in antidepressants compared to other medications, including stimulants. These trends highlight the critical nature of medication use in CMHCs and the necessity of coordination between service providers regarding individual or family psychological treatment and medication management.

CASE MANAGEMENT SERVICES

Consistent with a systems-of-care perspective, communities are beginning to increase financial support for community-based services for youth to remain in their natural environment rather than being placed in inpatient units. The shift from inpatient treatment to outpatient services, including case management, has been occasioned by a number of factors. For example, it has been shown that hospitalization can prove very costly to communities and there are data to suggest that inpatient treatment may be inappropriate and possibly harmful to some youth (Pfeiffer & Strzelecki, 1990). In addition, the length of stay for hospitalization is much shorter than in the past, requiring that crisis stabilization is often the primary goal rather than empowering families or making changes through behavioral interventions (Sondheimer, Schoenwald, & Rowland, 1994). Although youth diagnosis is predictive of hospital reentry (i.e., psychotic disorder more likely than other disorders), availability of community-based services also appears related to decreased rates of rehospitalization (Pavkov, Goerge, & Lee, 1997).

Case management services are frequently employed in CMHCs for youth identified as SED in need of more intensive services. A case manager may assist with service access and coordinating services across providers and systems. This task is seen as a core need in current systems-of-care thinking. As defined in a system-of-care model, case managers not only coordinate services but also monitor progress, facilitate communication across systems, help families plan services and identify strengths and needs, and rely on family input to guide the treatment process. Although case management is seen as critical, it is unusual for case managers to work independently with a family separate from a treatment team so it can be difficult to define this professional role and assess its effectiveness.

More about using case management within a team approach is described below.

There has been some empirical support obtained for Intensive Case Management (ICS) used in a team approach to increase participation in treatment services, use of wider range of services, and positive outcomes for SED youth (Burns, Farmer, Angold, Costello, & Behar, 1996). The strengths of case management services include providing a missing link to service access and coordination from traditional outpatient services, as well as being more intensive and comprehensive in meeting youth and family needs. A potential drawback to case management includes some difficulties defining what case managers actually do in the field since their role is so broadly defined. In addition, the case manager's role may become confusing to families in relation to other professionals from different sectors and there may be overlap or fragmentation in services if there is not continuous coordination among professionals regarding treatment goals.

WRAPAROUND SERVICES

A stronger focus on the individual needs of youth with SED and their families has developed in what are called wraparound services (Grundle, 2002; Huffine, 2002) in that the services are provided as needed by a child and family in a coordinated way, not fitting the child to services, but, in essence, "wrapping" services around the child. This model is centered on a strengths-based approach that looks to overcome difficulties by building on the youth and families' assets. Further, it is predicated on the dual assumptions that (1) children should be treated in the context of their community, and (2) that the family can work to improve their ability to function independently (Myaard, Crawford, Jackson, & Alessi, 2000; Malysiak, 1997).

Basic to the wraparound process is that a treatment team works together on goals developed by the family. These team members may include a therapist, case manager, and possible other members such as a youth specialist or parent support worker. The therapist or Qualified Mental Health Professional (QMHP) generally oversees the treatment plan and guides the other team members in their goals for a particular family. As described previously, a case manager typically assists in pulling together members of the team, developing goals, and coordinating treatment delivery. Team members may also include a youth specialist, who works directly with youth building skills in the community, and a parent support specialist, who may be another parent who has had a child with SED in services and supports the parent through the treatment process. The members of the team are identified by the family and, by definition, should not be predominantly professional staff. Therefore, although therapists and other professionals such as school personnel may be a part of the team, the family also identifies natural resources such as family, friends, neighbors, among others that can support them in meeting treatment goals.

Community-based care has taken national spotlight with the National Evaluation of the Comprehensive Community Mental Health Services for Children and their Families Program (Holden, Friedman, & Santiago, 2001; see Chapter 25 for more details). Controversial findings of community-based services (Burns, Hoagwood, & Mrazek, 1999; Bickman et al., 1995; Bickman, Summerfelt, & Noser, 1997), particularly in comparison to university-based treatment studies (Weisz, Donenberg, Han, & Weiss, 1995) have led to efforts to operationalize treatment services more effectively in order to stay true to a systems-of-care theory and assess improvements in this care compared to traditional care with potential cost savings. The Comprehensive Community Mental Health Services for Children and their Families Program provides federal monies to a range of communities to test the theory propositions. The treatment protocols are individualized to the communities but based on the principles of system-of-care. These principles include a focus on the individual needs of the family and youth, including the strengths in the system, input of the family into treatment goals and interventions, collaboration across settings to coordinate the family services, and use of the least restrictive treatment setting for the youth and family (Stroul & Friedman, 1986). The project has shown positive results for treatment fidelity and comparison with traditional services (Hernandez, Gomez, Lipien, Greenbaum, Armstrong, & Gonzalez, 2001), cost sustainability (Foster, Kelsch, Kamradt, Sosna, & Yang, 2001), and family participation at all levels of treatment (Osher, Kammen, & Zaro, 2001). In addition, improvements have been found across communities in children's behavioral and emotional symptoms as well as increases in their functioning (Manteuffel, Stephens, & Santiago, 2002).

FAMILY PRESERVATION

Family preservation models have been in existence for several decades in the social work area. Their function within these settings have traditionally been preventing out-of-home placement for children in dangerous settings where there may be the imminent threat of out-of-home placement due to such factors as physical or sexual abuse or neglect by caregivers. Such high risk often necessitates short-term, intensive services that may help the caregivers to learn skills to potentially avoid a costly and emotionally stressing placement. In addition, work is done in the home with the caregivers and child focusing on specific goals. Examining family strengths and working in the family system, such as the school and neighborhood is seen as key, which enhances theories concentrated on individual work with the youth.

Programs that come from a family preservation model may focus on brief (1–2 months) or longer-term (3–6 months) goals. Brief programs tend to focus on immediate crises and helping families to secure resources to avoid out-of-home placements. A challenge to these shorter programs is finding ways to make lasting changes with families. Intensive longer-term programs are seen as giving workers more time to provide comprehensive

services to change systems that may have perpetuated the problem behavior. Some outcome results of these programs show that the intensive
longer-term programs may show more lasting effects on changed behavior than the short-term crisis focused programs (Nelson, Landsman, &
Deutelbaum, 1990).

An example of a family preservation program that combines aspects of
brief and long-term programs is the Homebuilders Model (Haapala, 1996).
The program was initiated in 1974 as an intensive, in-home family- and
community-based crisis intervention program. Although the average length
of service in the program is 4–8 weeks, therapists have very small caseloads
of 1–2 families so that the service in the 2 months is very concentrated and
flexible for scheduling time that meet the family's needs. Six key principles
are used to guide the treatment, including building on the family strengths,
being mindful of the systems involved in change, creating a partnership
with the family for making change, individualizing services for the family,
developing short-term goals, and selecting staff that are able to engage
families and identify or focus on necessary change areas. During treatment, realistic goals are developed with the family focusing on a limited
number of target behaviors that can be changed so as to increase family
functioning and lessen the change of the youth's out-of-home placement.
The services range from meeting concrete needs of families such as food,
clothing, or shelter, to providing a range of therapeutic services for the
youth and family, which may include didactic training regarding child development, monetary budgeting, anger management, assertiveness, and
individual or family treatment. The primary goal is to teach the family new
skills so that they are able to function better and have longer-term positive
outcomes.

Family preservation programs have been housed in different community agencies, such as CMHCs and work closely with social service case
workers. Programs such as the Homebuilders Model have shown effectiveness in keeping children in homes (Haapala, 1996). However, there have
been limitations of other family preservation projects (e.g., poor implementation of the model by having high caseloads) that have called into question
the overall effectiveness of this service delivery approach, particularly for
long-term changes with children and families.

MULTISYSTEMIC TREATMENT (MST)

The MST program, which is similar to family preservation but with
a focus on juvenile offenders, may also be offered in CMHCs. MST is a
community-based, short-term, intensive program that was designed to reduce and prevent youth criminal activity, and decrease out-of-home placement of youth (Henggeler, Schoenwald, Borduin, Rowland, & Cunningham, 1998). Their model for evaluating and disseminating MST is unique
and has a special relevance to public community-based service settings.
MST works to empower caregivers and relies on the collaboration of all
systems (i.e., family, school, peer, and neighborhood) involved to meet

treatment goals. Although similar to a family preservation model, MST uses treatment theory and empirical research regarding multiple risk factors associated with delinquency. Treatment targets validated causes of delinquency, namely peer relationships, school performance, and community factors. MST treatment is crisis-oriented, working intensively with families, due to the high threat of out-of-home placement of the youth. Therapists hold lower caseloads in order to be able to provide a wide range of services to families, as well as be available for crisis intervention. In addition, treatment is short term, lasting an average of 3–5 months, focusing on the family's goals and strengths, and building supports in their natural environment.

Multiple outcome studies (summarized in Henggeler, 1999) have shown the effectiveness of this program for reducing recidivism and out-of-home placements for youths in the juvenile justice system. MST is also listed as an empirically validated program for conduct disorder (Kazdin & Weisz, 1998) as well as by the Surgeon General (U.S. Department of Health and Human Services, 2001). Clinical trials have shown short- and long-term positive outcomes for youth and particularly strong effects when compared with traditional treatment.

Previous treatment approaches for juvenile offenders include nondirective, client-centered counseling, psychodynamic therapy, and punitive programs such as intensive supervision, electronic monitoring, boot camps, and "scared straight" programs. Although most of these approaches have shown poor results and some even have shown some deleterious effects on juvenile offenders, many communities still use these approaches. However, with tighter budgets, and the support of effective programs by the Surgeon General, more communities may begin to adopt programs that have been supported by the research literature. MST has shown not only beneficial treatment results but also cost effectiveness when compared to other programs for juvenile offenders (Washington State Institute for Public Policy, 1998).

Based on clinical findings regarding its effectiveness and cost savings, MST Services, which is the main administrative oversight organization of the individual programs, has worked to disseminate the program into a variety of applied settings to evaluate whether similar results can be shown in these settings (Schoenwald, Brown, & Henggeler, 2000). A major feature of those dissemination trials has been an emphasis on the necessity of treatment adherence and other quality assurance procedures. Dissemination and treatment quality assurance for the MST program include an initial 1 week intensive training series that focuses on the principles and treatment with MST, followed by weekly consultations from MST Services, quarterly treatment workshops for MST staff, and regular review of clinical outcomes. This frequency and intensity of supervision and oversight is necessary in part because of the conceptual nature of MST treatment. Each case is analyzed individually with unique treatment goals and procedures to fit with the identified youth and family. This approach is distinguished from other dissemination projects of mental health services that have used a manualized, standardized set of treatment procedures because the MST procedures in particular are individualized for each family but follow the same set of nine MST principles.

Considering the effectiveness of MST with juvenile offenders, MST proponents have examined the use of similar principles for youth with SED presenting with psychiatric crises (Henggeler, Schoenwald, Rowland, & Cunningham, 2002). Preliminary research has shown this treatment as an effective alternative to inpatient hospitalization (Sondheimer et al., 1994). Since it has been shown that many youths cross different sectors of care (Garland et al., 2001), it is reasonable to assume that treatments effective for one set of youth may also work for another set. Therefore, much of the MST process is similar for youths in psychiatric crises as with juvenile offenders, but there are also unique aspects for this population. MST plans for youths in crisis are defined by the youth being potentially actively at risk to harm of self or others, as evidenced by suicidal, homicidal, or psychotic symptoms. Goals for these crisis plans involve keeping the youth safe, providing emergency services in the youth's natural environment, and empowering the caregivers to be able to respond to the crisis and to future difficulties. Added to the MST team is a crisis caseworker to respond to emergencies, implement crisis plans, and gather information to help prevent further crises. In addition, a child psychiatrist works closely with the team for medication maintenance. As with traditional MST, each team member is held responsible for the outcomes of the youth and family.

MST Services are also devising a continuum of care, which can follow the youth and family through stages of treatment (Henggeler et al., 2002). This helps to keep continuity between the family and MST therapists and theoretical orientation, but also fits the intensity of the program to the needs of the family, from very intensive interventions to less intensive outpatient care. This type of system works well in a CMHC, given the chronicity of most cases, particularly children identified as SED.

There are strengths and weaknesses of delivering MST in a community program based in a CMHC. The strengths, as stated earlier, involve empirical validation, potentially greater connection to families and community partners, and short-term intensive work that makes changes in the youth's natural environment to support further changes. Challenges with this program include how different it is to traditional outpatient services and to traditional team approaches that include having a therapist, case manager, and possibly other players such as a youth specialist and parent support worker. Because MST has one therapist performing many of these roles, it can be very different for most CMHCs to implement. In addition, the program is very "top-heavy" with many requirements for programs to maintain MST licensure, which includes not only the initial trainings but also ongoing consultation and booster trainings by MST consultants. Although it is understood how important these procedures are to protect dissemination, it can be very costly for individual centers to support. That is one of the reasons that MST Services initially assists communities to assess their commitment to the program theoretically and financially to find ways to sustain the program in the long term. However, in tough financial times, unless there is commitment from state and local communities for funding, it can be difficult to maintain the full program.

EVALUATING STRENGTHS OF CMHCS

From their initial inception, CMHCS have been federally mandated to evaluate the effectiveness of their treatment programs. Several different methods have been used to evaluate treatment programs, including assessing caregiver and child satisfaction with the program, examining child behavior change over time, and assessing the lack of negative outcomes, such as hospital reentry or criminal recidivism rates. In addition, cost-effectiveness studies can be critical components to see if the program cost outweighs outcomes that are obtained. However, an analysis of cost-effectiveness should be attempted only after it is known that the intervention is effective in some way (Naar-King, Siegel, Smyth, & Simpson, 2000).

There are some aspects of CMHCS that make them very rich areas for clinical research. As suggested by latest calls to research from the National Institute for Mental Health (NIMH) that focus on public health, the next generation of empirical investigation needs to be conducted in the "real world" with difficulties that families face day to day and focus on potential improvements in quality of life (Foxhall, 2000). This more naturalistic research approach will assist in making the assessed interventions powerful across settings and populations and make them more useful to everyday practitioners. Because CMHCS have a very diverse client population, studies can be done on the effectiveness of treatment programs with comorbid conditions, which would be an important expansion to the present research primarily done in academic settings with a very homogenous group, such as those with a single diagnosis. In addition, the range of different professionals working in the CMHC would assist in evaluating the "team approach" and insight that is gathered from the range of professionals working with a youth and family. Studies can also assess the range of treatments available from outpatient work such as individual, group, family, and medication treatment, to more intensive community-based services. Also, as stated before, CMHCS share a federal mandate to evaluate their work to assess if interventions lead to youth behavior change and endearing changes in the family system.

CHALLENGES FACING CMHCS

There are also some potential challenges to conducting research in a CMHC setting. Although CMHCS have been mandated to evaluate their services, much of this research has included state-funded basic evaluations such as assessing youth behavior change on a single questionnaire such as the CBCL (Achenbach, 1991) or client satisfaction with services. Unfortunately, these measures are not always seen as priorities by the CMHC staff and there may be much missing data unless funding sources attach importance to the information. In addition, the personnel at CMHCs often have a range of training that may, or may not, include training in research methods. This variance may influence the staff's acceptance of research procedures or therapist adherence to established protocols. Also, because CMHCs can be very distinct across the country, it may be very difficult to compare techniques or protocols across communities if they are providing services very differently. In fact, it can be difficult even statewide to adopt similar procedures unless there is a mandate to do so.

Wagner, Swenson, and Henggeler (2000) documented particular challenges in evaluating community-based interventions. These guidelines can be used to examine research completed in CMHCs. First, the authors discussed potential weak research design due to insufficient sample size, high attrition, low treatment fidelity, and difficulties in randomizing subjects. It is more difficult in a CMHC to randomize subjects to different control groups. However, some studies have used dropout lists of children who completed the initial assessment but then rejected further services or therapy wait-list comparisons (Dalton et al., 2000).

Second, difficulties can arise in designating treatment guidelines and evaluating therapist's adherence to developed protocols. This is a particular difficulty with operationalizing the wraparound process, because there are so many unique and individualized components to the treatment (Malysiak, 1997). However, the ongoing system-of-care study has developed implementation assessment strategies to examine the organizational arrangements and service delivery domains to see how it relates to family outcomes using qualitative and quantitative measures (Vinson, Brannan, Baughman, Wilce, & Gawron, 2001). The MST program uses their nine treatment principles as the foundation to have families evaluate the effectiveness of therapists in the program (Henggeler et al., 1998).

Third, participant issues can be an issue, particularly engaging community members as well as families into the treatment, obtaining informed consent, and increasing motivation for families to participate in the research portion of the treatment. This issue is not as difficult for CMHCs because often the program evaluation measures are integrated into the ongoing treatment programs. Therefore, measures such as the CBCL or the Child and Adolescent Functioning Assessment Scale (CAFAS; Hodges, 1990, 1994 revision; Hodges, Wong, & Latessa, 1998) may be used with families as normal procedures during treatment intake and then again at the completion of treatment. However, incorporating additional measures may be difficult due to not only community acceptance but also engagement of staff around the necessity of the measures. Therefore, didactic training can be important at all levels and feedback regarding outcomes can be very informative and motivating to staff.

Fourth, the clinical culture can be a barrier to treatment progress, including differing training of professionals and the range of treatment approaches used. Schoenwald, Brown, and Henggeler (2000) identified characteristics of therapists that are related to effective practice. These characteristics include openness to peer supervision, ability to have treatment approaches evaluated, a strong work ethic, an ability to be ecologically minded when treating the child and family, flexibility, intelligence, open-mindedness, and empathy with the client. The authors stated there is always a challenge of hiring appropriate staff for community-based work that is influenced by professional qualifications, therapist characteristics, and cultural understanding. This challenge could make or break the treatment outcomes, because research has shown that connection with therapist may explain a large part of treatment success.

Last, community challenges were noted, including obtaining the engagement of important community leaders and connections with agencies that have input on the characteristics of the youth and possible involvement with the youth's outcome. CMHCs interact with many different community members, including social services, adoption and foster placement agencies, schools, hospitals, and juvenile justice authorities. It is critical that they have the buy-in and commitment of these agencies to conduct program evaluation. In fact, information gathered from evaluating treatment practices can be used by these agencies to advocate for continued treatment or funding decisions.

REFERENCES

Aarons, G. A., Brown, S. A., Hough, R. L., Garland, A. F., & Wood, P. A. (2001). Prevalence of adolescent substance use disorders across five sectors of care. *Journal of the American Academy of Child and Adolescent Psychiatry, 40,* 419–426.

Achenbach, T. M. (1991). *Integrative guide to the 1991 cbcl/4-18, YSR, and TRF profiles.* Burlington, VT: University of Vermont, Department of Psychiatry.

American Psychiatric Association. (2000). *Diagnostic and statistical manual of mental disorders* (4th ed., Text Revision). Washington, DC: Author.

Bickman, L., Guthrie, P. R., Foster, E. M., Lambert, E. W., Summerfelt, W. T., Breda, C. S., & Heflinger, C. A. (1995). *Evaluating managed mental health services: The Fort Bragg experiment.* New York: Plenum.

Bickman, L., Summerfelt, W. T., & Noser, K. (1997). Comparative outcomes of emotionally disturbed children and adolescents in a system of services and usual care. *Psychiatric Services, 48,* 1543–1548.

Burns, B. J., Farmer, E. M. Z., Angold, A., Costello, E. J., & Behar, L. (1996). A randomized trial of case management for youths with serious emotional disturbance. *Journal of Clinical Child Psychology, 25,* 476–486.

Burns, B. J., Hoagwood, K., & Mrazek, P. J. (1999). Effective treatments for mental disorders in children and adolescents. *Clinical Child Psychology Review, 2,* 199–254.

Dalton, R., Pellerin, K., Carbone, V., Theriot, A., Thibodeauz, D., Stewart, L. et al. (2000). Treatment outcome among child psychiatric outpatients in a community mental health center. *Community Mental Health Journal, 36,* 195–203.

Foster, E. M., Kelsch, C. C., Kamradt, B., Sosna, T., & Yang, Z. (2001). Expenditures and sustainability in systems of care. *Journal of Emotional and Behavioral Disorder, 9,* 53–62.

Foxhall, K. (2000). Research for the real world. *Monitor on Psychology, 31,* 28–36.

Friedman, R. M., Katz-Leavy, J. W., Manderscheid, R. W., & Sondheimer, D. I. (1996). *Prevalence of serious emotional disturbance in children and adolescents. Mental Health. United States.* (DHHS Publication SMA 96-3098). Center for Mental Health Services. Washington, DC: Superintendent of Documents, U.S. Government Printing Office.

Garland, A. F., Hough, R. L., McCabe, K. M., Yeh, M., Wood, P. A., & Aarons, G. A. (2001). Prevalence of psychiatric disorders in youths across five sectors of care. *Journal of American Academy of Child and Adolescent Psychiatry, 40,* 409–418.

Grob, G. N. (1991). *From asylum to community: Mental health policy in modern America.* Princeton, NJ: Princeton University Press.

Grundle, T. J. (2002). Wraparound care. In D. I. Marsh, & M. A. Fristad (Eds.), *Handbook of serious emotional disturbance in children and adolescents* (pp. 323–333). New York: Wiley.

Haapala, D. A. (1996). The Homebuilders model: An evolving service approach for families. In M. C. Roberts (Ed.), *Model programs in service delivery in child and family mental health* (pp. 295–315). New York: LEA.

Henggeler, S. W. (1999). Multisystemic therapy: An overview of clinical procedures, outcomes, and policy implications. *Child Psychology and Psychiatry Review, 4,* 2–10.

Henggeler, S. W., Schoenwald, S. K., Borduin, C. M., Rowland, M. D., & Cunningham, P. B. (1998). *Multisystemic treatment of antisocial behavior in youth.* New York: Guilford.

Henggeler, S. W., Schoenwald, S. K., Rowland, M. D., & Cunningham, P. B. (2002). *Serious emotional disturbance in children and adolescents.* New York: Guilford.

Hernandez, M., Gomez, A., Lipien, L, Greenbaum, P. E., Armstrong, K. H., & Gonzalez, P. (2001). Use of the system-of-care practice review in the national evaluation: Evaluating the fidelity of practice to system-of-care practices. *Journal of Emotional and Behavioral Disorder, 9,* 43–52.

Hodges, K. (1990, 1994 revision). *Child and adolescent functional assessment scale.* Ypsilanti, MI: Eastern Michigan University, Department of Psychology.

Hodges, K., Wong, M. M., & Latessa, M. (1998). Use of the Child and Adolescent Functional Assessment Scale (CAFAS) as an outcome measure in clinical settings. *Journal of Behavioral Health Services and Research, 25,* 325–336.

Holden, E. W., Friedman, R. M., & Santiago, R. L. (2001). Overview of the national evaluation of the Comprehensive Community Mental Health Services for Children and their Families Program. *Journal of Emotional and Behavioral Disorders, 9,* 4–12.

Huffine, C. (2002). Current trends in the community treatment of seriously emotionally disturbed youths. *Psychiatric Services, 53,* 809–811.

Kazdin, A. E., & Weisz, J. R. (1998). Identifying and developing empirically supported child and adolescent treatments. *Journal of Consulting and Clinical Psychology, 66,* 19–36.

Malysiak, R. (1997). Exploring the theory and paradigm base for wraparound. *Journal of Child and Family Studies, 6,* 399–408.

Manteuffel, B., Stephens, R. L., & Santiago, R. (2002). Overview of the national evaluation of the Comprehensive Mental Health Services for Children and their Families Program and summary of current findings. *Children's Services: Social Policy, Research, and Practice, 5,* 3–20.

Mechanic, D. (1998). Emerging trends in mental health policy and practice. *Health Affairs, 17,* 82–98.

Myaard, M. J., Crawford, C., Jackson, M., & Alessi, G. (2000). Applying behavior analysis within the wraparound process: A multiple baseline study. *Journal of Emotional and Behavioral Disorders, 8,* 216–229.

Naar-King, S., Siegel, P. T., Smyth, M., & Simpson, P. (2000). A model for evaluating collaborative health care programs for children with special needs. *Children's Services: Social Policy, Research, and Practice, 3,* 233–245.

Nelson, K. E., Landsman, M. J., & Deutelbaum, W. (1990). Three models of family-centered placement prevention services. *Child Welfare, 69,* 3–19.

Osher, T. W., Kammen, W., & Zaro, S. M. (2001). Family participation in evaluating systems of care: Family, research, and service system perspectives. *Journal of Emotional and Behavioral Disorders, 9,* 63–70.

Pavkov, T. W., Goerge, R. M., & Lee, B. J. (1997). State hospital reentry among youth with serious emotional disturbance: A longitudinal analysis. *Journal of Child and Family Studies, 6,* 373–383.

Pfeiffer, S., & Strzelecki, S. (1990). Inpatient psychiatric treatment of children and adolescents: A review of outcome studies. *Journal of American Academy of Child and Adolescent Psychiatry, 29,* 847–853.

Safer, D. J. (1997). Changing patterns of psychotropic medications prescribed by child psychiatrists in the 1990s. *Journal of Child and Adolescent Psychopharmacology, 7,* 267–274.

Schoenwald, S. K., Brown, T. L., & Henggeler, S. W. (2000). Inside multisystemic therapy: Therapists, supervisory, and program practices. *Journal of Emotional and Behavioral Disorders, 8,* 113–127.

Shapiro, J. P., Welker, C. J., & Jacobson, B. J. (1997). A naturalistic study of psychotherapeutic methods and child in-therapy functioning in a child community setting. *Journal of Clinical Child Psychology, 26,* 385–396.

Sondheimer, D. L., Schoenwald, S. K., & Rowland, M. D. (1994). Alternatives to hospitalization of youth with a serious emotional disturbance. *Journal of Clinical Child Psychology, 23*(Suppl.), 7–12.

Storch, D. D. (1998). Outpatient pharmacotherapy in a community mental health center. *Journal of the American Academy of Child and Adolescent Psychiatry, 37,* 249–250.

Stroul, B. A., & Friedman, R. M. (1986). *A system-of-care for children and youth with severe emotional disturbances.* (Revised ed.). Washington, DC: Georgetown University Child Development Center, CASSP Technical Assistance Center.

U.S. Department of Health and Human Services. (2001). *Youth violence: A report of the Surgeon General.* Rockville, MD: U.S. Department of Health and Human Services, Centers for Disease Control and Prevention, National Center for Injury Prevention and Control, Substance Abuse and Mental Health Services Administration, Center for Mental Health Services, and National Institutes of Health, National Institute of Mental Health.

Vinson, N. B., Brannan, A. M., Baughman, L. N., Wilce, M., & Gawron, T. (2001). The systems-of-care model: Implementation in twenty-seven communities. *Journal of Emotional and Behavioral Disorders, 9,* 30–42.

Wagner, E. F., Swenson, C. C., & Henggeler, S. W. (2000). Practical and methodological challenges in validating community-based interventions. *Children's Services: Social Policy, Research, and Practice, 3,* 211–231.

Washington State Institute for Public Policy. (1998). *Watching the bottom line: Cost- effective interventions for reducing crime in Washington.* Olympia, WA: Evergreen State College.

Weisz, J. R., Donenberg, G. R., Han, S. S., & Weiss, B. (1995). Bridging the gap between laboratory and clinic in child and adolescent psychotherapy. *Journal of Consulting and Clinical Psychology, 63,* 688–702.

8

Outpatient–Private Practice Model[†]

BERNADETTE M. LANDOLF

In the United States, outpatient private practice emerged as a distinct model for delivering mental health services in the latter half of the 1800s. Prior to that time, the young discipline of psychiatry was concerned almost exclusively with the care of severely disturbed individuals confined to asylums, and other mental health disciplines had not yet evolved (Brown, n.d.; Reisman, 1991). Since then, private practice has become a major vehicle for delivering mental health services. A brief summary of some of the key setting factors and antecedent events that contributed to the development of, and eventual boom in, outpatient private practice in the United States will be presented followed by an examination of contemporary private practice as a model for delivering mental health services to children, adolescents, and families.

From the late 1700s to the middle 1800s, post-Enlightenment concern for the less fortunate coupled with a growing respect for rationality and science contributed to a shift away from superstitious, inhumane, and pessimistic views of psychological disturbance, which led to the warehousing (or worse) of afflicted individuals, to more scientific, humane, and optimistic views that fostered a search for effective treatments (Reisman, 1991). Between 1869 and 1879, neurologists George Miller Beard and S. Weir Mitchell helped legitimize less severe forms of psychological disturbance, and neurologist William A. Hammond published a paper entitled, "The Non-asylum Treatment of the Insane," thus helping to move the locus of mental health care from asylums to outpatient practices (Brown, n.d.).

BERNADETTE M. LANDOLF • Behavior Therapy Center of Greater Washington, Silver Spring, Maryland 20901.

[†]The author would like to thank Steven R. Fritsche, Associate Professor of Accounting, Howard University, for his suggestions and contributions to this chapter.

In 1879, scientific psychology coalesced as a discipline, and not long afterward, in 1896, Lightner Witmer initiated the field of clinical psychology by opening a psychological clinic, the first of its kind in the world, at the University of Pennsylvania. Witmer's clinic served primarily children and may be viewed as an early forerunner of child guidance clinics (Reisman, 1991). Adolf Meyer, a pathologist and director of the New York Psychiatric Institute, initiated the practice of psychiatric social work in 1904 (Reisman, 1991). Interest in psychoanalysis and other forms of psychological therapies rose in the United States after Sigmund Freud and Carl Jung delivered a series of lectures at Clark University in 1909 (Reisman, 1991). During the same year, social reformer, writer, and philanthropist Ethel Sturges Dummer, physician William Healy, and others created the Juvenile Psychopathic Institute in Chicago, considered by many to be the first child guidance clinic in the world (Jones, 1999; Reisman, 1991). Around 1917, states began legally recognizing psychologists as experts in mental retardation, much to the displeasure of psychiatrists and others in the medical profession interested in protecting what they considered their turf (Reisman, 1991). Demand for outpatient mental health services grew and then skyrocketed after World War II. The federal government responded by providing funding for graduate training in psychology, and predictably, the number of graduate programs increased. At about the same time (middle 1940s), states began enacting certification and licensing laws for psychologists, thereby allowing them to practice independently (Reisman, 1991).

The most recent boom in outpatient private practice began during the 1960s with the passage of "freedom-of-choice" legislation requiring third-party payers to provide reimbursement for services regardless of which licensed or certified professional (e.g., psychiatrist or psychologist) delivered the services (Routh, 1994). During the late 1970s and early 1980s, litigation resulted in at least two key court decisions that held that non-M.D. mental health practitioners were entitled to practice independently (i.e., without physician oversight) and to receive third-party reimbursement for their services (Reisman, 1991). Thus, during the 1960s, 1970s, and early 1980s, legislation and litigation provided another source of funding for psychologists in private practice; opened the doors of private practice to social workers, psychiatric nurses, professional counselors, marriage and family therapists, and others; and provided a major financial impetus for entrepreneurship in the delivery of mental health services.

Eventually, and not surprisingly, a tightening of the financial reigns became necessary when health care spending skyrocketed. With the rise of managed care in the 1990s, a new climate was created—a climate unsupportive of unfettered growth in the business of health care delivery. As a result, providers are now forced to compete for fewer dollars. During this period of adaptation, changes are bound to occur throughout the system that will alter the ways in which mental health services are delivered. For the time being, however, private practice continues to be an important and viable service delivery model.

DEFINITION AND ORGANIZATIONAL SCHEMES

For the purposes of this chapter, the outpatient private practice model includes single- and multi-owner professional practices that, within applicable legal parameters, function autonomously in the provision of outpatient mental health services for compensation and whose financial solvency depends on the compensation collected for those services. The model subsumes sole proprietorships and multi-owner practices in various forms regardless of size. In the current context, a sole proprietorship is a professional practice owned and managed by one person (i.e., the sole proprietor). The sole proprietor has unlimited liability with regard to any financial responsibilities and legal actions arising from the conduct of any agent of the proprietorship. That is, both personal assets of the proprietor and practice assets may be claimed by creditors or other parties to satisfy obligations of the practice. Chapman (1990) described several forms of sole proprietorships including solo practices with no support staff, single-owner practices with or without support staff or practitioner employees, and groups of two or more sole proprietors who share overhead expenses. All of these are subsumed under the definition of private practice above.

Similarly, multi-owner practices (i.e., partnerships) can be organized in a variety of ways and still qualify as private practices according to the definition above. Laws governing multi-owner organizations vary from state to state. In general, unless the partnership agreement specifically exempts one or more partners from liability (as would organizing as a limited liability partnership, professional corporation, or limited liability company), all partners are subject to the same financial and legal exposure as they would be if they practiced as independent sole proprietors.

Excluded from the definition of private practice above is any service delivery entity that derives a significant portion of its operating revenue from sources other than fees collected directly from clients for services rendered to those clients (e.g., publicly funded agencies or nonprofit agencies that rely on donations, grants, and other external sources of funding). Service delivery entities that are not financially or operationally independent of a larger organization that provides services other than direct mental health services to clients (e.g., universities, schools, hospitals, managed care organizations, etc.) also are excluded. Superficial features (e.g., size of the practice, appearance of the physical plant, ownership arrangements, etc.) are not what distinguishes private practice from other service delivery models. Autonomy is the defining feature—a private practice is self-directed and self-reliant. Thus, the distinction between private practice and employer-based practice blurs as involvement of third-party payers (insurance companies, managed care organizations) increases. That is, at some point along the continuum, the private practitioner is no longer financially or operationally independent and instead becomes a *de facto* employee of the third party.

POPULATIONS SERVED

There are no reliable data regarding the number of children, adolescents, and families seen for treatment exclusively in outpatient private practice settings. Citing research by Burns, Hoagwood, and Maultsby (1998), which estimated that between 5% and 10% of children and their families utilize outpatient mental health services annually, the 1999 Surgeon General's report on mental health identified outpatient treatment as the most common form of treatment for children and adolescents (Satcher, 1999). As is the case with other data sources, the term "outpatient" refers to many modes of outpatient service delivery, both public and private.

Private mental health professionals are not the leading source of outpatient mental health services to children and youth. Burns et al. (1995) found that nearly three quarters of the severely emotionally disturbed children they followed who received treatment received at least some mental health services from the education sector whereas fewer than half received some mental health services from the specialty mental health sector (psychiatric hospital, psychiatric unit in a general hospital, residential treatment center, group home, partial hospitalization, therapeutic foster care, mental health center, detoxification unit, outpatient drug and alcohol clinic, case management, or private mental health professional). These researchers and others (Hoagwood & Erwin, 1997) have concluded that schools are the primary source of outpatient mental health services to children (cf. Satcher, 1999). Thus, although private practitioners are financially and operationally independent, they must remain cognizant of the high probability that their child clients are receiving mental health services from other sources (such as schools) and must be able to coordinate services with other agencies when necessary.

Kazdin, Siegel, and Bass (1990) surveyed 1,162 psychologists and psychiatrists involved directly with the treatment of children, approximately half of whom were primarily employed in private practice settings. The psychologists and psychiatrists included in the sample reported that one third of their caseloads consisted of middle socioeconomic status (SES) children referred for treatment; the other two thirds were evenly split between upper-middle to upper SES and lower-middle to lower SES referred youngsters. Upper SES children accounted for the lowest percentage of cases (6.6% of psychologists' caseloads, and 7.2% of psychiatrists' caseloads). The racial composition of the average caseload, aggregated across the two provider groups, appeared comparable to census data for 1980 and 1990 (cf. Office of the Assistant Secretary for Planning and Evaluation, 1997). These data should not be interpreted to mean that the clientele of every outpatient private practice is representative of the U. S. population at large *vis-à-vis* economic and racial composition. What they do suggest is that the outpatient private practice model does not disproportionately include or exclude individuals from one or more economic or racial groups.

Just as outpatient private practice does not necessarily include or exclude individuals from particular SES or racial groups, neither does it necessarily include or exclude individuals with particular presenting problems. Kazdin et al. (1990) asked the psychologists and psychiatrists in their sample to rank the five problems most frequently seen in their practices. The problems most frequently reported were emotional (internalizing) problems, behavioral problems at home, behavioral problems at school, parent–child problems, and learning problems.

Private practice is, perhaps, the most flexible service delivery model. A private practitioner can locate anywhere there is sufficient demand for services. Considering that part-time practice is an option, private practitioners may be found where demand for services is not sufficient to support a larger or more complex service delivery model. Although the private practice model is able to serve a demographically diverse clientele and a broad range of presenting problems, its survival depends on the ability of its clients to financially support its operations. Apart from this economic constraint, the model places no restrictions on service delivery. Unless a private practitioner decides to limit the scope of the practice in some way, such limiting does not exist as it does, for example, when there is an institutional mandate to serve a particular population.

ECONOMICS OF PRIVATE PRACTICE

Members of the helping professions seem prone to subscribe to the dichotomy of helper versus businessperson. This dichotomy is neither logical nor useful. Regarding its logicality, the dichotomy fails to recognize that anyone who receives recompense for goods or services is *de facto* a participant in an economic transaction. Moreover, the dichotomy fails to recognize that in any endeavor involving the exchange of some form of compensation for goods or services, the source of compensation—whether from individual consumers, taxpayers, insurance companies, charities, or other sources—conveys no information at all about the helpfulness of the endeavor. Clearly then, the dichotomy is a false one.

Apart from its falseness, the dichotomy can and should be challenged for more utilitarian reasons. The dichotomy encourages the perception that helping occurs in isolation from a larger societal context. In so doing, helping is likely to be viewed only in terms of benefits provided. Unfortunately, focusing exclusively on benefits provided obscures the fact that helping, regardless of the form it takes (e.g., providing clinical services, consulting, teaching or training, conducting research, etc.), consumes limited human and financial resources. Thus, the dichotomy distracts from the critical activity of evaluating the benefits of helping relative to its costs and therefore does nothing to encourage accountability. Those paying for services provided by the helping professions should and will make judgments regarding the value of the services independent of whether the provider believes they are valuable, and this holds true regardless of the venue in which the services are rendered.

That private practice is both a service delivery enterprise and an economic enterprise does not make it unique relative to other settings in which members of the helping professions function. What makes private practice unique is that its practitioners function autonomously, are directly compensated by consumers for services provided, and depend on that compensation to allow them to continue providing services.

Private practices receive funding through fees paid by clients or clients' insurers (including managed care companies). Clients may include individuals or organizations. Services offered include psychotherapy (individual, family, and group therapies), consultation, staff training or continuing education, professional supervision, and contractual services (e.g., as an independent contractor for an employee assistance program). Research grants in private practice settings are not unheard of, but this source of funding is not a major one in most private practices.

In private practice settings, revenue generated from service delivery is used not only to compensate the provider or providers for services rendered but also to cover costs associated with operating the practice (e.g., office space, utilities, supplies, support staff salaries, malpractice insurance, general liability insurance, other forms of insurance, training or continuing education, licensing fees, taxes, etc.). For the practice to survive, the fees collected must match or exceed the cost of providing a standard of service that is acceptable to the owner or owners of the practice and also meets or exceeds applicable legal and ethical requirements. Although theoretical orientation, practice philosophy (e.g., the value placed on empirical research), and other ideological factors certainly impact decisions concerning which services to offer and the manner in which to offer them, the extent to which certain basic economic principles are followed will determine whether the practice continues to serve the community or goes out of business.

The variety of fee arrangements possible within private practice settings is constrained by laws, ethical guidelines, and economic reality. Therapists can offer services free of charge (*pro bono*), they can set fees based on a sliding scale (i.e., the fee charged a particular client is based on the client's income level), they can write off some portion of a fee or offer to provide some services free of charge or at a reduced rate, or they can charge full fee for all services. Full fee is usually comparable to the standard fee profile for similarly licensed professionals in a particular geographic location, but some providers may charge significantly more or less depending on their unique circumstances. Group practices may structure fees based on the experience level or licensure of the various service providers on staff. Private practices that serve as training sites for local educational institutions may offer reduced fees for services rendered by trainees. Participating in managed care or insurance plans usually means that a therapist agrees to see clients at a reduced fee (the managed care or insurance company's "usual and customary" fee) in exchange for a greater number of referrals from the manage care or insurance organization. Therapists may offer further fee reductions to clients with insurance, but any such fee reduction must be reflected on claims. It is both illegal and unethical to reduce a client's fee and submit a claim to a third-party payer indicating that the client paid a higher fee.

Because private practitioners are paid based on their time, and because there are a limited number of hours a therapist can work and still maintain a high level of quality, decisions regarding fee arrangements necessarily involve a balancing act. In setting fees, practitioners must consider a number of important issues including clients' needs, which services are required to meet their clients' needs, for which services to charge (e.g., responding to phone calls of varying lengths, responding to e-mail communications, reviewing reports and other sources of background information, completing treatment plans and satisfying other requests or requirements for interagency communication or coordination of services, extra-session time required to design intervention programs, transportation to and from *in vivo* sessions, etc.), amount of income required to keep the practice afloat, amount of compensation required to maintain therapist morale, range of available treatment options and the cost-effectiveness associated with each option, and many others.

Whether a practice can absorb reductions in fees depends at least in part on the financial health of the practice and the costs required to provide services. Services differ along a number of dimensions including their cost to practices (e.g., therapist time, support and material costs, etc.), their cost to clients (e.g., financial costs, time lost, etc.), and their effectiveness. Traditional in-office talk therapies place relatively few burdens on a practice's resources whereas other types of therapy can place extraordinary burdens on a practice's resources. The use of video self-modeling, for example, has been shown to be a potentially useful component in the treatment of selective mutism, but the initial investment in equipment (digital movie camera, video-editing software, computer with enough power to run video-editing software, and other hardware and software) and the resource costs associated with the time and expertise required to do the filming and subsequent editing (or paying someone else to do it), are massive compared to the resource costs of traditional in-office psychotherapy (Kehle, Madaus, Baratta, & Bray, 1998; Kehle, Owen, & Cressey, 1990). Similarly, Webster-Stratton's Incredible Year's Parent, Teacher, and Child Training program (Webster-Stratton & Reid, 2003) is impressive for its strong theoretical and empirical bases; numerous studies support both its efficacy and its effectiveness (Chambless & Ollendick, 2001; Taylor & Biglan, 1998). Those wishing to use the program will incur considerable start-up costs including the cost of materials, training, and supervision. There are many casual, relatively inexpensive ways to provide parent training that, although less likely than Webster-Stratton's program to be effective, may allow practitioners to lower the per unit fee as start-up costs associated with such approaches are negligible. As a further example, exposure-based interventions (e.g., reinforced practice, participant modeling, exposure and ritual prevention) enjoy strong theoretical and empirical support as components in the treatment of anxiety disorders in adults and children (Chambless & Ollendick, 2001; Weisz & Jensen, 2001). Clients may be able to manage exposures on their own or with the assistance of family members, but the therapist's presence is often necessary for an exposure to be successful. Out-of-office services, such as *in vivo* exposure, require an inordinate amount of therapist time in the form of travel to and from sessions (including the necessity to build in a reasonable cushion for unforeseen delays caused by traffic and road construction). Some of this time may not be billable, but it still reduces the amount of time available to schedule other clients. Furthermore, costs associated with the automobile (e.g., fuel and wear and tear) and other ancillary costs also need to be considered. In summary, because services differ along a number of dimensions including their cost to practices, some practices may have less freedom than others to negotiate lower per unit fees; however, services that are more costly to provide per unit or hour may actually shorten the length of therapy and therefore be more cost-effective for clients in the long run.

One of the most difficult decisions a private practitioner must make regarding financial arrangements is whether to participate in insurance plans or operate exclusively on a fee-for-service basis. On the one hand, participating makes the per unit cost of therapy more affordable for those who cannot pay the per unit cost out of pocket. On the other hand, participating in insurance plans places increased administrative burdens on practices (e.g., by requiring a greater proportion of administrative work from clinical staff or the addition of clerical staff to handle the processing of treatment plans and claims) and restricts service delivery in ways that do not necessarily lead to improved outcomes. In their excellent review of the empirical literature on behavioral family interventions, Taylor and Biglan (1998) discussed several insurance industry policies that limit practice arbitrarily and fail to support (and may actually exclude) the implementation of empirically supported treatments—an obvious quality-of-care issue. For example, many insurance companies will authorize for reimbursement only those services in which the "identified patient" (i.e., the child) is present even though the treatments with the strongest empirical support for some of the most commonly seen problems (e.g., conduct and oppositional problems) involve working primarily with the parents (see Brestan & Eyberg, 1998; Chambless et al., 1998; Chambless & Ollendick, 2001; Nathan & Gorman, 1998; Roth & Fonagy, 1996). Additionally, arbitrary caps on length of sessions or number of sessions allowed may force clinicians to omit key components (e.g., practice, role-playing, and *in vivo* exposure) of empirically supported treatments (see Ollendick & King, 1998; Webster-Stratton, 1984; Webster-Stratton, Kolpacoff, & Hollinsworth, 1988).

In addition to the policies discussed by Taylor and Biglan (1998), several other insurance industry policies fail to acknowledge and provide for differences between adult and child treatment. For example, third-party payers generally will not reimburse for meetings between a therapist and a child's school even though such meetings may be needed to coordinate treatment efforts. Additionally, most third-party payers will not reimburse for two different services provided to the same client on the same day even though providing both services on the same day may be clinically justifiable and cost-effective for the family. So, for example, if a child is being treated for obsessive–compulsive disorder and is seen for an exposure session, the parents cannot be seen on the same day (if the parents wish to be reimbursed for both sessions) even if treatment success depends on making sure the parents are not inadvertently reinforcing their child's avoidance or compulsive behavior and seeing all parties on the same day is cost-effective for the family.

Private practitioners may decide against participating in managed care or insurance plans for economic reasons (e.g., to avoid incurring additional administrative costs), to avoid having their practice limited in ways that could adversely impact the quality of services provided, or for both of these reasons. Insurance industry policies favor a pathology-based, linear model of treatment (i.e., the medical model). Unless policies change to accommodate field or systems thinking, many child, adolescent, and family therapists in private practice will find participating in managed care or insurance plans frustrating. Practitioners who elect to participate with insurance or managed care companies may wish to attempt to forge special contractual arrangements with those companies allowing them to obtain reimbursement for services not otherwise covered. Practitioners who are familiar with the scientific literature and can present a coherent case supported by data (i.e., data from the literature as well as program evaluation data from their own practices) may have some success in negotiating with third-party payers. Ultimately, however, policies must change to accommodate the special needs of children and empirically supported treatments that deviate from the simplistic pathology-based, linear model of treatment.

FACTORS INFLUENCING SERVICES OFFERED

As mentioned previously, the private practice model places no restrictions on service delivery. Within rather broad legal and ethical bounds, private practitioners are free to offer whatever services they deem appropriate. A practitioner's theoretical orientation, the setting in which the practice is located, and broader market forces all influence service delivery.

Theoretical orientation influences service selection and delivery in a number of ways. Whether a therapist subscribes to a behavioral orientation, psychodynamic orientation, eclectic orientation, family systems orientation, or any number of other orientations will affect selection of treatment goals and the means by which the therapist will attempt to achieve those goals. Theoretical orientation also affects therapists' receptivity to research findings. In their survey of 279 primarily adult therapists in private practice (all members of Division 29, Division of Psychotherapy, of the American Psychological Association), Morrow-Bradley and Elliott (1986) found that theoretical orientation was the strongest and most consistent correlate of research utilization with behavior or cognitive therapists rating therapy research as being more useful, and psychodynamic therapists rating it as being less useful. Research utilization by private practitioners did not differ from research utilization by nonprivate practitioners, nor did research utilization by academicians differ from research utilization by nonacademicians.

The unique demands of the setting in which a private practice is located, including the population served within the setting, influence which services are offered and shape the way in which services are delivered. For example, compared to traditional child-focused private practices, private practices in primary care settings see more clients, spend less time with each client, see a lower proportion of severely disturbed clients, and focus more on prevention and early intervention than on treatment of severe problems (Schroeder, 1997). For a more complete discussion of mental health services in primary care settings, see Chapter 6 of this volume.

Looking beyond the immediate setting, characteristics of the market in which a practice is located can also affect service delivery. Large population centers can support a range of practice types from general practices to highly specialized practices. Less populated areas cannot support a high degree of specialization; therefore, practices located in those areas tend to be more general (unless they are able to reach beyond their more immediate market and attract clients regionally or nationally). Moreover, highly competitive areas, that is, areas containing a high concentration of providers, encourage niche marketing as therapists attempt to gain a competitive edge over others in their area.

Unlike service delivery models that receive funding from government or other external sources, private practice is more directly influenced by market forces. Offering consumers a choice is the cornerstone of a free market, but in health care delivery, the public interest is best served by placing a priority on client safety even if doing so limits choices. Many fear that the current marketplace, characterized by an oversupply of psychotherapists competing for shrinking funds, is fertile ground for the proliferation of untested, fringe, or harmful therapies (Tavris, 2003). Indeed, Kazdin (2000) identified more than 550 different forms of child psychotherapy, most of which have no empirical support. Furthermore, several popular therapies (e.g., some peer-group interventions for conduct disordered youth and critical incident stress debriefing) have been shown to be potentially harmful (Dishion, McCord, & Poulin, 1999; Lohr, Hooke, Gist, & Tolin, 2003), and recent efforts to identify ineffective or iatrogenic therapies are bound to turn up more (Lilienfeld, Lynn, & Lohr, 2003). Finally, several recent cases involving the death of children at the hands of therapists utilizing treatments lacking sufficient scientific grounding (e.g., rage reduction therapy and rebirthing therapy) have received national attention (Cohen, 1996; Mercer, 2002). Clearly, compelling support exists for concerns regarding public heath risks associated with the proliferation of untested therapies. No service delivery system is inherently immune to factors capable of promoting the adoption of practices that push the boundaries of what is professionally and ethically defensible; however, because of the freedoms that characterize the private practice model, the economic pressures associated with an increasingly competitive market, and the expedience of differentiating one's practice from all others, private practice is perhaps more susceptible to such factors than other service delivery models.

OUTPATIENT PRIVATE PRACTICE AND THERAPEUTIC EFFECTIVENESS

The literature on the efficacy of child psychotherapy has grown to over 500 studies (Weisz & Jensen, 2001). Four meta-analyses encompassing a wide range of target problems and treatments are often cited to provide evidence for the efficacy of child psychotherapy (Weersing & Weisz, 2002; Weisz, Donenberg, Han, & Weiss, 1995; Weisz & Weiss, 1993). The four meta-analyses (Casey & Berman, 1985; Kazdin, Bass, Ayers, & Rodgers, 1990; Weisz, Weiss, Alicke, & Klotz, 1987; Weisz, Weiss, Han, Granger, & Morton, 1995) summarized the findings of more than 300 randomized controlled studies published between 1952 and 1993. The studies included in the four meta-analyses involved more than 11,000 subjects (Weisz & Weiss, 1993) between the ages of 2 and 18 years, and found that, on average, treated children had a better outcome than approximately 76% to 81% of control children. Moreover, two of the four meta-analyses showed that treatment effects were maintained at follow-up, which averaged 6 months across studies (Weisz et al., 1987, 1995).

In contrast to the large number of studies evaluating the efficacy of structured treatments administered under contrived conditions, very few studies exist that evaluate the effectiveness of child psychotherapy as it is practiced in real-world clinic situations. Weisz and Jensen (2001) found only 14 treatment versus control studies that involved clinic-referred children (rather than recruited subjects) treated in actual clinic settings (rather than nonclinical settings such as university labs) by practicing clinicians (rather than researchers and their assistants) using standard treatments typically practiced in those settings (rather than structured, research-based treatment protocols). Meta-analytic examination of these studies showed that, on average, treated children had no better outcome than untreated control children (Weisz et al., 1995; Weisz & Jensen, 2001). Weisz et al. (1995) concluded that two independent factors account for the difference in outcomes between research therapy and clinic therapy favoring the former: first, clinic-referred children are more difficult to treat than children recruited for research therapy, and, second, most research studies employ behavior or cognitive behavior therapies whereas most practicing clinicians favor nonbehavioral therapies.

The literature regarding outcomes of child psychotherapy as it is delivered in private practice settings is weaker yet. Of the 223 controlled outcome studies summarized by Kazdin et al. (1990), fewer than 1% involved treatment conducted in private practice settings. Weisz et al. (1995) commented that the effectiveness of treatment delivered in individual and group private practices is a question that is largely unaddressed in the literature.

Differences in outcomes between research therapy and clinic therapy (i.e., practice-as-usual) are not limited to psychosocial treatments but are also seen with pharmacologic treatments (Weisz & Jensen, 1999; MTA Cooperative Group, 1999). Moreover, as with psychosocial treatments, there is a dearth of evidence supporting the effectiveness of pharmacologic treatments as delivered in the community, for example, polypharmacy (Weisz & Jensen, 1999).

Clearly, the successful implementation of research findings in clinical practice is a matter of public safety, and efforts aimed at encouraging research-informed practice and practice-informed research are worthwhile. Articles suggesting ways to adapt empirically validated treatments to clinical practice are beginning to appear in the literature (Connor-Smith & Weisz, 2003). Although it is not yet clear to what extent manualized treatments can be modified without sacrificing therapeutic integrity, at least two conditions would seem to be essential to making successful modifications. First, the therapist should have a firm understanding of the theoretical underpinnings of the treatment so as to avoid the pitfalls associated with viewing treatment as a "bag of tricks" rather than the application of a coherent theoretical system; and second, the key components of the treatment must be preserved. The first condition presents the greatest hurdle for private practitioners as many will have to seek additional education, training, and supervision. Promoting the use of empirically supported treatments among practitioners is an extremely complex issue and one which requires the combined efforts of practitioners; researchers; professional organizations; education, training, or research institutions; funding sources (including third-party payers and granting agencies); journal editors; regulatory bodies; client advocacy groups; and others.

CONCLUSIONS

Outpatient private practice is an extremely flexible and adaptable service delivery model. It has survived for more than 125 years in this country and will continue to survive as long as there are clients willing and able to pay for services. The model accommodates work with children, adolescents, and families, but insurance industry policies often do not support clinically justifiable and empirically validated practices with this unique and complex population. Because private practices are self-directed, entrepreneurial enterprises, market forces will always have a significant impact on their operations, including service delivery. The mental health field's greatest challenge will be to help create an environment that supports private practitioners' desires to provide consistently high-quality, cost-effective services.

REFERENCES

Brestan, E. V., & Eyberg, S. M. (1998). Effective psychosocial treatments of conduct-disordered children and adolescents: 29 years, 82 studies, and 5,272 kids. *Journal of Clinical Child Psychology*, 27, 180–189.

Brown, E. M. (n.d.). *Neurology's influence on American psychiatry: 1865–1915.* Retrieved September 21, 2003, from Brown University, Division of Biology and Medicine Web site: http://bms.brown.edu/HistoryofPsychiatry/influence.html

Burns, B. J., Costello, E. J., Angold, A., Tweed, D., Stangl, D., Farmer, E. M. Z. et al. (1995). Children's mental health service use across service sectors. *Health Affairs, 14*(3), 147–159.

Burns, B. J., Hoagwood, K., & Maultsby, L. T. (1998). Improving outcomes for children and adolescents with serious emotional and behavioral disorders: Current and future directions. In M. H. Epstein, K. Kutash, & A. J. Duchnowski (Eds.), *Outcomes for children and youth with emotional and behavioral disorders and their families: Programs and evaluation best practices* (pp. 686–707). Austin, TX: Pro-Ed.

Casey, R. J., & Berman, J. S. (1985). The outcome of psychotherapy with children. *Psychological Bulletin, 98,* 388–400.

Chambless, D. L., Baker, M., Baucom, D. H., Beutler, L. E., Calhoun, K. S., Crits-Christoph, P. et al. (1998). Update on empirically validated therapies, II. *The Clinical Psychologist, 51,* 3–16. Chambless, D., & Ollendick, T. H. (2001). Empirically supported interventions: Controversies and evidence. *Annual Review of Psychology, 52,* 685–716.

Chapman, R. (1990). Sole proprietorship. In E. A. Margenau (Ed.), *The encyclopedic handbook of private practice* (pp. 5–17). New York: Gardner.

Cohen, E. (1996, October 24). Rage reduction therapy: Help or abuse? *CNN Interactive.* Retrieved June 15, 2003, from http://www.cnn.com/US/9610/24/rage.reduction.therapy/

Connor-Smith, J. K., & Weisz, J. R. (2003). Applying treatment outcome research in clinical practice: Techniques for adapting interventions to the real world. *Child and Adolescent Mental Health, 8,* 3–10.

Dishion, T., McCord, J., & Poulin, F. (1999). When interventions harm: Peer groups and problem behavior. *American Psychologist, 54,* 755–764.

Hoagwood, K., & Erwin, H. D. (1997). Effectiveness of school-based mental health services for children: A 10-year research review. *Journal of Child and Family Studies, 6,* 435–454.

Jones, K. W. (1999). *Taming of the troublesome child: American families, child guidance, and the limits of psychiatric authority.* Cambridge, MA: Harvard University Press.

Kazdin, A. E. (2000). *Psychotherapy for children and adolescents: Directions for research and practice.* New York: Oxford University Press.

Kazdin, A. E., Bass, D., Ayers, W. A., & Rodgers, A. (1990). Empirical and clinical focus of child and adolescent psychotherapy research. *Journal of Consulting and Clinical Psychology, 58,* 729–740.

Kazdin, A. E., Siegel, T. C., & Bass, D. (1990). Drawing on clinical practice to inform research on child and adolescent psychotherapy: Survey of practitioners. *Professional Psychology: Research and Practice, 21,* 189–198.

Kehle, T. J., Madaus, M. R., Raratta, V. S., & Bray, M. A. (1998). Augmented self-modeling as a treatment for children with selective mutism. *Journal of School Psychology, 36,* 247–260.

Kehle, T. J., Owen, S. V., & Cressy, E. T. (1990). The use of self-modeling as an intervention in school psychology: A case study of an elective mute. *School Psychology Review, 19,* 115–121.

Lilienfeld, S. O., Lynn, S. J., & Lohr, J. M. (2003). Science and pseudoscience in clinical psychology: Initial thoughts, reflections, and considerations. In S. O. Lilienfeld, S. J. Lynn, & J. M. Lohr (Eds.), *Science and pseudoscience in clinical psychology* (pp. 1–14). New York: Guilford.

Lohr, J. M., Hooke, W., Gist, R., & Tolin, D. F. (2003). Novel and controversial treatments for trauma-related stress disorders. In S. O. Lilienfeld, S. J. Lynn, & J. M. Lohr (Eds.), *Science and pseudoscience in clinical psychology* (pp. 243–272). New York: Guilford.

Mercer, J. (2002). Attachment therapy: A treatment without empirical support. *The Scientific Review of Mental Health Practice, 1,* 105–112.

Morrow-Bradley, C., & Elliott, R. (1986). Utilization of psychotherapy research by practicing psychotherapists. *American Psychologist, 41,* 188–197.

MTA Cooperative Group. (1999). A 14-month randomized clinical trial of treatment strategies for attention-deficit/hyperactivity disorder. *Archives of General Psychiatry, 56,* 1073–1086.

Nathan, P., & Gorman, J. (Eds.). (1998). *A guide to treatments that work.* New York: Oxford University Press.

Office of the Assistant Secretary for Planning and Evaluation, U.S. Department of Health and Human Services (1997). *Trends in the well-being of America's children and youth: 1997 Edition.* Retrieved October 15, 2003, from http://aspe.hhs.gov/hsp/97trends/PF1-4.htm

Ollendick, T. H., & King, N. J. (1998). Empirically supported treatments for children with phobic and anxiety disorders: Current status. *Journal of Clinical Child Psychology, 27,* 156–167.

Reisman, J. M. (1991). *A history of clinical psychology.* New York: Hemisphere Publishing Corp.

Roth, A., & Fonagy, P. (1996). *What works for whom? A critical review of psychotherapy research.* New York: Guilford.

Routh, D. K. (1994). *Clinical psychology since 1917: Science, practice, and organization.* New York: Plenum.

Satcher, D. (1999). *Mental health: A report of the surgeon general.* Retrieved June 23, 2003, from http://www.surgeongeneral.gov/library/mentalhealth/home.html

Schroeder, C. S. (1997). Conducting an integrated practice in a pediatric setting. In R. J. Illback, C. T. Cobb, & H. M. Joseph, Jr. (Eds.), *Integrated services for children and families: Opportunities for psychological practice* (pp. 221–255). Washington, DC: American Psychological Association.

Tavris, C. (2003). The widening scientist–practitioner gap: A view from the bridge. In S. O. Lilienfeld, S. J. Lynn, & J. M. Lohr (Eds.), *Science and pseudoscience in clinical psychology* (pp. ix–xvii). New York: Guilford.

Taylor, T. K., & Biglan, A. (1998). Behavioral family interventions for improving child-rearing: A review of the literature for clinicians and policy makers. *Child and Family Psychology Review, 1,* 41–60.

Webster-Stratton, C. (1984). Randomized trial of two parent-training programs for families with conduct-disordered children. *Journal of Consulting and Clinical Psychology, 52,* 666–678.

Webster-Stratton, C., Kolpacoff, M., & Hollinsworth, T. (1988). Self-administered videotape therapy for families with conduct-problem children: Comparison with two cost-effective treatments and a control group. *Journal of Consulting and Clinical Psychology, 56,* 558–566.

Webster-Stratton, C., & Reid, M. J. (2003). The incredible years parents, teachers, and children training series: A multifaceted treatment approach for young children with conduct problems. In A. E. Kazdin & J. R. Weisz (Eds.), *Evidence-based psychotherapies for children and adolescents.* New York: Guilford.

Weersing, V. R., & Weisz, J. R. (2002). Mechanisms of action in youth psychotherapy. *Journal of Child Psychology & Psychiatry & Allied Disciplines, 43,* 3–29.

Weisz, J. R., Donenberg, G. R., Han, S. S., & Weiss, B. (1995). Bridging the gap between laboratory and clinic in child and adolescent psychotherapy. *Journal of Consulting and Clinical Psychology, 63,* 688–701.

Weisz, J. R., & Jensen, P. S. (1999). Efficacy and effectiveness of child and adolescent psychotherapy and pharmacotherapy. *Mental Health Services Research, 1*(3), 125–157.

Weisz, J. R., & Jensen, A. L. (2001). Child and adolescent psychotherapy in research and practice contexts: Review of the evidence and suggestions for improving the field. *European Child & Adolescent Psychiatry, 10*(Suppl.), 12–18.

Weisz, J. R., & Weiss, B. (1993). *Effects of psychotherapy with children and adolescents.* New York: Sage.

Weisz, J. R., Weiss, B., Alicke, M. D., & Klotz, M. L. (1987). Effectiveness of psychotherapy with children and adolescents: A meta-analysis for clinicians. *Journal of Consulting and Clinical Psychology, 55,* 542–549.

Weisz, J. R., Weiss, B., Han, S., Granger, D. A., & Morton, T. (1995). Effects of psychotherapy with children and adolescents revisited: A meta-analysis of treatment outcome studies. *Psychological Bulletin, 117,* 450–468.

9

Inpatient Treatment Models[†]

LUIS A. VARGAS and ARTEMIO DE DIOS BRAMBILA

Inpatient psychiatric services for youth[1] have undergone significant changes since inpatient units were established in the 1920s and 1930s to treat children with autism and schizophrenia and to manage children with postencephalitic brain damage (American Psychiatric Association [APA], 1957; Hendren & Berlin, 1991). Over time, inpatient psychiatric services developed multimodal, integrated programs in the context of a therapeutic milieu for children whose mental disorders could not be treated on an outpatient basis (Berlin, 1978). Inpatient treatment was similar to residential care in treatment philosophy and length of stay (Jemerin & Philips, 1988). Both were influenced by developmental psychodynamic perspectives on treatment of youth that were dominant at the time (e.g., Bettelheim, 1950, 1974; Berlin, 1978; Noshpitz, 1982; Redl, 1959, 1966) and emphasized psychosocial interventions within a safe and protected environment in which the demands of and stresses from the family and the community were reduced. For the period from 1970 to 1986, the average length of stay in state psychiatric hospitals and psychiatric units in general hospitals decreased whereas the length of stay for youth in private psychiatric hospitals increased from 1980 to 1986 (Mandersheid & Millazzo-Sayre as cited in Ponton, 1991). Further, during the 1970s and 1980s, hospital-based psychiatric units grew significantly in number (Harper & Geraty, 1987) and admission rates rose from the 1980s to the 1990s (Weller, Cook, Hendren, & Woolston, 1995).

LUIS A. VARGAS and ARTEMIO DE DIOS BRAMBILA • Division of Child and Adolescent Psychiatry, Department of Psychiatry, University of New Mexico School of Medicine, Albuquerque, New Mexico 87131.

[†]We would like to acknowledge Grace Bolanos, B. A., for her assistance and diligence in the library research and preparation of this chapter.

[1]The term "youth" will be used to refer to both children and adolescents.

The change toward shorter lengths of stay has been attributed to a number of factors that include: (1) the increased knowledge and development of psychotropic medications, along with the emergence of biological psychiatry in which the biological aspects of mental disorders are emphasized; (2) growing interest in and need for rapid and safe treatments (Jemerin & Philips, 1988); (3) decreased coverage by third-party payers due to rising costs and increased numbers of youth hospitalized (Harper & Geraty, 1987); (4) growing public and professional concern that youth were being inappropriately hospitalized (Knitzer, 1982; Weithorn, 1988; Weller et al., 1995); (5) the emergence of managed care organizations (MCOs) and behavioral health organizations (BHOs); (6) the "systems-of-care" movement that promotes the idea that the mental health needs of youth are best met in community-based, family-centered, and prevention-oriented services that are integrated and coordinated across providers (Friedman, 1994; Stroul & Friedman, 1986); and (7) the development of recommendations and policies by professional groups to "tighten up" the criteria for hospitalization of youth using the notions of "acuity," "danger to self or others," and "least restrictive environment" (American Academy of Child and Adolescent Psychiatry [AACAP], 1989; APA, 1976; Joint Commission on Accreditation of Hospitals, 1988).

Under pressures to both reduce admissions to inpatient units and decrease lengths of stay, the child- and adolescent-oriented models based on establishing therapeutic environments as the primary vehicles of change were abandoned or modified in preference of inpatient models that focus on symptom alleviation and improvement in functional impairment sufficient to move the youth to a lower level of care as quickly as possible. However, acute inpatient services and residential treatment centers are appropriate for some youth with severe mental disorders. It is estimated that 9–13% of youth experience serious mental disorders that substantially interfere with or limit their ability to function at home, school, and community and 5–9% have disorders with extreme functional impairment (Manderscheid & Sonnenschein, 1996).

ORGANIZATION OF ACUTE INPATIENT SERVICES

Inpatient hospitalization is the most restrictive level of care for youth. It consumes the largest part of the mental health resources, about half of the funding for children and adolescent mental health (Burns, Hoagwood, & Mrazek, 1999). In addition, it is the clinical intervention with the weakest evidence base, particularly in relation to the resources consumed and the risks associated with hospital-based treatment for youth (U.S. Department of Health and Human Services [USDHHS,], 1999). Nevertheless, because some children with severe mental disorders require a restrictive treatment environment, hospitals remain an integral component of a system of care (Singh, Landrum, Donatelli, Hampton, & Ellis, 1994).

Current acute psychiatric inpatient facilities incorporate an array of medical and behavioral health services for the primary purpose of "stabilizing" the mental condition or crisis of a youth sufficiently so that the youth no longer poses an imminent risk of harm to self or others or is no longer severely functionally impaired. Many providers offering acute inpatient services aspire to provide treatment within a "biopsychosocial" model in which the array of interventions integrates the biological, psychological, and social aspects of mental disorders. In a biopsychosocial model, treatment is implemented by multidisciplinary teams that provide comprehensive assessments and an array of services that includes medication, psychotherapy, allied therapies (speech and language, occupational, art, and recreational therapies), and milieu treatment. Inpatient services are clinically directed by an attending psychiatrist. The inpatient milieu is viewed as a critical component of the therapeutic intervention. These multimodal therapies are meant not only to address and resolve the underlying issues of presenting clinical problems, but also to teach more socially adaptive skills to maintain the youth in their homes, schools, and communities. The implementation of the biopsychosocial model has been demonstrated to be costly, of long duration, and its effectiveness difficult to ascertain. As a result of the emphasis on medical or crisis stabilization under managed care, the treatment focus in inpatient services is primarily on symptom alleviation and interventions that improve functional impairment to reduce "acuity."

Criteria for Hospitalization

Most MCOs and BHOs have clinical criteria that require that acute inpatient care for youth provide multidisciplinary assessments and multimodal interventions in secure units that have daily medical care, defined as 24-hour nursing care and daily medical care by a psychiatrist or, for children under the age of 12 years, a child psychiatrist (see, e.g., AACAP, 1989). Lengths of stay are usually short (from days to a few weeks) because of the focus on "stabilization." Acute inpatient units must be prepared to provide special treatment that includes physical or mechanical restraints, seclusion, use of PRN medications, and locked units.

Acuity is usually defined by the MCO or BHO as including: (1) a DSM-IV Axis I diagnosis and (2) evidence of imminent danger to self or others or severe functional impairment. The latter typically includes a serious suicide attempt or suicidal ideation and intent; serious threats or assaultive behavior due to a mental disorder; self-mutilation; risk-taking behavior that poses danger to self or others; violence due to a mental disorder, delusions or hallucinations that pose a risk of danger to self or others; bizarre or disorganized behavior, disorientation, or psychomotor agitation or retardation that grossly impairs the youth's ability to function at a less restrictive level of care; inability to maintain age-appropriate self-care or responsibilities due to a mental disorder; and the experience of severe or life-threatening side effects of or atypical responses to psychotropic medication. Continued stays in acute inpatient psychiatric units must be reviewed at every few days and discharge planning must be evident from the time of admission. MCOs or BHOs have discharge criteria that typically include meeting treatment goals and objectives, no longer meeting admission criteria, lack of participation of youth or family in treatment, or lack of indication of likelihood to benefit from treatment.

In spite of documented admission criteria, their interpretation and implementation varies across the United States, as well as among MCOs and BHOs, and service providers. The variability in adherence to these admission criteria demonstrates how difficult it is to apply them to a diverse, complex, and idiosyncratic clinical child and adolescent population. Dalton, Mueller, and Forman (1989) noted that the problem with rigid criteria for hospitalization is that admission is determined by other factors, particularly the resources available to the referrer. Decisions to hospitalize are dependent upon the nature and quality of mental health services within the continuum of care in the community. Thus, the admission threshold cannot be an absolute, based on factors restricted to the specific case; rather it has to allow for the expertise and resources within the referrer's array of services, and in other local services (Maskey, 1998).

Safeguards for Unnecessary Admissions

To prevent unnecessary admissions and promote safe care when hospitalization is necessary, a policy statement was developed and recommended by the AACAP (1989). The AACAP standards state that hospitalizations should be used only when treatment in a less intensive setting is not possible or has failed and that patients should be placed in the least intensive and least restrictive level of care compatible with safe and effective treatment (APA, 1989). Such standards can only be attained when (1) less restrictive services are available; (2) criteria for access to each level of care are clearly delineated; and (3) a strategy is in place for easy transfer from one level of restrictive care to a less restrictive one (Burns et al., 1999). In addition to these standards, state mental health statutes specify criteria that must be met for a youth to be voluntarily or involuntarily hospitalized (e.g., that the youth suffers from a mental disorder that needs treatment, that the youth is likely to benefit from treatment, and that the treatment is consistent with the "least drastic means principle"), and may require assignment of guardians *ad litem* for hospitalized youth to ensure that that admissions are appropriate. Furthermore, parent support and advocacy groups provide youth and their families with information and assistance in understanding and meeting the rights of youth within the mental health system.

Economic Factors Influencing Use of Inpatient Hospitalization

According to Blanz and Schimdt (2000), pressure from insurance companies influences decisions as to whether a hospital inpatient admission is a viable option. Based on insurance claims, Patrick, Padgett, Burns, Schlesinger, and Cohen (1993) showed that a cut in inpatient benefits that occurred between 1978 and 1983 led to a 22% drop in the rate of inpatient hospitalization for youth. The role of insurance companies has become more integral in the decision-making processes for inpatient hospitalization for children and youth. Towbin and Campbell (1995) noted that referrals for inpatient admission have been subject to greater prescreenings and authorizations. This increased complexity in the decision-making process involved in the hospitalization of youth has resulted in less seriously impaired patients being diverted to other levels of care.

Other Factors Influencing Use of Inpatient Hospitalization

On one hand, the degree of impairment, acuity, and severity of disorder displayed by patients entering inpatient services has increased (Towbin & Campbell, 1995). On the other hand, as Martin and Leslie (2003) reported, the number of youth admitted to inpatient psychiatric services decreased by almost 24% from 1997 to 2000. Further, they noted that there was a 20% reduction in inpatient days. Although economic factors associated with managed care might explain these consequences, there are other factors that appear to predict psychiatric hospitalization. Pottick, Hansell, Gutterman, White, and Raskin (1995) noted that psychiatric hospitalization of youth is predicted by "(1) public or private insurance coverage versus no insurance; (2) previous hospitalization; (3) psychiatric diagnosis of affective or psychotic disorders versus conduct disorders, adjustment disorders, drug and alcohol abuse, and other disorders; and (4) age, with adolescents more likely to be hospitalized than children" (p. 425).

FACTORS AFFECTING THE DELIVERY OF INPATIENT SERVICES

Although many inpatient units aspire to provide interventions within a biopsychosocial model, short lengths of stay often encourage use of medications and discourage psychotherapies that do not have an immediate impact on crisis stabilization. The movement toward biological psychiatry, the increased knowledge and development of psychotropic medications, and the pressure from funding sources to employ interventions that are aggressive and have rapid results have encouraged the conceptualization of the presenting problem as a medical illness in which the first line of treatment is medication.

However, another movement, systems-of-care (Stroul & Friedman, 1986), has promoted greater attention to the conceptualization of brief inpatient hospitalization as only one level of care within a continuum of other services. Deriving from a core tenet that youth should be treated in their community whenever possible, one of the goals of inpatient care is to prepare the family, school, and community to better meet the discharged patients' needs. Thus, inpatient units influenced by the system-of-care philosophy are more likely to incorporate very active case management and ecologically oriented interventions to develop the necessary supports and resources in the family, school, and community to better meet the patients' needs. Many MCOs and BCOs, along with state departments or divisions of children's behavioral health services, also have encouraged the development of mental health delivery systems that include intensive and comprehensive outpatient programs to maintain youth with serious mental disorders in their communities. These include wraparound services that incorporate case management, home-based treatment, behavior management specialists in the home or school, multisystemic treatment approaches such as Multisystemic Therapy (Henggeler, Schoenwald, Borduin, Rowland, & Cunningham, 1998), treatment foster care, and day treatment programs, any of which may be arranged prior to the patient's discharge to optimize the likelihood of successful re-integration back into the home and community.

Use of Medications

One of the concerns about the pressure by MCOs and BCOs to keep inpatient care as brief as possible has been the potential overemphasis on the use of medication during the inpatient stay. There are not sufficient data at this point to indicate if this is, in fact, the case. The use of medication across all levels of care has increased. In a study using data from two nationally representative surveys of the general population focusing on youth 18 years of age or younger, the overall rate of the use of psychotropic medications increased from 1.4 per 100 youth in 1987 to 3.9 in 1996 (Olfson, Marcus, Weissman, & Jensen, 2002). In the 1990s, psychotropic medication use for youth under 20 years of age reached a level close to adult utilization rates; the prevalence of psychotropic medication use for these youth increased two- to three-fold (Zito et al., 2003). This is consistent with a study by the Center for Health Care Policy and Evaluation (2000), which showed that the use of selective serotonin reuptake inhibitors (SSRIs) increased 62% and other antidepressants, excluding tricyclic antidepressants, increased 195% during the period of 1995–1999. Use of central nervous system stimulants also increased from 23.8 to 30.0 per 1000 youth.

Although it is not clear how inpatient psychiatric services fared, as compared to outpatient services, in the use of psychotropic medications over this time period, another study using a national database on privately insured youth sheds some light on this issue (Martin & Leslie, 2003). The authors concluded that reductions in the intensity of and reimbursement in inpatient and outpatient psychiatric services continued through the late 1990s. Along with these declines were concurrent increases in the use and costs associated with psychotropic medications, especially for youth with mood and anxiety disorders, and a shift toward medication-based outpatient treatment. They noted that, as lengths of stay in inpatient settings decreased and there was also a reduction in outpatient visits (about 11%) and a decline in payments per outpatient visits (about 6%) from 1997 to 2000, the number of youth receiving medication increased by almost 5% and the mean medication-related costs per outpatient increased by about 21%.

Accessibility to Inpatient Services

It is estimated that more than 7 out of 10 adolescents who suffer from mental health problems are not receiving any services (U.S. Public Health Service, 2000). Access to inpatient services for youth with serious mental disorders is particularly problematic (President's New Freedom Commission on Mental Health, 2003). Many states have closed acute inpatient beds due to budget cuts. Families complain that they must hospitalize their children in facilities that are distant from their homes. Families in crisis are reluctant to seek care in hospital emergency rooms that are not well equipped or staffed to handle the needs of youth with serious mental disorders. Others complain that insurance companies are only willing to pay for stays that are too short to allow for stabilization. The lack of health insurance poses yet another obstacle to access. In 1999, 14% of children in the United States did not have health insurance (Annie E. Casey Foundation, 2002).

The problem for ethnic minority youth is likely to be even greater. About one fourth of African Americans, about 21% of Asian Americans and Pacific Islanders, and about 37% of Latinos are uninsured (Brown, Ojeda, Wyn, & Levan, 2000). About 20% of American Indians report having access to the Indian Health Service and 24% of American Indians and Alaska Natives do not have health insurance (Brown et al., 2000). There are very few data currently available on ethnic or racial disparities on the use of inpatient psychiatric services for youth. However, there is evidence that many ethnic minority youth, with the possible exception of African Americans (Cohen & Hesselbart, 1993), receive even fewer mental health services than European Americans. African American youth are less likely than European American youth to have made a mental health outpatient visit (Cunningham & Freiman, 1996) and less likely than European American youth to receive mental health care (Zahner & Daskalakis, 1997). Few African American youth receive psychiatric inpatient care (Chabra, Chavez, Harris, & Shah, 1999) but many African American youth are treated in residential treatment centers (RTCS) (Firestone, 1990). This is possibly due to African American youth lacking health insurance, because RTCS are often funded from public sources, and to the fact that child welfare agencies often initiate treatment for African American youth (USDHHS, 2001). The few studies that are available show that Latino youth are underrepresented in mental health services (USDHHS, 2001). Zwillich (2000) noted that 80% of Latino youth with mental health problems do not receive any services. Among other barriers that many ethnic minorities face in accessing mental health care, in general, and inpatient services, in particular, are: limited financial resources or poverty, limited awareness on how to negotiate mental health systems, limited providers who speak their languages, and, for some, immigration status.

EVALUATION OF INPATIENT SERVICES

Although there is a paucity of controlled studies on the outcome of inpatient psychiatric care of youth, some studies suggest the usefulness of inpatient care. Blotcky, Dimperio, and Gossett (1984) reviewed 24 uncontrolled follow-up studies of children under the age of 12 years who were treated in psychiatric hospitals. The follow-up period in these studies ranged from 6 months to 24 years. They found that all follow-up studies reported some positive treatment outcomes, with more than half demonstrating positive long-term outcome. They further found that a favorable prognosis was positively correlated with three broad groups of variables: (1) patient variables (e.g., adequate intelligence, later onset of symptoms, nonpsychotic and nonorganic diagnoses, absence of antisocial features or bizarre symptoms), (2) family variables (e.g., healthy family functioning), and (3) treatment variables (e.g., adequate lengths of stay, specialized treatment programs and involvement in aftercare).

Applying a more rigorous methodology and statistical procedure, Pfeiffer and Strzelecki (1990) identified 34 studies, published between 1975 and 1991, focusing on the outcome of inpatient treatment of child and adolescent mental disorders. They concluded that psychiatric hospitalization of youth is often beneficial, particularly if special aspects of treatment are fulfilled; for example, a good therapeutic alliance (Clarkin, Hurst, & Crilly, 1987), treatment with a cognitive-based, problem-solving skills training package (Kazdin, Esveldt-Dawson, French, & Unis, 1987), completion of treatment program (Gossett, Barnhart, Lewis, & Phillips, 1977, planned discharge (White, Benn, Gross, & Schaffer-Lopez, 1979) and aftercare services (Gossett et al., 1977) are present. Outpatient aftercare (Gossett et al., 1977), availability of foster home placements (Stewart, Adams, & Meardon, 1978), and low level of psychosocial stress in the postdischarge environment (Cohen-Sandler, Berman, & King, 1982; Koret, 1980) have been identified as necessary to ensure the transfer and generalization of treatment gains to the discharged patient's environment and to minimize the risk for rehospitalization.

As may be expected, healthier patients respond more favorably to inpatient psychiatric treatment (Pfeiffer & Strzelecki, 1990), especially youth with adequate intelligence, later onset of symptoms, nonpsychotic and nonorganic diagnoses, absence of antisocial features or bizarre symptoms, or a pure anxiety or affective disorder (Blotcky et al., 1984; Pfeiffer & Strzelecki, 1990; Sourander & Phia, 1998). Severe parent or family pathology and poor family functioning, as evidenced by parental substance abuse, child abuse or maltreatment, or parents' previous psychiatric hospital treatment, appear to be negative elements in the outcome of many hospitalized youth (Gabel & Schindledecker, 1990; Sourander et al., 1996). In general, adverse family circumstances change less during hospitalization than the child's symptoms do (Robertson & Friedberg, 1979).

A report by the Surgeon General on mental health (USDHHS, 1999) indicated that only three controlled studies have examined the outcome of inpatient care and all three studies, which date prior to 1990, showed that community care was at least as effective as inpatient care. Blanz and Schmidt (2000) pointed out that only a few studies of inpatient child and adolescent treatment outcome have been published since the Pfeiffer and Strzelecki (1990) review. Two recent studies show conflicting outcomes. In an uncontrolled study of one inpatient facility, Mayes et al. (2001) found that children improved significantly in their psychological functioning at discharge and follow-up at 1 and 6 months. Furthermore, they found that children who were more impaired at admission showed greater progress during their hospital stays but did not maintain their gains at follow-up, when compared to children with less serious problems. Children with emotional disorders, as opposed to those with behavior disorders, had a better outcome. A controlled study compared two German child and adolescent inpatient settings with home-based treatment (Mattejat, Hirt, Wilken, Schmidt, & Remschmidt, 2001). Although both treatment groups improved and had similar effect sizes, there was no difference in the two treatment groups at discharge from the program and at follow-up periods of 8 months and 3 years. The authors suggest that home-based treatment should be used more frequently due to its effects and cost.

ORGANIZATION OF RESIDENTIAL TREATMENT CENTERS (RTCS)

RTCS are the second most restrictive level of care for youth. They provide services to about 5–8% of treated youth; however, they consume almost one fourth of the resources for mental health services for youth (Burns, Hoagwood, & Maultsby, 1998; Warner & Pottick, 2003). RTCS can vary greatly, from settings that are similar to inpatient psychiatric services to those that are similar to group homes; they may be located in hospitals, on small campuses, or embedded in communities. Consequently, they do not have a uniform organization. However, RTCS are often developed around the "therapeutic milieu." The key elements of a therapeutic milieu consist of the maintenance of a safe and containing environment, a highly structured program, physical and emotional support, collective involvement of the child, family, and staff in the RTC regimen, and continuous evaluation of all therapeutic interventions (Gunderson, 1978). A therapeutic milieu "emphasizes the therapeutic manipulation of time and space and of individual and group experiences in order to make the children's living situation itself a comprehensive therapeutic intervention" (Cotton, 1993, p. 5). Although theoretical orientations utilized in RTCS vary, a psychosocial model is often espoused within the therapeutic milieu that includes, for example, use of a peer culture to change individual and group behaviors, the implementation of multimodal therapies, development of alternative strategies of modulating emotions and impulses, psychoeducation to prepare the resident for reentry into the community, and development self-awareness and relapse prevention strategies for the children's and adolescents' mental disorders.

There is also great variability in the staffing and training of staff in RTCS. Some RTCS provide a full array of services similar to those offered in inpatient psychiatric services and include psychiatrists, psychologists, social workers, nurses, counselors, and allied therapists, along with the paraprofessional staff members who supervise the youth on a 24-hour basis. In these types of RTCS, all of these staff members take part in administering the treatment program. In other RTCS, professional staff provides services primarily in the context of the paraprofessional staff's work with the youth; psychiatrists, psychologists, or other professional staff may serve as consultants to those actually administering the treatment program. RTCS vary considerably in their staff-to-resident ratio and in their ability to adequately monitor and supervise their residents. One notable trend in RTC care is the shift toward greater family and community participation in the transition of the residents into their homes and communities. RTCS are making greater use of wraparound services to decrease lengths of stay and recidivism and to improve the residents' functioning in their home environments.

Concerns about the Use of RTCs

There have been a number of concerns expressed about the use of RTCS: (1) the lack of admission criteria (Wells, 1991); (2) the lack of uniform standards for RTCS (e.g., with regard to organization, structure, staffing); (3) the variability in the training of line staff; (4) the cost of these programs (Burns et al., 1999; Friedman & Street, 1985; USDHHS, 1999); (5) the placement of youth in RTCS that are outside of their communities and sometimes even in other states (Stroul & Friedman, 1986); and (6) the risk that youth may be adversely affected by placement in RTCS (Barker, 1998). Nonetheless, RTCS must now treat much more seriously disturbed youth than previously (Leichtman, Leichtman, Cornsweet Barber, & Neese, 2001; Warner & Pottick, 2003). Unlike psychiatric inpatient services, the resident population of RTCS can vary considerably. Youth are placed in RTCS for a variety of reasons: severe emotional problems; inability of the youth to adequately function at home and in the community; violent and aggressive behavior; continued but not imminent risk of harm to self or high likelihood of victimization; delinquent or severely oppositional and defiant behavior; substance abuse; and runaway risk. Some of these populations may not be likely to benefit from placement in an RTC. For example, youth with violent and aggressive behavior do not appear to respond positively to RTC placement (Joshi & Rosenberg, 1997).

Changes in Lengths of Stay

Historically, RTCS were long-term facilities that ranged from 6 months to 18 months, and sometimes even longer. Under managed care, the youth seen in these facilities are more psychiatrically disturbed and often come from multiproblem families; often they do not have consistent or available natural support systems (USDHHS, 1999). The shift in RTC populations toward youth with enduring and pervasive mental disorders reflects the cascade effects of having the more disturbed and, at times, medically fragile or diagnostically complicated patients being referred from acute psychiatric hospitals (due to increasingly shorter lengths of stay) for further stabilization and treatment in RTC settings. Currently, RTC lengths of stay may range from 2 weeks to 3 months, depending on the patient's severity of psychiatric symptoms, degree of functional impairment, and the adult caretaker's capacity to maintain the emotionally disturbed youth at home and in the community.

EVALUATION OF RESIDENTIAL TREATMENT CENTERS

Youth placed in RTCs constitute a difficult-to-treat population. Unfortunately, there is a lack of RTC outcome studies in the last 20 years. Further, the results of not providing residential care are unknown. Most of the outcome studies are uncontrolled and were published in the 1970s and 1980s (Curry, 1991; USDHHS, 1999). Burns et al. (1999) reported that there were only three controlled studies of RTCs. Two of these studies were of a program ("Project Re-Education") that is not typical of most RTC programs, based on a treatment model developed in the 1960s, which used teacher-counselors supported by mental health consultants and Outward Bound-type camping activities. Adolescents completing this program improved in self-esteem, showed a decrease in impulsiveness, and demonstrated greater internal control as compared to the untreated group (Weinstein, 1974). A follow-up study of this program showed that, when outcomes in adjustment were maintained 6 months post discharge, those outcomes were better predicted by community factors, which led the researchers to suggest that this RTC program was as effective as interventions in the adolescent's community (Lewis, 1988). The third study, which compared RTC with therapeutic foster care, showed that the two treatment programs were equally effective but RTC was twice as expensive (Rubenstein, Armentrout, Levin, & Herald, 1978).

The uncontrolled studies of RTC suggest that 60–80% show gains in areas that included clinical status, academics, and peer relationships (Burns et al., 1999; USDHHS, 1999). Some uncontrolled RTC studies, subsequent to the Surgeon General's report (USDHHS, 1999), have followed its recommendations to further examine differential outcomes and the coordination of between RTC staff and community services. Lyons, Terry, Martinovich, Peterson, and Bouska (2001) reviewed 285 care records at multiple intervals for youth placed in eight RTCs in a western state. They found that youth improved during their stay in all of the RTCs and that there were differential changes in the residents. Specifically, youth in all eight RTCs showed improvement in high-risk behaviors (suicidal ideation, self-mutilation, and aggression toward people). Depression and reality testing improved, while disobedience, impulsivity and sexualized behavior remained the same. They suggest that RTC placement may be more effective for youth with posttraumatic stress and other emotional disorders as opposed to those with attention-deficit or hyperactivity or disruptive behavior disorders. Leichtman et al. (2001) reported on an intensive short-term residential program at the Menninger Clinic created in response to managed care. They conducted an analysis of follow-up data on 123 adolescents who were admitted between March 1994 and January 1998. The emphasis in this short-term program was on helping youth transition from RTC into the community, where children and their families could continue to work on problems at home. Leichtman and his colleagues found that the adolescents showed substantial improvement at discharge and that improvement was sustained for the year following discharge. They suggest that gains can be maintained only if discharge planning includes an emphasis on working with families, participation in community activities, and discharge planning.

Although these studies reflect a favorable outcome for RTCs, the findings of these RTC studies should be viewed as tentative due to their methodological flaws, such as the absence of control groups and diagnostic heterogeneity in the RTC populations. The sustainability of gains in RTC appears to depend on the supports available in the child's or adolescent's environment after discharge from RTC, involvement of the adolescents' families, participation in community activities, and discharge planning (Burns et al., 1999; Leichtman et al., 2001; USDHHS, 1999; Wells, 1991).

CULTURAL RESPONSIVENESS OF THE INPATIENT SERVICES AND RTCS

Despite the increasing amount of literature on cultural competence standards and guidelines in the provision of services to youth, there is little written about how to actually carry out culturally responsive interventions in inpatient settings and RTCs. A few authors (Canino & Spurlock, 2002; Hendren & Berlin, 1991) have given attention to the need to address culture within the psychiatric inpatient or RTC milieu. It is likely that ethnic minority youth experience the inpatient environment as quite foreign and emotionally destabilizing (Vargas & Berlin, 1991). The inpatient units in which seriously emotionally disturbed youth are placed and in which they must live for a period of time are often based on the values and beliefs of the dominant culture. These values and beliefs are represented in the way the units of structured, in the way staff interact with the youth, in the types of rules staff has for the youth, and on the types of behaviors that are overtly and covertly encouraged or discouraged or rewarded or punished. Placement of an ethnic minority youth into an American mainstream psychiatric inpatient unit or RTC may be likened to the experience of an emotionally fragile exchange student living in a family with unfamiliar customs, beliefs, and attitudes. For the seriously emotionally disturbed, ethnic minority youth who already are experiencing significant stresses, the placement experience may not facilitate or promote improvement unless these cultural issues are addressed or integrated into the treatment program.

CONCLUSION

The research literature on the outcomes of psychiatric hospitalization and residential care of youth remains methodologically flawed and limits any causal inferences on the effectiveness of inpatient psychiatric treatment. Furthermore, because most studies on inpatient care and residential care have been conducted prior to 1990 and the delivery of inpatient care has changed dramatically since then, the effectiveness of inpatient care, as it is delivered today, is unknown. Acute psychiatric inpatient hospitalization and RTCs will very likely continue to have a place in child and adolescent mental health services. Regardless of the innovative, intensive, community-based outpatient treatment models that are being developed and are showing positive results in the treatment of youth with serious mental disorders, some youth will still have crises or exacerbation of their mental disorders that do not respond to or cannot be treated in intensive community-based outpatient services. However, the success of inpatient services and RTCs is, in part, dependent on the coordination and integration with "discharge partners" (e.g., families, community-based services, medical services, and schools).

REFERENCES

American Academy of Child and Adolescent Psychiatry. (1989). *Policy statement: Inpatient hospital treatment of children and adolescents.* Washington, DC: Author.

American Psychiatric Association. (1957). *Psychiatric inpatient treatment of children.* Baltimore: Lord Baltimore Press.

American Psychiatric Association. (1976). *Manual of psychiatric peer review.* Washington, DC: APA Committee on Peer Review.

American Psychiatric Association. (1989). *Concepts and definitions in psychiatric quality assurance and utilization review.* Washington, DC: Author.

Annie E. Casey Foundation. (2002). *Kids count data book: 2002.* Baltimore: Author.

Barker, P. (1998). The future of residential treatment for children. In *C. Schaefer & A. Swanson (Eds.), Children in residential care: Critical issues in treatment.* (pp. 1–16). New York: Van Nostrand Reinhold.

Berlin, I. N. (1978). Developmental issues in the psychiatric hospitalization of children. *American Journal of Psychiatry, 135,* 1044–1048.

Bettelheim, B. (1950). *Love is not enough.* New York: Free Press.

Bettelheim, B. (1974). *A home for the heart.* New York: Knopf.

Blanz, B., & Schimdt, M. H. (2000). Practitioner review: Preconditions and outcome of inpatient treatment in child and adolescent psychiatry. *Journal of Child Psychology and Psychiatry, 41,* 703–712.

Blotcky, M. J., Dimperio, T. J., & Gossett, J. T. (1984). Follow-up of children treated in psychiatric hospitals: A review of studies. *American Journal of Psychiatry, 141,* 1499–1507.

Brown, E. R., Ojeda, V. D., Wyn, R., & Levan, R. (2000). *Racial and ethnic disparities in access to health insurance and health care.* Los Angeles: UCLA Center for Health Policy Research and The Henry J. Kaiser Family Foundation.

Burns, B. J., Hoagwood, K., & Maultsby, L. T. (1998). Improving outcomes for children and adolescents with serious emotional and behavioral disorders: Current and future directions. In M. H. Epstein, K. Kutash, & A. J. Duchnowski (Eds.), *Outcomes for children and youth with emotional and behavioral disorders and their families: Programs and evaluation best practices* (pp. 685–707). Austin, TX: Pro-Ed.

Burns, B. J., Hoagwood, K., & Mrazek, P. J. (1999). Effective treatment for mental disorders in children and adolescents. *Clinical Child and Family Psychology Review, 2*(4), 199–254.

Canino, I. A., & Spurlock, J. (2000). *Culturally diverse children and adolescents: Assessment, diagnosis, and treatment, second edition.* New York: Guilford.

Center for Health Care Policy and Evaluation. (2002, March). How prevalent is the use of psychotropic medications by children and adolescents? *Research Findings, 8*(1). Retrieved April 19, 2003, from http://www.centerhcpe.com/researchfindings/rfmar2002.pdf

Chabra, A., Chavez, G. F., Harris, E. S., & Shah, R. (1999). Hospitalization for mental illness in adolescents: Risk groups and impact on the health care system. *Journal of Adolescent Health, 24,* 349–36.

Clarkin, J. F., Hurst, S. W., & Crilly, J. L. (1987). Therapeutic alliance and hospital treatment outcome. *Hospital Community Psychiatry, 38,* 871–875.

Cohen, P., & Hesselbart, C. (1993). Demographic factors in the use of children's mental health services. *American Journal of Public Health, 83,* 49–52.

Cohen-Sandler, R., Berman, A. L., & King, R. A. (1982). A follow-up study of hospitalized suicidal children. *Journal of American Academy of Child Psychiatry, 21,* 398–402.

Cotton, N. S. (1993). *Lessons from the lion's den.* San Francisco: Jossey-Bass.

Cunningham, P. J., & Freiman, M. P. (1996). Determinants of ambulatory mental health service use for school-age children and adolescents. *Mental Health Services Research, 31,* 409–427.

Curry, J. F. (1991). Outcome research on residential treatment: Implications and suggested directions. *American Journal of Orthopsychiatry, 61,* 348–357.

Dalton, A., Mueller, B., & Forman, M. A. (1989). The psychiatric hospitalization of children: An overview. *Child Psychiatry & Human Development, 19,* 231–244.

Firestone, B. (1990). *Information packet on use of mental health services by children and adolescents.* Rockville, MD: Center for Mental Health Services Survey and Analysis Branch.

Friedman, R. M., & Street, S. (1985). Admission and discharge criteria for children's mental health services: A review of the issue. *Journal of Clinical Child Psychology, 14,* 229–235.

Friedman, R. M. (1994). Restructuring of systems to emphasize prevention and family support. *Journal of Clinical Child Psychology, 23*(Suppl.), 40–47.

Gabel, S., & Schindledecker, R. (1990). Parental substance abuse and suspected child abuse/maltreatment predict outcome in children's inpatient treatment. *Journal of the American Academy of Child and Adolescent Psychiatry, 29,* 919–224.

Henggeler, S. W., Schoenwald, S. K., Borduin, C. M., Rowland, M. D., & Cunningham, P. B. (1998). *Multisystemic treatment of antisocial behavior in children and adolescents.* New York: Guilford.

Gossett, J. F., Barnhart, S. W., Lewis, J. M., & Phillips, V. A. (1977). Follow-up of adolescents treated in a psychiatric hospital. *Archives of General Psychiatry, 34,* 1037–1042.

Green, J., & Burke, M. (1998). The ward as a therapeutic agent. In J. Green & B. Jacobs (Eds.), *Inpatient child psychiatry: Modern practice, research and the future* (pp. 93–109). London: Routledge.

Gunderson, J. G. (1978). Defining the therapeutic processes in psychiatric milieus. *Psychiatry, 41,* 327–335.

Harper, G., & Geraty, R. (1987). Hospital and residential treatment. In R. Michels & J. Cavenar, Jr. (Eds.), *Psychiatry* (Vol. 2, Chapter 64). New York: Basic.

Hendren, R. L., & Berlin, I. N. (Eds.) (1991). *Psychiatric inpatient care of children and adolescents: A multicultural approach.* New York: Wiley.

Hersov, L. (1994). Inpatient and day hospital units. In J. M. Rutter, E. Taylor, & L. Hersov (Eds.), *Child and adolescent psychiatry: Modern approaches* (pp. 993–995). Oxford: Blackwell Science.

Jemerin, J. M., & Philips, I. (1988). Changes in inpatient child psychiatry: Consequences and recommendations. *Journal of the American Academy of Child and Adolescent Psychiatry, 27,* 397–403.

Joint Commission on Accreditation of Hospitals. (1988). *Accreditation manual for psychiatric facilities serving children and adolescents.* Chicago: Author.

Joshi, P. K., & Rosenberg, L. A. (1997). Children's behavioral response to residential treatment. *Journal of Clinical Psychology, 53,* 567–573.

Kazdin, A. E., Esveldt-Dawson, K., French, N. H., & Unis, A. S. (1987). Problem-solving skills training and relationship therapy in the treatment of antisocial child behavior. *Journal of Consulting and Clinical Psychology, 55,* 76–85.

Knitzer, J. (1982). *Unclaimed children: The failure of public responsibility to children and adolescents in need of mental health services.* Washington, DC: Children's Defense Fund.

Koret, S. (1980). Follow-up study on residential treatment of children, ages six through twelve. *Journal of the National Association of Private Psychiatric Hospitals, 11,* 43–47.

Leichtman, M., Leichtman, M. L., Cornsweet Barber, C., & Neese, D. T. (2001). Effectiveness of intensive short-term residential treatment with severely disturbed adolescents. *American Journal of Psychiatry, 71*(2), 227–235.

Lewis, W. W. (1988). The role of ecological variables in residential treatment. *Behavioral Disorders, 13,* 98–107.

Lyons, J. S., Terry, P., Martinovich, Z., Peterson, J., & Bouska, B. (2001). Outcome trajectories for adolescents in residential treatment: A statewide evaluation. *Journal of Child and Family Studies, 10*(3), 333–345.

Manderscheid, R., & Sonnenschein, M. A. (1996). *Mental health, United States. Meta-analysis study.* U.S. Department of Health and Human Services, Substance Abuse and Mental Health Services Administration, Center for Mental Health Services.

Martin, A., & Leslie, S. (2003). Psychiatric inpatient, outpatient, and medication utilization and costs among privately insured youth, 1997–2000. *American Journal of Psychiatry, 160*(4), 757–764.

Maskey, S. (1998). The process of admission. In J. Green & B. Jacob (Eds.), Inpatient child psychiatry. *Modern practice, research and the future* (pp. 39–50). London: Routledge.

Mattejat, F., Hirt, B. R., Wilken, J., Schmidt, M. H., & Remschmidt, H. (2001). Efficacy of inpatient and home treatment in psychiatrically disturbed children and adolescents: Follow-up assessment of the results of a controlled treatment study. *European Child and Adolescent Psychiatry, 10*(1), 71–79.

Mayes, S. D., Krecko, V. F., Calhoun, S. L., Vesell, H. P., Schuch, S., & Toole, W. R. (2001). Variables related to outcome following child psychiatric hospitalization. *General Hospital Psychiatry, 23,* 278–284.

Noshpitz, J. D. (1982). Toward a history of the role of milieu in the residential treatment of children. *Family and Child Mental Health Journal, 8,* 5–25.

Olfson, M, Marcus, S. C., Weissman, M. M., & Jensen, P. S. (2002). National trends in the use of psychotropic medications by children. *Journal of the American Academy of Child and Adolescent Psychiatry, 41,* 514–521.

Patrick, C., Padgett, D. K., Burns, B. J., Schlesinger, H. J., & Cohen, J. (1993). Use of inpatient services by a national population: Do benefits make a difference? *Journal of the American Academy of Child and Adolescent Psychiatry, 32,* 144–152.

Pfeiffer, S. I., & Strzelecki, S. C. (1990). Inpatient psychiatric treatment of children and adolescents: A review of outcome studies. *Journal of the American Academy of Child and Adolescent Psychiatry, 29,* 847–853.

Ponton, L. E. (1991). Short-term psychiatric hospitalization of children. In R. L. Hendren & I. N. Berlin (Eds.), *Psychiatric inpatient care of children and adolescents: A multicultural approach* (pp. 176–193). New York: Wiley.

Pottick, K., Hansell, S. Gutterman, E. & White, H. R. (1995). Factors associated with inpatient and outpatient treatment for children and adolescents with serious mental illness. *Journal of the American Academy of Child and Adolescent Psychiatry, 34*(4), 425–433.

President's New Freedom Commission on Mental Health. (2003, January 10). *A report of the public comments submitted to the President's New Freedom Commission on Mental Health.* Retrieved February 10, 2003, from http://www.mentalhealthcommission.gov/reports/reports.htm

Redl, F. (1959). The concept of a therapeutic milieu. *American Journal of Orthopsychiatry, 29,* 721–736.

Redl, F. (1966). *When we deal with children: Selected writings.* New York: Free Press.

Robertson, B. A., & Friedberg, S. (1979). Follow-up study of children admitted to a psychiatric day center. *South African Medical Journal, 56,* 1129–1131.

Rubenstein, J. S., Armentrout, J. A., Levin, S., & Herald, D. (1978). The parent therapist program: Alternative care for emotionally disturbed children. *American Journal of Orthopsychiatry, 48,* 654–662.

Singh, N. N., Landrum, T. J., Donatelli, L. S., Hampton, C., & Ellis, C. R. (1994). Characteristics of children and adolescents with serious emotional disturbance in systems of care. Part I: Partial hospitalization and inpatient psychiatric services. *Journal of Emotional and Behavioral Disorders, 2,* 13–20.

Sourander, A., Helenius, H., Leijala, H., Heikkilä, T., Bergroth, L., & Phia, J. (1996). Predictors of outcome of short-term child psychiatric inpatient treatment. *European Child and Adolescent Psychiatry, 5,* 75–82.

Sourander, A., & Phia, J. (1998). Three year follow-up of child psychiatric inpatient treatment. *European Child and Adolescent Psychiatry, 7,* 153–162.

Stewart, M. A., Adams, C. C., & Meardon, J. K. (1978). Unsocialized aggressive boys. *Journal of Clinical Psychiatry, 39,* 797–799.

Stroul, B. A., & Friedman, R. M. (1986). *A system of care for severely emotionally disturbed children and youth.* Washington, DC: CASSP Technical Assistance Center, Georgetown University Child Developmental Center.

Towbin, K. E., & Campbell, P. A. (1995). Ethical conflicts and their management, inpatient child and adolescent psychiatry. *Child and Adolescent Psychiatric Clinics of North America, 4,* 747–767.

U.S. Department of Health and Human Services. (1999). *Mental health: A report of the Surgeon General. Chapter 3: Children and mental health.* Rockville, MD: U.S. Department of Health and Human Services, Substance Abuse and Mental Health Services Administration, Center for Mental Health Services, National Institutes of Health, National Institute of Mental Health.

U.S. Department of Health and Human Services. (2001). *Mental health: Culture, race, and ethnicity—A supplement to mental health: A report of the Surgeon General.* Rockville, MD: U.S. Department of Health and Human Services, Public Health Service, Office of the Surgeon General.

U.S. Public Health Service. (2000). *Report of the Surgeon General's conference on children's mental health: A national action agenda.* Washington, DC: Department of Health and Human Services.

Vargas, L. A., & Berlin, I. N. (1991). Culturally responsive inpatient care of children and adolescents. In R. L. Hendren & I. N. Berlin (Eds.), *Psychiatric inpatient care of children and adolescents: A multicultural approach* (pp. 14–33). New York: Wiley.

Warner, L. A., & Pottick, K. J. (2003, Summer). Nearly 66,000 youth live in U.S. mental health programs. *Latest Findings in Children's Mental Health, Policy Report submitted to the Annie E. Casey Foundation* (Vol. 2, No. 1). New Brunswick, NJ: Institute for Health, Health Care Policy, and Aging Research, Rutgers University.

Weinstein, L. (1974). *Evaluation of a program for re-educating disturbed children: A follow-up comparison with untreated children.* Washington, DC: Department of Health, Education, and Welfare, Bureau for the Education of the Handicapped.

Weithorn, L. A. (1988). Mental hospitalization of troublesome youth: An analysis of skyrocketing admission rates. *Stanford Law Review, 40,* 773–838.

Weller, E. B., Cook, S. C., Hendren, R. L., & Woolson, J. L. (1995). *On the use of mental health services by minors: Report to the American Psychiatric Association Task Force to study the use of psychiatric hospitalization of minors: A review of statistical data on the use of mental health services by minors.* Washington, DC: American Psychiatric Association.

Wells, K. (1991). Placement of emotionally disturbed children in residential treatment: A review of placement criteria. *American Journal of Orthopsychiatry, 61,* 339–347.

White, T. A., Benn, R., Gross, D., & Shaffer-Lopez, C. (1979). Assessing the need for follow-up. *Child Psychiatry Human Development, 10,* 91–102.

Zahner, G. E. P., & Daskalakis, C. (1997). Factors associated with mental health, general health, and school-based service use for child psychopathology. *American Journal of Public Health, 87*(9), 1440–1448.

Zito, J. M., Safer, D. J., dosReis, S., Gardner, J. F., Magder, L., Soeken, K. et al. (2003). Psychotropic practice patterns for youth: A 10-year perspective. *Archives of Pediatric and Adolescent Medicine, 157,* 17–25.

Zwillich, T. (2000, September 20). U.S. healthcare system missing most mentally ill children and adolescents. *Reuters Medical News.* Retrieved April 15, 2003, from http://psychiatry.medscape.com/reuters/prof/2000/09/09.20/200009publ009.html

10

Child Abuse Prevention and Intervention Services

MICHELLE R. KEES and BARBARA L. BONNER

The abuse and neglect of children and adolescents continues to be a major social, legal, health, and mental health problem in the United States. The most recent figures for 2002 show that more than 3 million children were reported for suspected child maltreatment. An estimated 896,000 children were determined to be victims of abuse or neglect by Child Protective Services (CPS), establishing an abuse rate of 12.3 per 1,000 children (U.S. Department of Health and Human Services, 2004). These cases include children who were neglected, physically abused, sexually abused, and psychologically maltreated. Research studies over the past 30 years have clearly documented the short- and long-term effects of abuse and neglect, and the degree to which maltreated children are at risk for psychological, psychiatric, and delinquency problems that call for effective mental health interventions (e.g., Egeland, Yates, Appleyard, & van Dulmen, 2002; Felitti et al., 1998; Kolko & Swenson, 2002).

For children in foster care, 50–80% experience developmental and mental health problems, a rate significantly higher than matched socioeconomic comparisons (Landsverk & Garland, 1999; Pilowsky, 1995). Children and adolescents in the child welfare system are increasingly being referred for mental health services as part of a family's treatment plan; however, recent figures indicate that less than half of all children whose families were being investigated for physical or sexual abuse actually receive mental health services (Kolko, Selelyo, & Brown, 1999). Children who have been sexually or physically abused are more likely to receive services than children who have experienced neglect or other types of maltreatment (Garland, Landsverk, Hough, & Ellis-Macleod, 1996). Racial and ethnic

MICHELLE R. KEES and BARBARA L. BONNER • Center on Child Abuse and Neglect, Department of Pediatrics, University of Oklahoma Health Sciences Center, Oklahoma City, Oklahoma 73104.

differences have also been suggested as a factor influencing whether children receive mental health services. In a sample of foster care children,
Garland et al. (2000) found that White American children were more likely
to receive mental health services than were African American or Latino
children, even when controlling for age, gender, type of maltreatment, and
need for services.

In the past, child maltreatment services centered on interventions for
families in which abuse had occurred, typically including case management by the CPS workers and referrals for outpatient health and mental
health services. As the number of child abuse and neglect cases continued
to increase and studies reported that federally funded abuse treatment
programs had limited effectiveness (e.g., Cohn & Daro, 1987), a strong
movement emerged to focus on preventing maltreatment before it occurred.
Interestingly, this movement developed from the private sector through
nongovernmental organizations rather than the public sector, which is
atypical for major social and health problems. Early leadership in the primary prevention of child maltreatment came from the National Committee
to Prevent Child Abuse and Neglect, now known as Prevent Child Abuse
America (PCA). A recent national initiative, "The National Call to Action to
End Child Abuse," is designed as a major, collaborative, long-term effort to
end child abuse in the next generation (Chadwick, 2002; Hensler, 2000).

Currently, service provision in the field of child maltreatment is designed to reduce the harm caused by child maltreatment, strengthen the
family's ability to care for their children, and prevent future incidences of
abuse and neglect. However, it is not always clear how to accomplish these
objectives. Specifically, a number of questions require answers, such as at
what point should services be offered, what type of services should be provided and in what setting, who should receive services, how should these
services be organized and delivered, and which services are effective across
the various types of abuse.

The services to prevent child abuse and to intervene with children and
families affected by child abuse hold unique characteristics in comparison to other mental health services. Services in this area are delivered
to both parents and children, but with different treatment goals. Parenting services are designed to alter potentially abusive parenting behaviors,
whereas services for children are focused on treating abuse-specific symptoms. Child maltreatment interventions also exist on a continuum, starting
at the level of primary prevention or public education, to prevention services for at-risk populations, investigation of child abuse, and intervention
services for children and parents. Across the continuum, these services
are organized in different structures and delivered in a variety of settings,
including the family's home, schools, and traditional mental health settings such as outpatient agencies, group homes, residential, and inpatient
settings.

This chapter will address service delivery for parents and children in
the field of child maltreatment across the continuum of need, from prevention to intervention. The chapter will utilize a public health model (i.e.,
primary prevention, secondary intervention, and tertiary intervention) to

review and describe the types of services and the various settings in which abused children and their families receive services.

PRIMARY PREVENTION: PUBLIC HEALTH MODEL

The primary prevention of child maltreatment is a relatively new area of focus and generally follows a public health model. This model of prevention is designed to raise public awareness about a problem and provide information to the general public, in this case about healthy parenting and preventing abuse before it occurs. The primary prevention of child maltreatment is conducted at the local, state, and national levels, and often includes prevention messages via the media, as well as community resources to contact for help. The information is typically provided through television public service announcements, brochures in doctors' offices, announcements on radio talk shows, advertisements in newspapers and magazine articles, billboards, and more recently, through the Internet. Although this approach has been viewed as less important than other more targeted approaches to at-risk populations, research studies have found that public awareness and education programs may be critical components in implementing major changes in behavior such as attitudes and values regarding parenting (Daro & Donnelly, 2002).

Adult-Focused Prevention

Most primary prevention programs in child maltreatment have been aimed at adults and have focused on the prevention of physical abuse. These include programs such as "Don't Shake Your Baby," which is designed to prevent shaken baby syndrome (Showers, 1992). Few primary prevention programs have been developed or described in the literature to prevent neglect, although the majority of substantiated cases of maltreatment each year are of neglect. Even with the major focus on child sexual abuse over the past 15 years, only one public health campaign targeting potential adult sexual abusers has been described in the literature. This program included a broad-based media campaign targeting adults, a one-to-one communications strategy that provides information to agencies working with at-risk families, a toll-free helpline for adults in sexually abusive situations, and strategies to educate decision makers and leaders (see Chasan-Taber & Tabachnick, 1999).

Child-Focused Prevention

Primary prevention programs have also targeted children. Programs have been implemented in schools, day care settings, and churches and have focused primarily on the prevention of sexual abuse, although some programs focus on overall safety skills. The primary prevention of sexual abuse is unique in that it has focused almost exclusively on potential victims (i.e., children), rather than potential abusers (i.e., primarily adolescent and adult males). This approach is the opposite of prevention efforts in physical abuse that focus solely on potential abusers. There are no child-focused prevention programs for physical abuse, neglect, or psychological maltreatment currently described in the literature.

Sexual abuse prevention programs for children are typically group-based instructional programs that teach children what sexual abuse is, how to protect themselves, and what to do if abuse occurs. A meta-analysis of research studies evaluating these types of programs found significant follow-up effect sizes, indicating that sexual victimization prevention programs are successful in teaching children concepts related to sexual abuse and self-protection skills (Rispens, Aleman, & Goudena, 1997). The advisability of this approach (i.e., that children are capable of preventing their own abuse) has been questioned and whereas studies have documented that children's knowledge is increased (Berrick & Barth, 1992; Finkelhor, Asdigian, & Dziuba-Leatherman, 1995a, 1995b), no studies have documented the effectiveness of the programs in reducing the sexual victimization of children. The disturbing findings from a national survey of children who participated in school-based, comprehensive sexual victimization prevention programs were that these children were not less likely to experience sexual abuse, but were slightly more likely to be injured if victimized (Finkelhor et al., 1995a, 1995b). One positive finding, however, has been that sexual abuse prevention programs provide an opportunity for children to disclose sexual abuse and thus prevent continued abuse. Two studies found that both an intensive media-based program and a school-based intervention resulted in significantly more disclosures of sexual abuse (Hoefnagels & Baartman, 1997; Oldfield, Hays, & Megel, 1996).

SECONDARY PREVENTION: SERVICES WITH AT-RISK POPULATIONS

Major efforts and a range of programs have been implemented with parents thought to be at risk for child maltreatment over the past 30 years, with varying levels of success in preventing abuse and neglect. The programs have targeted various populations, including teenage parents, parents with substance abuse problems, single parents living in poverty, first-time parents, and parents with limited cognitive abilities. The programs are often described as early intervention rather than child abuse prevention to convey a more positive focus. These programs have been implemented in schools for teenage parents, in hospitals for new parents thought to be at risk, in outpatient mental health and family support agencies, and in the family's home.

Family Support Programs

In the past decade, there has been a growing trend to provide early, comprehensive, and individualized services to families with young children and millions of dollars of public and private funds have been utilized for community-based family support programs, home visitation programs, respite care, and crisis child care services. Family support programs are designed to empower people by increasing the individual's and family's capabilities. The programs are voluntary and are based on a family-centered philosophy, which states that services to children and families should (1) be offered to the entire family and not to children and parents separately, (2) build on the strengths of the family, (3) allow families to make decisions about the kind and extent of services they receive, (4) include a wide array of comprehensive and individualized services for families, and (5) be offered preventatively (Kagan, 1994). This model of service delivery has become increasingly popular with human service providers, including home visitors, social workers, and professionals providing early intervention services.

In spite of the rapid expansion of the model nationally, there is minimal evidence as to the effectiveness of the programs (St. Pierre, Layzer, & Barnes, 1995). To date, few empirical studies have been conducted to determine the proper implementation of the model, which families are likely to utilize the services, and what techniques could be used to successfully engage and retain the families in the programs. Previous research has indicated that this type of voluntary, prevention-oriented program has high rates of attrition and low levels of participation (Daro & Donnelly, 2002).

The small number of studies that have examined the service delivery process has found that the tenets of the family-centered approach are not being consistently implemented with families, that service providers are focusing almost exclusively on the child, and that much less time is being spent dealing with family issues or modeling appropriate behavior for the parent (Downey, Hebbler, & Lopez, 1996). A more recent study echoed these earlier findings in that there was little evidence that services were being delivered to address the individual needs of the families. On a positive note, however, families seen as being at high risk for negative child outcomes remained in the programs longer and received more types and more intensive services than families seen as being at low risk (Green, Johnson, & Rodgers, 1999).

Home Visitation Programs

Early intervention programs have been found to have significant effects on parental behavior and child well-being and home visitation has been advocated as being a service delivery model with the potential to effect a wide range of family issues, including child abuse (Margie & Phillips, 1999). Several home visitation models have been developed, implemented, and studied to varying degrees for their effectiveness. Two of the programs that are particularly relevant for abused and neglected children are Healthy Families America and the Olds Nurse Home Visitation Model. Several rigorously controlled studies of the nurse home visitation model suggest that home visits started during pregnancy have positive effects on maternal behavior, abuse potential, and the long-term development of the child (Kitzman et al., 1997; Olds et al., 1997, 1998, 1999).

The Healthy Families America (HFA) model uses a variety of nonprofessionals to provide services in the homes and has been adopted and implemented by several states to provide services statewide. In 1997, approximately 18,000 families were participating in HFA intensive home visitation services provided by more than 270 HFA programs in 38 states and the District of Columbia (Daro & Harding, 1999). Preliminary results of HFA program evaluations suggest that HFA programs may be most successful at improving parent–child relationships, but have limited success in the prevention of child maltreatment, improving the mother's life course outcomes, and in health care status and utilization (Daro & Harding, 1999).

Despite the widespread adoption and implementation of home visitation programs to prevent child maltreatment, the results of recent studies have not found positive results (Chaffin, Bonner, & Hill, 2001). To date, none of the major home visitation models being implemented nationwide have documented consistent positive effects in important areas such as increased social support for families, improved child development, or reduced child abuse and neglect, leading to the conclusion that home visitation may not be the most effective intervention for a broad set of goals and that additional research is needed to determine which specific factors the model can effect (Daro & Donnelly, 2002).

School-Based Programs

Other intervention programs for families viewed to be at risk for abuse have been conducted through comprehensive school-based services. In these programs, a variety of issues are addressed, including parenting skills, family socialization, and educational development, with child abuse prevention being one of the many associated positive outcomes. For example, Chicago's Child–Parent Centers (CPC), provide preschool education for low-income children, continued education programs after preschool, and a range of school-based family support and education services. In a large-scale ($N = 1408$ children) evaluation of CPC, participants in the preschool program showed significantly lower rates of court petitions for child maltreatment in comparison to children in alternative kindergarten interventions (5% vs. 10.5%; Reynolds & Robertson, 2003). Families participating in the extended education program up to third grade also showed significantly lower rates of child maltreatment reports versus the comparison group (3.6% vs. 6.9%; Reynolds & Robertson, 2003). These findings suggest that ecologically based early intervention programs offering a range of service components may prove to be a promising approach to child abuse prevention.

TERTIARY INTERVENTION: INVESTIGATION AND TREATMENT

Investigation

Child Protective Services (CPS)

For cases of suspected child maltreatment, services are initially provided by state, county, or city Child Protective Service agencies. The overarching mission of CPS is to protect children from harm. The activities of CPS center on investigation and protection, which may include intensive home services to prevent the removal of children from their homes, placement in foster care, or later adoption. Service delivery occurs in the home and community for investigation, in-home or agency-based services for family preservation, and in foster care homes.

CPS agencies across the nation have been fraught with complaints about limited resources, too few workers, and excessively high caseloads. CPS workers are in the position of having to make important decisions about the safety of children, yet their training and expertise varies widely and they are often criticized for making inconsistent or inappropriate decisions. Research in this area has shown that decision making about the safety of children does vary across workers, even among those considered to be child welfare experts (Rossi, Schuerman, & Budde, 1996). Based on similar case information, one child welfare worker may decide that removal is in the best interest of the child, whereas another worker could advocate for in-home services to prevent removal. Efforts to cope with limited resources, high caseload demand, and increased liability for errors have resulted in some states seeking new strategies for investigation and implementation of services.

One model supported by the Office of Child Abuse and Neglect and the Children's Research Center, a division of the National Council on Crime and Delinquency, is that of Structured Decision Making (SDM; Children's Research Center [CRC], 1999). SDM is a new approach to service organization and delivery that impacts decision making at all points of service within CPS, including removal, placement, family reunification, termination of parental rights, and adoption. The goals of SDM are to increase the structure of decision making, improve the consistency and validity of decisions, target the available resources to children at most risk of harm, and improve service delivery within CPS (CRC, 1999).

The SDM approach consists of several components, the most important of which is a highly structured and detailed assessment protocol that then determines case priorities and all subsequent services and recommendations. SDM has been implemented in several states, including Michigan, where randomized trials of SDM versus services as usual has shown that SDM is associated with positive changes in decision making, greater participation in services by families, improved service provision, and lower rates of new abuse substantiations (Baird, Wagner, Caskey, & Neuenfeldt, 1995; Baird, Wagner, Healy, & Johnson, 1999).

After CPS has investigated a child abuse allegation via the SDM model or other approaches, services may be recommended as a preventive intervention, or when abuse is clearly substantiated, a treatment plan will be court-mandated for families. In most states, mental health services are not provided by CPS to the child or to the parent; rather services are provided through linkages to mental health agencies. For example, CPS may recommend parenting classes to a parent or individual therapy for a child as a condition of reunification. CPS often contracts with community agencies or recommends outpatient agencies, paid through Medicaid, self-pay, or other insurance, that would deliver these services and provide reports back to CPS and the court on the child's and family's progress. At this point, services offered by CPS primarily take the form of monitoring the parent for treatment completion and the child for safety and progress in treatment. If the child is returned to the parent, CPS typically continues to monitor the family for a period of time. Other services offered by CPS may include treatment or service referrals for other issues (i.e., substance abuse, housing, employment), placement in foster care, or adoptive placement for children permanently removed from their families.

Child Advocacy Centers

Another avenue of investigation for child abuse allegations is that of Child Advocacy Centers (CACs). The establishment of CACs was a major development in the field of child maltreatment occurring in the mid 1980s. The centers were developed primarily in response to cases of child sexual abuse to streamline and more comprehensively address the investigation and prosecution of these cases. CACs are staffed by multidisciplinary teams of professionals with personnel from CPS, law enforcement, medicine, mental health, and the legal system. Multidisciplinary teams are increasingly more common in cases of child abuse and neglect for both investigation and intervention. The benefits of a multidisciplinary team approach include that multiple sources of knowledge, skill, and expertise are available to collaborate on cases of child abuse and can provide more accurate and complete information.

CACs are located in the community or are hospital-based in child-friendly settings where the child can be interviewed, medically examined, and triaged or treated for mental health problems, thereby reducing the number of places and times a child is interviewed. CACs are generally funded by private donations, and state and federal grants. There are currently over 200 centers operating nationally, and the National Children's Alliance (www.nca-online.org) has been organized to set criteria for team structure and provide ongoing training and technical support. A study conducted in California (California Attorney General's Office, 1994) has documented the effectiveness of the centers in reducing the number of child interviews.

Intervention Services with Parents

Child maltreatment interventions vary in their intended population and may be designed either for parents in an attempt to prevent future abuse, or for children to address abuse-specific symptoms. The services are provided in various settings, including the family home, community-based mental health centers, and specialized centers that provide services to families referred for maltreatment. For parents with serious mental health or substance abuse problems, short-term inpatient treatment may be necessary before outpatient interventions can be effective.

Outpatient Services

For physically abusive parents, interventions primarily occur in an outpatient setting and have historically been provided through a psycho-educational group or parenting class format in community agencies. Curriculum and content in parenting groups and classes often vary, and there is minimal empirical research to support any specific program content in preventing future child physical abuse.

Innovative treatment approaches in the area of physical abuse have been emerging in the past 5–10 years. These programs are conducted in an outpatient setting and include both the parent and child in treatment. Kolko (1996) published one of the few empirical studies in recent years on treatment of physically abusive parents and their children. The families were randomly assigned to either cognitive-behavioral treatment (CBT) or Family Therapy (FT) and were assessed weekly over 12 sessions. Although the results indicated continuing high levels of physical discipline, parental anger, and family problems, the CBT children and parents reported lower levels of physical discipline and parental anger than FT parents. Kolko suggested that the results might be improved through increasing the length of treatment and the comprehensiveness of the treatment interventions.

Another promising intervention designed to modify abusive parental behavior, Parent–Child Interaction Therapy (PCIT), is based on the work of Eyberg (Eyberg, 1979; Eyberg & Boggs, 1989). PCIT is a dyadic parent–child training program that teaches parents specific behavioral skills through direct coaching from therapists via a "bug-in-the-ear" wireless device. (For a full description of the program, see Hembree-Kigin & McNeil, 1995.) PCIT was initially developed to address child behavior problems but has recently been applied to prevent physical abuse recurrence. Unlike group therapy or parenting classes, new parenting skills are practiced *in vivo*, are behaviorally specific, and are learned to set criteria. In a randomized clinical trial, Chaffin et al. (2004) compared a community parenting group to a combined PCIT and motivation intervention for parents where physical abuse was an issue. Families in the combined PCIT and motivation condition had significantly lower physical abuse recurrence at 3-year follow-up in comparison to the community parenting group (20% recurrence for PCIT vs. 60% for parenting groups). The effects of PCIT and the motivation intervention were inherently intertwined in the research design, and a current project by Chaffin and colleagues is focusing on dismantling these intervention components to assess the independent, long-term effects of PCIT versus a motivational intervention on physical abuse recurrence (M. Chaffin, Personal communication, July 8, 2004). This new project is being implemented through a local community agency as a dissemination trial, with a special interest in enhancing treatment retention and participation.

Home Visiting Programs

To address physical or emotional neglect of children, interventions have centered more on a home visiting model. Despite robust national statistics indicating that neglect is the most prevalent form of child mal-treatment with a high rate of recurrence, few studies have focused on evidenced-based models for specifically addressing neglect. Perhaps one of the best-documented treatment programs for abusive and neglectful families is Project 12-Ways (Lutzker & Newman, 1986). The program provides *in vivo* treatment (e.g., in homes) in an effort to improve generalization and reduce the stigma that may be attached to clinic-based programs. The services provided include training in parenting, stress reduction, assertiveness, self-control, leisure time activities, job placement, money management, health maintenance and nutrition, home safety, and behavior management across multiple settings. Other program components include basic skills training for children, marital counseling, social support groups, alcohol treatment and referral, and unwed mother services.

Based on recurrence data from 352 families receiving services from Project 12-Ways and 358 comparison families, Project 12-Ways appears to be successful in reducing future child abuse and neglect (Lutzker & Rice, 1987). However, abuse and neglect were not separated in this study, and it is unclear what percentage of the treatment families or families with repeated offenses were neglectful families. Currently, a randomized trial of a modified version of Project 12-Ways, SafeCare, is being implemented through statewide community dissemination and rigorously evaluated with high-risk neglectful families (D. Hecht, Personal communication, July 8, 2004). SafeCare is being evaluated through the combined efforts of local treatment providers, the Oklahoma Department of Human Services, the National Institutes of Health, and the Centers for Disease Control and Prevention.

Family Preservation Services (FPS)

Intensive, in-home family preservation services are sometimes offered to parents as an intervention to maintain children in the home and prevent future abuse. Most families referred to FPS are not new to the child welfare system and have one or more previously confirmed reports of abuse or neglect (Littell & Schuerman, 2002). FPS may include a variety of services, including outpatient therapy for the parent or child, parenting classes, in-home services, and referrals to other treatment providers. Unfortunately, controlled research studies on FPS have not been promising, with FPS showing minimal impact on the prevention of out-of-home placement or recurrence of child maltreatment (Schuerman, Rzepnicki, & Littell, 1994). Even when looking at specific subgroups of child welfare families receiving FPS (i.e., those with substance abuse, new to child welfare, teen parents, housing problems only), FPS versus regular child welfare services was not associated with a decrease in subsequent maltreatment or risk of out-of-home placement (Littell & Schuerman, 2002). In addition, the duration of services, intensity of services, and breadth of services had no discernible impact on outcomes. Advocates have suggested that greater matching between family presenting problems and the FPS offered may be more promising.

Interventions with Children

Interventions have typically focused on the physically abusive or neglectful parents and until recently, failed to assess and provide treatment for children. Preventing child abuse is only one aspect of intervention, and treating child victims of abuse must also be considered (Kaplan, Pelcovitz, & Labruna, 1999). Attention to the treatment needs of children has recently increased, with new efforts to develop and validate interventions that address abuse-specific symptoms in children. Interventions for child abuse victims should be tailored to the child's presenting symptomatology, recognizing that not all abused children will require mental health services (Chaffin, 2000).

Outpatient Services

Services for child victims of abuse are most often provided in outpatient settings, either in individual or group format, and with varying degrees of parental involvement in the treatment. Play therapy approaches have pervaded the literature and clinical practice; however, the effectiveness of this type of intervention has not been well supported (Kaplan et al., 1999). Research suggests that structured behavioral and cognitive-behavioral interventions may be more effective than less directive approaches in treating child victims of abuse (Cohen & Mannarino, 1998; O'Donohue & Elliot, 1992). Treatment interventions should focus on the child's specific symptoms and draw from the clinical research literature on evidenced-based treatments for those symptoms, such as exposure-based therapy for posttraumatic stress and anxiety symptoms, cognitive interventions for depression, and behavioral parent training for children with behavior problems (Chaffin, 2000).

Looking at specific types of abuse, intervention research has focused predominantly on children who have been sexually abused. In a randomized clinical trial with child sexual abuse victims comparing cognitive-behavioral group treatment versus nondirective supportive group therapy, Cohen and Mannarino (1998) found that cognitive-behavioral group treatment was the strongest predictor of preschoolers' positive behavioral and emotional outcome at posttreatment and at 12-month follow-up. In another randomized design, Celano, Hazzard, Webb, and McCall (1996) found a structured intervention was more effective in increasing caregiver support of the child and decreasing negative attributions by the caregiver (e.g., self-blame). Parents' reactions to the sexual abuse and support given to the child are strongly associated with children's behavioral and emotional treatment outcomes (Cohen & Mannarino, 1996, 1998). Thus, teaching parents how to respond to their children in a developmentally appropriate, nurturing manner about abuse issues is a valuable goal of treatment. In summary, clinical research findings suggest that services for child sexual abuse victims should be structured, can be conducted effectively on an outpatient basis, and should include nonoffending parents and their response and attributions regarding the abuse.

School-Based Services

Few interventions for child abuse victims have been developed and initiated within the school setting. Group or individual treatment of abuse-related trauma symptoms in a school setting poses a variety of problems including questions about confidentiality, problems of reintegrating into the classroom after a difficult session, and missing valuable class time. School-based programs have been developed to address children's externalizing and disruptive behaviors in general, which are more typical in abused and neglect children than nonabused children. Effective behavioral approaches to classroom difficulties have emphasized the modification of teacher attention, differential reinforcement of appropriate behaviors, use of tokens, teaching or self-management strategies, and consequences for inappropriate behaviors (see review by McGoey, Eckert, & DuPaul, 2002).

A variety of other issues related to child abuse can also arise in a school setting. Horton (1996) describes the appropriate steps for school psychologists to take when responding to a child's disclosure of abuse, including reporting the suspected abuse to child welfare personnel, consulting with the parents when appropriate, and making referrals for therapeutic services. School personnel also need to carefully consider how to respond to a child with aggressive sexual behaviors, including parent consultation, making classroom placement decisions, and establishing adequate supervision while the child is in a school setting (Horton, 1996).

Foster Care

Children removed from their homes and placed in the state's custody have access to services delivered in nontraditional settings. Removed children may be placed in traditional foster care, kinship care with relatives, a temporary shelter, a group home, a residential center, or an inpatient psychiatric facility. Children with health, developmental, or mental health needs may be placed in treatment or therapeutic foster care (TFC) homes, where the foster parent has received additional training in mental health, developmental, or health issues. TFC homes were initially recommended to meet the needs of children in foster care, reframing foster care as an active intervention instead of just a living situation (Ruff, Blank, & Barnett, 1990). TFCs are more therapeutic in nature and allow a child with significant emotional, behavioral, developmental, or medical problems to remain in a family setting instead of being placed in a residential or an inpatient facility. In addition to TFC placement, these children often participate in outpatient therapy or other therapeutic programs.

Children who cannot be placed in homes immediately or where homes are not available may be temporarily placed in shelters with other children who have been removed from their homes. Other children with significant behavioral or mental health problems, including adolescents who are more difficult to place, may be placed in residential centers or group homes. Residential centers and group homes include other children in similar circumstances, but have fewer children than shelters and are often structured in a semi-home environment. In many shelters and residential centers, the center staff and counselors provide some form of mental health treatment either on a group basis, such as a survivor's group (child victims of sexual abuse) or social skills training, or through individual therapy. Children with significant mental health problems (i.e., suicidality, psychosis) will likely be placed in short-term inpatient hospitalization until they are stabilized.

SUMMARY AND CONCLUSIONS

In summary, children and families can be involved in several levels of services related to child maltreatment, from primary prevention programs that focus on all children and adults, to early interventions that target populations at risk for maltreatment, and finally, investigative services and interventions for children and their families after abuse or neglect has occurred. The current research and program evaluations studying the effects of primary prevention and early intervention programs reveal few positive, long-term outcomes in actually reducing abuse and neglect. Considerable research is needed to determine which aspects of which programs are effective with which parents.

There is a major lack of research on mental health service utilization by maltreating families and their children. The limited research available indicates that only about 50% of these children receive mental health services. Despite the overwhelming data on the negative psychological effects of maltreatment, the current system is not effectively meeting the needs of these children. Moreover, the literature currently offers a limited understanding of what treatments are most effective with children who have experienced abuse. After abuse has occurred, there are studies that document the effectiveness of cognitive-behavioral interventions with sexually abused children. However, these studies have been conducted in academic settings and have not been disseminated widely in the field. More work is necessary to develop and validate treatments for children who have experienced physical abuse, psychological maltreatment, and neglect. Efforts to then disseminate these evidence-based treatments into practice will be a critical step in the field.

REFERENCES

Baird, C., Wagner, D., Caskey, R.,& Neuenfeldt, D. (1995). *The Michigan Department of Social Services Structured Decision Making System: An evaluation of its impact on child protection services.* Madison, WI: Children's Research Center.

Baird, C., Wagner, D., Healy, T., & Johnson, K. (1999). *Reliability and validity of risk assessment in child protective services: A comparison of three systems.* Madison, WI: Children's Research Center.

Berrick, J., & Barth, R. (1992). Child sexual abuse prevention training: What do they learn? *Child Abuse & Neglect, 12,* 543–553.

California Attorney General's Office. (1994). *Child victim witness investigative pilot projects: Research and evaluation final report.* Sacramento, CA: State of California.

Celano, M., Hazzard, A., Webb, C., & McCall, C. (1996). Treatment of traumagenic beliefs among sexually abused girls and their mothers: An evaluation study. *Journal of Abnormal Child Psychology, 24,* 1–17.

Chadwick, D. (2002). Community organization of services to deal with and end child abuse. In J. E. B. Meyers, L. Berliner, J. Briere, C. T. Hendrix, C. Jenny, & T. A. Reid (Eds.), *The APSAC handbook on child maltreatment* (2nd ed., pp. 509–523). Thousand Oaks: Sage.

Chaffin, M. (2000). What types of mental health treatment should be considered for maltreated children? In H. Dubowitz & D. DePanfilis (Eds.), *Handbook for child protection practice* (pp. 409–413). Thousand Oaks: Sage.

Chaffin, M., Bonner, B. L., & Hill, R. F. (2001). Family preservation and family support programs: Child maltreatment outcomes across client risk levels and program types. *Child Abuse & Neglect, 25,* 1269–1289.

Chaffin, M. Silovsky, J., Funderburk, B., Valle, L. A., Brestan, E. V., Balachova, T., Jackson, S., Lensgraf, J., & Bonner, B. L. (2004). Parent-child interaction therapy with physically abusive parents: Efficacy for reducing future abuse reports. *Journal of Consulting and Clinical Psychology, 72,* 491–499.

Chasan-Taber, L., & Tabachnick, J. (1999). Evaluation of a child sexual abuse prevention program. *Sexual Abuse: Journal of Research & Treatment, 11,* 279–292.

Children's Research Center. (1999).*The improvement of child protective services with Structured Decision Making: The CRC model.* San Francisco, CA: National Council on Crime and Delinquency.

Cohen, J., & Mannarino, A. (1996). Factors that mediate treatment outcome of sexually abused preschool children. *Journal of the American Academy of Child and Adolescent Psychiatry, 34,* 1402–1410.

Cohen, J., & Mannarino, A. (1998). Factors that mediate treatment outcome of sexually abused preschool children: Six and 12-month follow-up. *Journal of the American Academy of Child and Adolescent Psychiatry, 37,* 44–51.

Cohn, A., & Daro, D. (1987). Is treatment too late? What ten years of evaluative research tells us. *Child Abuse and Neglect, 11,* 433–442.

Daro, D., & Donnelly, A. C. (2002). Child abuse prevention: Accomplishments and challenges. In J. E. B. Meyers, L. Berliner, J. Briere, C. T. Hendrix, C. Jenny, & T. A. Reid (Eds.), *The APSAC handbook on child maltreatment* (2nd ed., pp. 431–448). Thousand Oaks: Sage.

Daro, D., & Harding, K. (1999). Healthy Families America: Using research in going to scale. *Future of Children, 9(1),* 152–176.

Downey, S., Hebbler, K., & Lopez, M. (1996, June). *Where is the family in a child-centered Parents as Teachers program? An analysis of one PAT site.* Paper presented at Head Start's Third National Research Conference, Washington, DC.

Egeland, B., Yates, T., Appleyard, K., & van Dulmen, M. (2002). The long-term consequences of maltreatment in the early years: A developmental pathway model to antisocial behavior. *Children's Services: Social Policy, Research, and Practice, 5,* 249–260.

Eyberg, S. M. (1979, April). *A parent–child interaction model for the treatment of psychological disorders in early childhood.* Paper presented at the annual meeting of the Western Psychological Association, San Diego, CA.

Eyberg, S. M., & Boggs, S. R. (1989). Parent training for oppositional-defiant preschoolers. In C. E. Schafer & J. M. Briesmeister (Eds.), *Handbook of parent training: Parents as co-therapists for children's behavior problems* (pp. 105–132). New York: Wiley.

Felitti, V. J., Anda, R. F., Nordenberg, D., Williamson, D. F., Spitz, A. M., Edwards, V., et al. (1998). Relationship of childhood abuse and household dysfunction to many of the leading causes of death in adults. *American Journal of Preventive Medicine, 14,* 245–258.

Finkelhor, D., Asdigian, N., & Dziuba-Leatherman, J. (1995a). Victimization prevention program for children: A follow-up. *American Journal of Public Health, 85,* 1684–1689.

Finkelhor, D., Asdigian, N., & Dziuba-Leatherman, J. (1995b). The effectiveness of victimization prevention instruction: An evaluation of children's responses to actual threats and assaults. *Child Abuse & Neglect, 19,* 141–153.

Garland, A. F., Hough, R. L., Landsverk, J. A., McCabe, K. M., Yeh, M., & Ganger, W. C. et al. (2000). Racial and ethnic variations in mental health care utilization among children in foster care. *Children's Services: Social Policy, Research, and Practice, 3,* 133–146.

Garland, A. F., Landsverk, J. L., Hough, R. L., & Ellis-Macleod, E. (1996). Type of maltreatment as a predictor of mental health service use for children in foster care. *Child Abuse & Neglect, 20,* 675–688.

Green, B. L., Johnson, S. A., & Rodgers, A. (1999). Understanding patterns of service delivery and participation in community-based family support programs. *Children's Services: Social Policy, Research, and Practice, 2,* 1–22.

Hembree-Kigin, T., & McNeil, C. (1995). *Parent–child interaction therapy.* New York: Plenum.

Hensler, D. J. (2000). *The national call to action to eliminate child abuse* [Online]. Retrieved July 19, 2003, from http://www.nationalcalltoaction.com

Hoefnagels, C., & Baartman, H. (1997). On the threshold of disclosure: The effects of a mass medical field experiment. *Child Abuse & Neglect, 21,* 557–573.

Horton, C. B. (1996). Children who molest other children: The school psychologist's response to the sexually aggressive child. *School Psychology Review, 25,* 540–557.

Kagan, S. L. (1994). Defining and achieving quality in family support. In S. L. Kagan & B. Weissbourd (Eds.), *Putting families first* (pp. 375–400). San Francisco: Jossey-Bass.

Kaplan, S. J., Pelcovitz, D., & Labruna, V. (1999). Child and adolescent abuse and neglect research: A review of the past 10 years. Part I: Physical and emotional abuse and neglect. *Journal of the American Academy of Child & Adolescent Psychiatry, 38,*1214–1222.

Kitzman, H., Olds, D., Henderson, C., Hanks, C., Cole, R., & Tatelbaum, R. et al. (1997). Effects of prenatal and infancy home visitations by nurses on pregnancy outcomes, childhood injuries and repeated childbearing. *Journal of American Medical Association, 278*(22), 644–652.

Kolko, D. J. (1996). Child physical abuse. In J. Briere, L. Berliner, J. A. Bulkley, C. Jenny, & T. Reid (Eds.), *The APSAC handbook on child maltreatment* (pp. 21–50). Thousand Oaks, CA: Sage.

Kolko, D. J., Selelyo, J., & Brown, E. J. (1999). The treatment history and service involvement of physically and sexually abusive families: Description, correspondence, and clinical correlates. *Child Abuse & Neglect, 23,* 459–476.

Kolko, D. J., & Swenson, C. C. (2002). *Assessing and treating physically abused children and their families: A cognitive-behavioral approach.* Thousand Oaks, CA: Sage.

Landsverk, J., & Garland, A. (1999). Foster care pathways to mental health services. In P. Curtis, G. Dale, Jr., & J. C. Kendall (Eds.), *The foster care crisis: Translating research into practice and policy* (pp. 193–210). Omaha: University of Nebraska Press.

Littell, J. H., & Schuerman, J. R. (2002). What works best for whom? A closer look at intensive family preservation services. *Child Abuse & Neglect, 24,* 673–699.

Lutzker, J. R., & Newman, M. R. (1986). Child abuse and neglect: Community problem, community solutions. [Special issue: Health promotion in children: A behavior analysis and public health perspective]. *Education and Treatment of Children, 9,* 344–354.

Lutzker, J. R., & Rice, J. M. (1987). Using recidivism data to evaluate Project 12-Ways: An ecobehavioral approach to the treatment and prevention of child abuse and neglect. *Journal of Family Violence, 2,* 283–290.

Margie, N. G., & Phillips, D. A. (1999). *Revisiting home visiting: Summary of a workshop.* Washington, DC: National Research Council and Institute of Medicine.

McGoey, K. E., Eckert, T. L., & DuPaul, G. J. (2002). Early intervention for preschool-age children with ADHD: A literature review. *Journal of Emotional & Behavioral Disorders, 10,* 14–28.

O'Donohue, W., & Elliott, A. (1992). Treatment of the sexually abused child: A review. *Journal of Clinical Child Psychology, 21,* 218–228.

Oldfield, D., Hays, B. J., & Megel, M. E. (1996). Evaluation of the effectiveness of project TRUST: An elementary school-based victimization prevention program. *Child Abuse & Neglect, 20,* 821–832.

Olds, D., Eckenrode, J., Henderson, C. R., Jr., Kitzman, H., Powers, J., Cole, R. et al. (1997). Long-term effects of home visitation on maternal life course, child abuse and neglect and children's arrests: Fifteen-year follow-up of a randomized trial. *Journal of the American Medical Association, 278,* 637–643.

Olds, D., Henderson, C., Cole, R., Eckenrode, J., Kitzman, H., Luckey, D. et al. (1998). Long-term effects of nurse home visitation on children's criminal and antisocial behavior. *Journal of the American Medical Association, 280,* 1238–1244.

Olds, D., Henderson, C., Kitzman, H., Eckenrode, J., Cole, R., & Tatelbaum, R. (1999). Prenatal and infancy home visitation by nurses: Recent findings. *Future of Children, 9(1),* 44–65.

Pilowsky, D. (1995). Psychopathology among children placed in family foster care. *Psychiatric Services, 46,* 906–911.

Reynolds, A. J., & Robertson, D. L. (2003). School-based early intervention and later child maltreatment in the Chicago Longitudinal Study. *Child Development, 74,* 3–26.

Rispens, J., Aleman, A., & Goudena, P. P. (1997). Prevention of child sexual abuse victimization: A meta-analysis of school programs. *Child Abuse & Neglect, 21,* 975–987.

Rossi, P., Schuerman, J., & Budde, S. (1996). *Understanding child maltreatment decisions and those who make them.* Chicago: Chapin Hall Center for Children, University of Chicago.

Ruff, H. A., Blank, S., & Barnett, H. L. (1990). Early intervention in the context of foster care. *Journal of Developmental and Behavioral Pediatrics, 11,* 265–268.

Schuerman, J. R., Rzepnicki, T. L., & Littell, J. H. (1994). *Putting families first: An experiment in family preservation.* Hawthorne, NY: Aldine de Gruyter.

Showers, J. (1992). "Don't shake the baby": The effectiveness of a prevention program. *Child Abuse and Neglect, 16,* 11–18.

St. Pierre, R., Layzer, J., & Barnes, H. (1995). Two generation programs: Design, cost and short-term effectiveness. *The Future of Children: Long-term outcomes of early childhood programs, 5(3),* 76–93.

U.S. Department of Health and Human Services, Administration on Children, Youth and Families. (2004). *Child Maltreatment 2002.* Washington, DC: U.S. Government Printing Office.

11

Services to Prevent Sexually Transmitted Diseases in Adolescents

BETH A. AUSLANDER, MARY B. SHORT, and SUSAN L. ROSENTHAL

Sexually transmitted diseases (STDs) are a significant health problem for adolescents. Each year approximately 3 million adolescents acquire an STD (Cates, 1999). Of adolescents who are sexually active, one in four will get an STD before the age of 18 (Cates, 1999). In general, adolescents have higher rates of STDs than adults. More specifically, adolescent girls have the highest rates of gonorrhea and chlamydia, and young adult women have the highest risk for human papilloma virus (HPV) in comparison to other age groups and males (Centers for Disease Control and Prevention [CDC], 2002).

For biological, social, and behavioral reasons, adolescents may be at risk for acquiring STDs. For example, a young girl is at biological risk for HPV and its carcinogenic effects, due to her developing cervix (Biro, 1992). Further, adolescents may not have the same level of immunity as older individuals (Aral & Holmes, 1990). In addition to the greater susceptibility, there may be high rates of STDs among their partner pool (Biro, 1992). Given the asymptomatic nature of many STDs (Wang, Burstein, & Cohen, 2002), adolescents may be unaware of their infection and ability to transmit to others. The sexual behaviors of some adolescents place them at further risk; for example, approximately 16% of sexually experienced adolescents have four or more partners by the time they are 18 years old (CDC, 1998) and only 58% of teenagers reported using a condom the last time they had intercourse (CDC, 1998).

BETH A. AUSLANDER, MARY B. SHORT, and SUSAN L. ROSENTHAL • University of Texas Medical Branch at Galveston, Galveston, Texas 77555.

The medical problems associated with acquiring an STD can be significant for adolescents and their offspring. Some STDs, such as herpes simplex virus (HSV) and human immunodeficiency virus (HIV), can be life-long infections, making one at continued risk for transmitting infection to others. Long-term negative health outcomes of other STDs such as involuntary infertility, cervical cancer, pelvic inflammatory disease, and ectopic pregnancy are of particular concern for females (Aral, 2001). Infections can be passed to neonates leading to devastating consequences including blindness, neurological complications, and even death (Institute of Medicine, 1997).

In addition to the medical consequences of these infections, adolescents may experience a variety of emotions in response to the acquisition of STDs. These reactions can include depression, anxiety, or concerns about potential medical and interpersonal consequences. Adolescents typically employ a number of coping strategies that vary in terms of effectiveness (e.g., problem solving, emotional regulation). Interestingly, it appears that adolescent coping responses do not vary based on age, STD history, or type of infection (i.e., bacterial vs. viral); rather, they vary based on the strengths the adolescent brings to the situation (Rosenthal & Biro, 1991; Rosenthal, Biro, Cohen, Succop, & Stanberry, 1995b). Perception of an STD may be related to coping. Adolescents who view STD acquisition as being more negative are more likely to use a greater number of coping strategies (Rosenthal et al., 1995b). Those adolescents who do not think about their STD, wish that their STD would just magically resolve, or attribute their STD acquisition to their interpersonal character rather than their behavior (Baker et al., 2001; Rosenthal & Biro, 1991) may have greater difficulty implementing health-promoting actions (e.g., seeking treatment and using STD protection in the future). This is consistent with the findings that adolescents who have a history of an STD are not more likely to seek care promptly (Fortenberry, 1997) and many go on to have a second STD episode (Burstein et al., 1998).

Another important aspect of coping is managing the interpersonal sequelae of telling current and future partners. Little is known about how adolescents manage to have these discussions, which are difficult even for adults who presumably are more experienced in discussing sexually intimate matters (Liu, Detels, Li, Ma, & Yin, 2002). Adolescents anticipate telling their parents and expect that their parents will be helpful. Consistent with developmental changes in other areas of psychological development, younger adolescents are more likely to think they would tell their parents, but adolescents of all ages believe that their parents would be helpful if told (Rosenthal, Biro, Cohen, Succop, & Stanberry, 1995a).

In addition to the medical and psychological consequences of STDs, there are societal consequences as well. The financial burden to society is estimated at $8 billion yearly for diagnosis and treatment of non-HIV STDs and their complications (American Social Health Association [ASHA], 1998).

It takes both behavioral strategies and biomedical approaches to reduce the number of new STD cases. Current research on individually based interventions (i.e., condoms, topical microbicides, and vaccines) will be presented first followed by a review of research on programmatic interventions (i.e., health care, community or schools, and parent).

INDIVIDUALLY BASED INTERVENTIONS

Condoms

For people who choose to be sexually active, the male condom is considered to be the most effective method of preventing STDs. If properly used, male condoms protect the couple against infection by providing a barrier. A recent review of condom effectiveness studies found that condoms decrease the risks associated with STDs. The evidence is strongest for condom effectiveness in the protection of HIV and other "discharge" diseases (i.e., gonorrhea, chlamydia, and trichomoniasis). Condoms may provide some protection against HPV-associated diseases, in particular cervical neoplasia in women and genital warts in men. The evidence was less conclusive for the other STDs (i.e., syphilis) due to insufficient data and sparsity of well-controlled published studies (National Institute of Allergy and Infectious Diseases, 2001). Studies, published since the review, have found that condoms offer significant protection against genital herpes (Wald et al., 2001).

Condoms are only effective in preventing STDs if used consistently and correctly. Adolescents do not use condoms consistently; one study noted that 63% of sexually experienced adolescents reported inconsistent condom use (Boyer et al., 2000). This inconsistent use of condoms by an individual can occur for several reasons including dislike for the feel of condoms during intercourse, lack of condom availability, lack of perceived susceptibility, and lack of knowledge about the protective effect of condoms against STDs (Donald, Lucke, Dunne, O'Toole, & Raphael, 1994; Jadack, Fresia, Rompalo, & Zenilman, 1997). Condom use also can be affected by relationship characteristics, such as level of partner trust, length of relationship, and sexual communication (Ellen, Cahn, Eyre, & Boyer, 1996; Jadack et al., 1997). For example, condoms are used more frequently with "one-night stands" or in shorter relationships than they are with steady partners (Ellen et al., 1996).

For girls, one obvious obstacle to male condom use is that it requires negotiation and communication skills. Many people do not develop these skills until early adulthood. In addition, carrying condoms may result in perceptions of girls as promiscuous or "easy" (Hiller, Harrison, & Warr, 1998). Concerns about the lack of female control have led to the development of the female condom. Acceptability studies of the female condom found that when enrolled in studies, females and their partners find the female condom acceptable to use. Many adult women state a preference and intentions to use female-controlled barrier methods because they feel more in control of disease protection (Cecil, Perry, Seal, & Pinkerton, 1998). Positive partner attitudes, familiarity with use, discussions with other women, belief that the female condom provided better prophylactic efficacy than the male condom, and perception that the device increases sexual pleasure are associated with acceptability (Choi, Gregorich, Anderson, Grinstead, & Gomez, 2003; Witte, El-Bassel, Wada, Gray, & Wallace, 1999).

Only a few studies have been conducted on adolescent's acceptability of the female condom. As seen with adults, the device was acceptable, not as difficult as first perceived, and more likely to be used with more familiarity (Marshall, Giblin, Simpson, & Backos, 2002). However, clinical experience shows that it is not a widely used method, and care providers rarely suggest its use to adolescents, perhaps because it is anticipated that adolescent females will find it cumbersome, expensive, nondiscrete, and is not easily commercially available in most areas.

Topical Microbicides

One future exciting new female-controlled option would be topical microbicides, which are chemical products that would be used intravaginally or intrarectally to prevent STD infection. Currently, there are several types of microbicide products that are in various stages of development; however, they may not be available to the public for many years (Rosenthal, Cohen, & Stanberry, 1998).

If these products are to have an impact on infection rates, they need to be safe, effective, and acceptable to potential users. Acceptability studies have shown that topical microbicides theoretically are acceptable to a significant number of female users, and most females believe that the product would be an important option for women. Predictors of acceptability included women's current use of condoms, perception of exposure to risk, relationship status, race, and product characteristics, such as attractiveness of the product, ease of insertion, degree of messiness, amount of vaginal wetness, and ability to insert the product several hours before coitus (Darroch & Frost, 1999; Hammett et al., 2000; Short, Mills, Majkowski, Stanberry, & Rosenthal, 2003). Unique issues for adolescents may include developmental barriers to any STD protective method including anticipating intercourse, perception of susceptibility to STDs, and perceptions of efficacy based on concrete characteristics of the product (Short et al., 2003).

Vaccines

A method that would help protect adolescents from STDs and would not require negotiation skills is vaccines. Vaccines are one of medicine's primary methods of eradicating disease (CDC, 1999). At the present time, there is only one vaccine for a sexually transmitted pathogen (hepatitis B). Vaccines for HPV, HSV, and HIV are in clinical trials (Cao et al., 2003; Koutsky et al., 2002; Stanberry et al., 2002) and vaccines for other STDs are in development.

Experiences with non-STD-related vaccines indicate that the existence of a vaccine does not always lead to acceptance. Due to the possible stigma associated with STDs, acceptance of STD vaccines may be even more difficult. However, research has indicated that STD vaccine acceptability is affected by the same factors that influence vaccines for non-STDs, such as access issues, vaccine efficacy, health beliefs, and fears associated with needles and adverse effects (Liau, Zimet, & Fortenberry, 1998; Zimet, Fortenberry, & Blythe, 1999).

Efforts have been made to increase immunizations. Perhaps the most effective effort has been the school entry laws and free vaccines under the Vaccine for Children program. Individual-level interventions focusing on adolescents have included peer incentives, such as class pizza parties, to increase the return of vaccine consent forms at school (Unti, Coyle, Woodruff, & Boyer-Chuanroong, 1997). Others have found that telephone plus mail reminders (Sellors et al., 1997) and postal reminders with health belief information (e.g., susceptibility to STDs, benefits of vaccine) as opposed to appointment card reminders (Hawe, McKenzie, & Scurry, 1998) increased vaccine compliance rates. Additional recommendations, which have not been formally tested, include providing individual incentives (Guajardo, Middleman, & Sansaricq, 2002), reducing costs by not charging for the office visit, recording immunization status, and offering immunizations to adolescents during health care visits (Kollar, Rosenthal, & Biro, 1994).

PROGRAMMATIC INTERVENTIONS

Medical Treatment

Health care providers can make a difference through routine screening, prompt treatment, fostering partner notification, and educational efforts. For a review of the medical management of STDs, the reader is referred to the Sexually Transmitted Diseases Guidelines 2002 (CDC, 2002). Routine screening can be a very effective way to identify adolescents with asymptomatic infections (Cohen, Nsuami, Martin, & Farley, 1999). It is recommended that sexually experienced adolescents be screened annually for chlamydia (CDC, 2002). Even when adolescents are symptomatic, they may delay care-seeking. Adolescents who perceive greater barriers to care, have lower self-efficacy in their response to an STD, view STDs more seriously, have a prior history of STDs, feel more stigmatized by STDs, are symptomatic, are female, and take longer to seek health care for an STD (Fortenberry, 1997). Partner notification and treatment can help to decrease STDs in the adolescent population. Despite the fact that adolescents report that they prefer to notify their partners on their own (self-referral), and self-referral may be an easier method of locating partners, research suggests that provider notification is more effective (Oh et al., 1996). Self-referral may be facilitated by confidence in their ability to notify partners and greater relationship quality (e.g., supportive, emotionally connected) with their partners (Fortenberry, Brizendine, Katz, & Orr, 2002).

Health care providers also can serve as a resource for adolescents as they learn to make healthy sexual decisions. Although adolescents sometimes feel uncomfortable or embarrassed discussing sexual issues

(Klein, Wilson, McNulty, Kapphahn, & Collins, 1999), some evidence suggests that they are motivated to discuss sexuality with their health care providers, and they want their health care providers to ask about their sexual history directly (Rosenthal et al., 1999). One study found that adolescents were more likely to discuss risk-taking behaviors, including sexual risk behaviors, with their health care providers when they met without a parent present, had more overall risk factors (e.g., alcohol use, sex without contraception, smoking), had sought health information, and had a female health care provider (Klein & Wilson, 2002). Studies indicate that education and counseling about STDs and prevention methods during office visits can increase condom use (Boekeloo et al., 1999).

Parents also serve as an important resource for adolescents, although concerns about confidentiality may provide a barrier to care for some. A number of youth have reported that they do not seek health care because they do not want their parents to know about their sexual behaviors (Burack, 2000; Klein et al., 1999). Other adolescents reported that they would stop accessing care if parental notification was required (Reddy, Fleming, & Swain, 2002). Research indicates that adolescents want their health care providers to explain confidentiality in detail, in a language that they can understand, and in a manner that communicates care and trust (Ford, Thomsen, & Compton, 2001). Given the concerns regarding confidentiality, all 50 states and the District of Columbia have laws granting adolescents the right to consent to and receive confidential STD-related health care, with 30 states explicitly identifying HIV testing as one of the services (The Alan Guttmacher Institute, 2003). Providers should be aware of their state laws regarding STD prevention and treatment so that they can protect adolescents' rights to confidentiality while at the same time foster adolescent–parent communication.

Community and School-Based Interventions

Community and school-based interventions (both, school-based clinic interventions, and service learning programs) may play important roles in reducing the STD epidemic.

STD/HIV Programs

STD/HIV programs include both those labeled "abstinence-only" and those labeled "abstinence plus safer sex" programs. Both types of programs promote abstinence (particularly among young adolescents) as being the safest way to protect persons from STDs and unwanted pregnancy. Abstinence-only education teaches that sexual activity should occur only within the context of a marital relationship, that abstinence has social, psychological, and health benefits, and that sexual activity outside of marriage leads to negative consequences, such as STDs, unwanted pregnancy, and psychosocial difficulties (Section 510, Title V of the Social Security Act, 1998). Abstinence plus safer sex programs do not designate a specific time or context in which sexual activity is appropriate. Unlike the abstinence-only programs, abstinence plus safer sex programs also teach alternative methods to prevent STDs/HIV (e.g., condom use).

Some studies evaluating abstinence-only programs have reported positive effects (Goldfarb et al., 1999). However, many of these studies have significant methodological flaws, making their results difficult to interpret, replicate, and draw conclusions (Kirby, 2002). For example, an evaluation of two abstinence-only programs of middle school-age children found that the intervention significantly reduced the onset of sexual behavior and decreased sexual intercourse and intentions to have intercourse at a 1-year follow-up (Goldfarb et al., 1999). Though these results may seem encouraging, age was not distributed evenly across the groups. Significantly fewer control participants were in the highest age category, and therefore the results could have simply reflected age differences. Other outcome studies with better designs have failed to demonstrate positive results of abstinence-only programs (Kirby, 2002) and some have even demonstrated undesirable effects (Christopher & Roosa, 1990). For example at 1- and 2-year follow-up the *Success Express Program*, which is a 5-week program for low-income, middle school-age children, found no significant improvements in self-esteem, family communication, sexual attitudes, and sexual behaviors. Moreover, males participating in the intervention showed an increase in precoital sexual activity after 1 year (Christopher & Roosa, 1990).

In contrast, several well-designed outcome studies of abstinence plus safer sex programs have yielded positive results. These programs have been shown to decrease age of sexual initiation, reduce unprotected sexual activity, decrease the number of sexual partners, increase use of condoms and other contraceptives, and increase knowledge about STDs or AIDS. Moreover, there has been no evidence that teaching adolescents about safer sex is associated with increased sexual activity (Kirby, 2002). An example is *Becoming a Responsible Teen*. This 8-week program is aimed at providing adolescents with knowledge and behavioral skills to help them reduce their risk of acquiring HIV/AIDS. Participants engage in weekly group sessions on AIDS education, sexual decision-making skills, technical competency skills, refusal and condom negotiation skills, problem-solving skills, and social support and empowerment. At 1-year follow-up, intervention participants were more likely than control participants to delay sexual initiation, show reductions in unprotected intercourse, display increases in protected intercourse with condoms, and exhibit increases in behavior skills (e.g., refusal skills) (St. Lawrence, Brasfield, Jefferson, Alleyne, & O'Bannon, 1995).

When several programs with well-designed studies were reviewed by Kirby (2002), those programs that reduced unprotected sex were found to: (1) use approaches based on theories of health behavior; (2) allow sufficient time to accomplish the objectives; (3) provide accurate information about the consequences of unprotected sexual behavior; (4) use teaching methods that were varied, allowing the adolescent to personalize information in a meaningful manner; (5) directly address social pressures to engage in sexual behavior; (6) provide models of and opportunities to practice sexual communication including refusal and condom negotiation skills; (7) recruit facilitators who were proponents of the program and provide them with adequate training; (8) use behavioral goals and teaching methods that were appropriate to age, sexual experience, and culture of the participants; (9) address specific sexual behaviors; and (10) make a clear connection between sexual activity and contraceptive or condom use.

School-Based Health Clinics

The first school-based health clinic (SBHC) opened in Texas in 1970 (Kirby, Waszak, & Ziegler, 1991) and as of 2002, approximately 1,500 SBHCS throughout the United States were in existence (The Center for Health and Health Care in Schools, n.d.). SBHCS provide various health services, including routine physical exams, primary care, and mental health services. They are located conveniently within or near a school and are adolescent-friendly and inexpensive (Gullotta & Noyes, 1995). SBHCS often provide care to those who are uninsured (Kisker & Brown, 1996), which is important given the large number of adolescents and children who are uninsured (Elixhauser et al., 2002).

Soon after SBHCS came into existence, providers recognized the role SBHCS could play in the sexual health of adolescents and there was evidence that offering reproductive health care through SBHCS may help reduce teen pregnancy rates (Edwards, Steinman, Arnold, & Hakanson, 1980). Not all agree that SBHCS should provide reproductive health services, contraceptives, and condoms to adolescents (Peak & Hauser McKinney, 1996). Yet at the very least, studies indicate that providing reproductive health services and prevention methods to adolescents does not increase adolescent sexual behaviors (Kirby et al., 1999). At the very most, studies show that providing condoms to adolescents decreases rates of unprotected sex (Schuster, Bell, Berry, & Kanouse, 1998).

Service Learning Programs

Service learning programs are based on the belief that there are common causes for risk-taking behaviors. As such, these programs develop broad interventions that target these causes, so that several different risk-taking behaviors, such as school failure and sexual health-comprising behaviors, can be reduced (Allen, Philliber, Herrling, & Kupermine, 1997).

Adolescents in these programs typically volunteer in a variety of community settings (e.g., nursing homes, hospitals, schools). Afterward they reflect on their volunteer experience and participate in group conversations or education about adolescent-related issues (e.g., life skills, physical, social, and emotional development, drug use, sexually transmitted diseases). These programs hope to teach adolescents adult-like responsibilities that will help them develop competencies and autonomy, make better decisions for themselves, form positive relationships with peers and adults, learn to cope with their emotions, and develop long-term goals. Service learning programs have been shown to reduce adolescent sexual behaviors and pregnancy rates (Allen et al., 1997; O'Donnell et al., 1999).

Parent Interventions

As noted below, parents clearly play an important role in the development of healthy sexual behaviors; however, less is known about how to help parents be more effective in this role. When parents communicate with adolescents about sexuality and STD prevention, adolescents tend to have greater sexual knowledge, delay sexual initiation, engage in less risky behavior, have greater skill in communicating about sex and condom use, and display more conservative attitudes about sexual issues (Diiorio, Kelley, & Hockenberry-Eaton, 1999; Dittus & Jaccard, 2000; Miller & Whitaker, 2001). Further, parental monitoring is associated with the adolescent having a lower incidence of STDs, pregnancy, and high-risk partners, and increased condom and contraception use (Baker et al., 1999; Crosby et al., 2002; DiClemente et al., 2001). Interventions have focused on having the parents and children simultaneously getting information, learning a skill, or doing an activity. In these studies, adolescents and parents gained knowledge and the skills that were taught (e.g., condom use skill and problem-solving skills) (Blake, Simkin, Ledsky, Perkins, & Calabrese, 2001; Winett et al., 1993). However, one study examining the effects of the intervention on actual risky behaviors found no behavioral changes in the adolescent (Xiaoming et al., 2002). It may be that unless programs also provide behavioral skills for adolescents, there may be limited impact on risk behaviors.

CONCLUSION

Sexually transmitted diseases are a critical public health problem for our teens, and the problem is something that we cannot afford to leave "hidden" and ignored (Institute of Medicine, 1997). The medical and psychological effects of STDs and their sequelae and the costs associated with STD-related care can be devastating for individuals and society. A wide range of interventions (e.g., fostering condom use, developing new biomedical methods, routine screening, and school-based programs) are needed to help reduce the initial acquisition and further transmission and sequelae of STDs. Interventions will need to be comprehensive and implemented at a variety of levels. For example, it is always easy to assume that new biomedical approaches, such as vaccines will provide an instant, easy, and complete solution, but this is not realistic. Vaccines only will be effective if behavioral approaches are used to enhance their acceptance. In addition, through community or school-based programs and parent interventions, adolescents can learn about their susceptibility to STDs/AIDS, develop skills to implement safer sex behaviors (e.g., abstinence, condoms, care-seeking behavior), and learn about new methods of protection as they become available. Thus, health care professionals (e.g., nurses, physicians, psychologists), policy makers, members of the community, and adolescents and their families must work together to reduce the acquisition and cost of STDs to our youth and society.

REFERENCES

Allen, J. P., Philliber, S., Herrling, S., & Kupermine, G. P. (1997). Preventing teen pregnancy and academic failure: Experimental evaluation of a developmentally based approach. *Child Development, 64*, 729–742.

American Social Health Association. (1998, December). *Sexually transmitted diseases in America: How many cases and at what cost.* Retrieved August 26, 2003, from http://www.ashastd.org/pdfs/std_rep.pdf

Aral, S. O. (2001). Sexually transmitted diseases: Magnitude, determinants and consequences. *International Journal of STD & AIDS, 12*, 211–215.

Aral, S. O., & Holmes, K. K. (1990). Epidemiology of sexual behavior and sexually transmitted diseases. In K. K. Holmes, P. M. Mardh, P. F. Sparling, & P. J. Wiesner (Eds.), *Sexually transmitted diseases* (2nd ed., pp. 19–36). New York: McGraw-Hill.

Baker, J. G., Rosenthal, S. L., Leonhardt, D., Kollar, L. M., Succop, P. A., Burklow, K. A. et al. (1999). Relationship between perceived parental monitoring and young adolescent girls' sexual and substance use behaviors. *Journal of Pediatric and Adolescent Gynecology, 12*, 17–22.

Baker, J. G., Succop, P. A., Boehner, C. W., Biro, F. M., Stanberry, L. R., & Rosenthal, S. L. (2001). Adolescent girl's coping with an STD: Not enough problem solving and too much self-blame. *Journal of Pediatric and Adolescent Gynecology, 14*, 85–88.

Biro, F. M. (1992). *Adolescents and sexually transmitted diseases* (Maternal and Child Health Technical Information Bulletin). Washington, DC: National Center for Education in Maternal and Child Health.

Blake, S. M., Simkin, L., Ledsky, R., Perkins, C., & Calabrese, J. M. (2001). Effects of a parent–child communications intervention on young adolescents' risk for early onset of sexual intercourse. *Family Planning Perspectives, 33*, 52–61.

Boekeloo, B. O., Schamus, L. A., Simmens, S. J., Cheng, T. L., O'Connor, K., & D'Angelo, L. J. (1999). A STD/HIV prevention trial among adolescents in managed care. *Pediatrics, 103*, 107–115.

Boyer, C. B., Shafer, M., Wibbelsman, C. J., Seeberg, D., Teitle, E., & Lovell, N. (2000). Associations of sociodemographic, psychosocial, and behavioral factors with sexual risk and sexually transmitted diseases in teen clinic patients. *Journal of Adolescent Health, 27*, 102–111.

Burack, R. (2000). Young teenagers' attitudes towards general practitioners and their provisions of sexual health care. *British Journal of General Practice, 50*, 550–554.

Burstein, G. R., Gaydos, C. A., Diener-West, M., Howell, M. R., Zenilman, J. M., & Quinn, T. C. (1998). Incident Chlamydia trachomatis infections among inner-city adolescent females. *Journal of the American Medical Association, 280*, 521–526.

Cao, H., Kaleebu, P., Hom, D., Flores, J., Agrawal, D., Jones, N. et al. (2003). Immunogenicity of a recombinant human immunodeficiency virus (HIV)—Canarypox vaccine in HIV-seronegative Uganda volunteers: Results of the HIV network for prevention trials 007 vaccine study. *The Journal of Infectious Diseases, 187*, 887–895.

Cates, W. (1999). Estimates of incidence and prevalence of sexually transmitted diseases in the United States. *Sexually Transmitted Diseases, 26*(Suppl. 4), S2–S7.

Cecil, H., Perry, M., Seal, D., & Pinkerton, S. (1998). The female condom: What we have learned thus far. *AIDS and Behavior, 2*, 241–256.

Centers for Disease Control and Prevention. (1998). Trends in sexual risk behavior among high school students—United States, 1991–1997. *Journal of the American Medical Association, 280*, 1819–1820.

Centers for Disease Control and Prevention. (1999). Achievements in public health, 1900–1999 Impact of Vaccines Universally Recommended for Children—United States, 1990–1998. *Morbidity and Mortality Weekly Report, 48*, 243–248.

Centers for Disease Control and Prevention. (2002). Sexually transmitted diseases treatment guidelines 2002. *Morbidity and Mortality Weekly Report, 51*, 1–80.

Choi, K., Gregorich, S. E., Anderson, K., Grinstead, O. A., & Gomez, C. A. (2003). Patterns and predictors of female condom use among ethnically diverse women attending family planning clinics. *Sexually Transmitted Diseases, 30*, 91–98.

Christopher, F. S., & Roosa, M. W. (1990). An evaluation of an adolescent pregnancy prevention program: Is "Just say No" enough? *Family Relations, 39*, 68–72.

Cohen, D. A., Nsuami, M., Martin, D. H., & Farley, T. A. (1999). Repeated school-based screening for sexually transmitted diseases: A feasible strategy for reaching adolescents. *Pediatrics, 104*, 1281–1285.

Crosby, R. A., DiClemente, R. J., Wingood, G. M., Harrington, K., Davies, S., Hook, E. W. et al. (2002). Low parental monitoring predicts subsequent pregnancy among African-American adolescent females. *Journal of Pediatric Adolescent Gynecology, 15*, 43–46.

Darroch, J. E., & Frost, J. J. (1999). Women's interest in vaginal microbicides. *Family Planning Perspectives, 31*, 16–23.

DiClemente, R. J., Wingood, G. M., Crosby, R. A., Sionean, C., Cobb, B. K., Harrington, K. et al. (2001). Parental monitoring: Association with adolescents' risk behaviors. *Pediatrics, 107*, 1363–1368.

Diiorio, C., Kelley, M., & Hockenberry-Eaton, M. (1999). Communication about sexual issues: Mothers, fathers, and friends. *Journal of Adolescent Health, 24*, 181–189.

Dittus, P. J., & Jaccard, J. (2000). Adolescents' perceptions of maternal disapproval of sex: Relationship to sexual outcomes. *Journal of Adolescent Health, 26*, 268–278.

Donald, M., Lucke, J., Dunne, M., O'Toole, B., & Raphael, B. (1994). Determinants of condom use by Australian secondary school students. *Journal of Adolescent Health, 15*, 503–510.

Edwards, L. E., Steinman, M. E., Arnold, K. A., & Hakanson, E. Y. (1980). Adolescent pregnancy prevention services in high school clinics. *Family Planning Perspectives, 12*, 6–7+11–14.

Elixhauser, A., Machlin, S. R., Zodet, M. W., Chevarley, F. M., Patel, N., McCormick, M. C. et al. (2002). Health care for children and youth in the United States: 2001 annual report on access, utilization, quality, and expenditures. *Ambulatory Pediatrics, 2*, 419–437.

Ellen, J. M., Cahn, S., Eyre, S. L., & Boyer, C. B. (1996). Types of adolescent sexual relationships and associated perceptions about condom use. *Journal of Adolescent Health, 18*, 417–421.

Ford, C. A., Thomsen, S. L., & Compton, B. (2001). Adolescents' interpretations of conditional confidentiality assurances. *Journal of Adolescent Health, 29*, 156–159.

Fortenberry, J. D. (1997). Health care seeking behaviors related to sexually transmitted diseases among adolescents. *American Journal of Public Health, 87*, 417–420.

Fortenberry, J. D., Brizendine, E. J., Katz, B. P., & Orr, D. P. (2002). The role of self-efficacy and relationship quality in partner notification by adolescents with sexually transmitted infections. *Archives of Pediatrics and Adolescent Medicine, 156*, 1133–1137.

Goldfarb, E. S., Donnelly, J., Duncan, D. F., Young, M., Eadie, C., & Castiglia, D. (1999). Evaluation of an abstinence-based curriculum for early adolescents: First year changes in sex attitudes, knowledge, and behavior. *North American Journal of Psychology, 1*, 243–254.

Guajardo, A. D., Middleman, A. B., & Sansaricq, K. M. (2002). School nurses identify barriers and solutions to implementing a school-based hepatitis B immunization program. *Journal of School Health, 72*, 128–130.

Gullotta, T. P., & Noyes, L. (1995). The changing paradigm of community health: The role of school-based health centers. *Adolescence, 30*, 107–115.

Hammett, T. M., Mason, T. H., Joanis, C. L., Foster, S. E., Harmon, P., Robles, R. R. et al. (2000). Acceptability of formulations and application methods for vaginal microbicides among drug involved women: Results of product trials in three cities. *Sexually Transmitted Diseases, 27*, 119–126.

Hawe, P., McKenzie, N., & Scurry, R. (1998). Randomised controlled trial of the use of a modified postal reminder card on the uptake of measles vaccination. *Archives of Disease in Childhood, 79*, 136–140.

Hiller, L., Harrison, L., & Warr, D. (1998). "When you carry condoms all the boys think you want it: Negotiating competing discourses about safe sex." *Journal of Adolescence, 21*, 15–29.

Institute of Medicine. (1997). *The hidden epidemic: Confronting sexually transmitted diseases.* Washington DC: National Academy Press.

Jadack, R. A., Fresia, A., Rompalo, A. M., & Zenilman, J. (1997). Reasons for not using condoms of clients at urban sexually transmitted diseases clinics. *Sexually Transmitted Diseases, 24*, 402–408.

Kirby, D. (2002). Effective approaches to reducing adolescent unprotected sex, pregnancy, and childbearing. *The Journal of Sex Research, 39*, 51–57.

Kirby, D., Brener, N. D., Brown, N. L., Peterfreund, N., Hillard, P., & Harrist, R. (1999). The impact of condom distribution in Seattle schools on sexual behavior and condom use. *American Journal of Public Health, 89*, 182–187.

Kirby, D., Waszak, C., & Ziegler, J. (1991). Six school-based clinics: Their reproductive health services and impact on sexual behavior. *Family Planning Perspectives, 23*, 6–16.

Kisker, E., & Brown, R. S. (1996). Do school-based health centers improve adolescents' access to health care, health status, and risk-taking behavior. *Journal of Adolescent Health, 18*, 335–343.

Klein, J. D., & Wilson, K. M. (2002). Delivering quality care: Adolescents' discussion of health risks with their providers. *Journal of Adolescent Health, 30*, 190–195.

Klein, J. D., Wilson, K. M., McNulty, M., Kapphahn, C., & Collins, K. S. (1999). Access to medical care for adolescents: Results from the 1997 Commonwealth Fund Survey of the health of adolescent girls. *Journal of Adolescent Health, 25*, 120–130.

Kollar, L. M., Rosenthal, S. L., & Biro, F. M. (1994). Hepatitis B vaccine series compliance in adolescents. *Pediatric Infectious Disease Journal, 13*, 1006–1008.

Koutsky, L. A., Ault, K. A., Wheeler, C. M., Brown, D. R., Barr, E., Alvarez, F. B. et al. (2002). A controlled trial of a human papillomavirus type 16 vaccine. *New England Journal of Medicine, 347*, 1645–1651.

Liau, A., Zimet, G. D., & Fortenberry, J. D. (1998). Attitudes about human immunodeficiency virus immunization: The influence of health beliefs and vaccine characteristics. *Sexually Transmitted Diseases, 25*, 76–81.

Liu, H., Detels, R., Li, X., Ma, E., & Yin, Y. (2002). Stigma, delayed treatment, and spousal notification among patients with sexually transmitted disease in China. *Sexually Transmitted Diseases, 29*, 335–343.

Marshall, S., Giblin, P., Simpson, P., & Backos, A. (2002). Adolescent girls' perception and experiences with the reality female condom. *Journal of Adolescent Health, 31*, 5–6.

Miller, K. S., & Whitaker, D. J. (2001). Predictors of mother–adolescent discussions about condoms: Implications for providers who serve youth. *Pediatrics, 108*, e28.

National Institute of Allergy and Infectious Diseases. (2001). *Scientific evidence on condom effectiveness for sexually transmitted disease (STD) prevention.* Herndon, VA: National Institute of Allergy and Infectious Diseases.

O'Donnell, L., Stueve, A., Doval, A. S., Duran, R., Haber, D., Atnafou, R. et al. (1999). The effectiveness of the reach for health community youth service learning program in reducing early and unprotected sex among urban and middle school students. *American Journal of Public Health, 89*, 176–181.

Oh, M. K., Boker, J. R., Genuardi, F. J., Cloud, G. A., Reynolds, J., & Hodgens, J. B. (1996). Sexual contact tracing outcome in adolescent chlamydial and gonococcal cervicitis cases. *Journal of Adolescent Health, 18*, 4–9.

Peak, G. L., & Hauser McKinney, D. L. (1996). Reproductive and sexual health at the school-based/school-linked health center: An analysis of services provided by 180 clinics. *Journal of Adolescent Health, 19*, 276–281.

Reddy, D. M., Fleming, R., & Swain, C. (2002). Effective mandatory parental notification on adolescent girls' use of sexual health care services. *Journal of the American Medical Association, 288*, 710–714.

Rosenthal, S. L., & Biro, F. M. (1991). A preliminary investigation of the psychological impact of sexually transmitted diseases in adolescent females. *Adolescent and Pediatric Gynecology, 4*, 198–201.

Rosenthal, S. L., Biro, F. M., Cohen, S. S., Succop, P. A., & Stanberry, L. R. (1995a). Parents, peers, and the acquisition of an STD. Developmental changes in girls. *Journal of Adolescent Health, 16*, 45–49.

Rosenthal, S. L., Biro, F. M., Cohen, S. S., Succop, P. A., & Stanberry, L. R. (1995b). Strategies for coping with sexually transmitted diseases by adolescent females. *Adolescence, 30*, 655–666.

Rosenthal, S. L., Cohen, S. S., & Stanberry, L. R. (1998). Topical microbicides: Current status and research considerations for adolescent girls. *Sexually Transmitted Diseases, 25*, 368–377.

Rosenthal, S. L., Lewis, L. M., Succop, P. A., Burklow, K. A., Nelson, P. R., Shedd, K. D. et al. (1999). Adolescents' views regarding sexual history taking. *Clinical Pediatrics, 38*, 227–233.

Schuster, M. A., Bell, R. M., Berry, S. H., & Kanouse, D. E. (1998). Impact of a high school condom availability program on sexual attitudes and behaviors. *Family Planning Perspectives, 30*, 67–88.

Section 510, Title V of the Social Security Act, 42 U.S.C. §710. (1998).

Sellors, J., Pickard, L., Mahony, J. B., Jackson, K., Nelligan, P., Zimic-Vincetic, M. et al. (1997). Understanding and enhancing compliance with the second dose of hepatitis B vaccine: A cohort analysis and a randomized controlled trial. *Canadian Medical Association Journal, 157*, 143–148.

Short, M. B., Mills, L., Majkowski, J. M., Stanberry, L. R., & Rosenthal, S. L. (2003). Topical microbicide use by adolescent girls: Concerns about timing, efficacy, and safety. *Sexually Transmitted Diseases, 30*, 854–858.

St. Lawrence, J. S., Brasfield, T. L., Jefferson, K. W., Alleyne, E., & O'Bannon, R. E., III (1995). Cognitive-behavioral intervention to reduce African American adolescents' risk for HIV infection. *Journal of Consulting and Clinical Psychology, 63*, 221–237.

Stanberry, L., Spruance, S., Cunningham, A., Bernstein, D., Mindel, A., Sacks, S. et al. (2002). Glycoprotein-D-adjuvant vaccine to prevent genital herpes. *New England Journal of Medicine, 347*, 1652–1661.

The Alan Guttmacher Institute. (2003, April 1). *State policies in brief: Minors access to STD services*. Retrieved August 8, 2003, from http://www.guttmacher.org/pubs/spib_MASS.pdf

The Center for Health and Health Care in Schools. (n.d.). *2002 State survey of school-based health center initiatives*. Retrieved August 8, 2003, from http://www.healthinschools.org/sbhcs/narrative02.asp

Unti, L. M., Coyle, K. K., Woodruff, B. A., & Boyer-Chuanroong, L. (1997). Incentives and motivators in school-based hepatitis B vaccination programs. *Journal of School Health, 67*, 265–268.

Wald, A., Langenberg, A. G., Link, K., Izu, A. E., Ashley, R., Warren, T. et al. (2001). Effects of condoms on reducing the transmission of herpes simplex virus Type-2 from men to women. *Journal of the American Medical Association, 285*, 3100–3106.

Wang, L. Y., Burstein, G. R., & Cohen, D. A. (2002). An economic evaluation of a school-based sexually transmitted disease screening program. *Sexually Transmitted Diseases, 29*, 737–745.

Winett, R. A., Anderson, E. S., Moore, J. S., Taylor, C. D., Hook, R. J., Webster, D. A. et al. (1993). Efficacy of a home-based human immunodeficiency virus prevention video program for teens and parents. *Health Education Quarterly, 20*, 555–567.

Witte, S. S., El-Bassel, N., Wada, T., Gray, O., & Wallace, J. (1999). Acceptability of female condom use among women exchanging street sex in New York City. *International Journal of STD & AIDS, 10*, 162–168.

Xiaoming, L., Stanton, B., Galbraith, J., Burns, J., Cottrell, L., & Pack, R. (2002). Parental monitoring intervention: Practice makes perfect. *Journal of the National Medical Association, 94*, 364–369.

Zimet, G. D., Fortenberry, J. D., & Blythe, M. J. (1999). Adolescents' attitudes about HIV immunization. *Journal of Pediatric Psychology, 24*, 67–75.

12

Treatment Services for Adolescent Substance Abuse*

BEVERLY PRINGLE and JERRY FLANZER

Adolescent substance abuse has been a public health concern for decades, but the scientific knowledge base on the services engaged to treat this problem is comparatively new. This nascent knowledge base is poised to expand exponentially, as researchers and treatment providers struggle to meet a rising demand for evidence-based treatment services. Until recently, research on adolescent substance abuse consisted primarily of a limited set of large-scale national studies of adults that included adolescent samples (e.g., Drug Abuse Reporting Program, Treatment Outcome Prospective Study, National Treatment Improvement Evaluation Study), small studies with methodological problems, and program evaluations. Within the past decade, adolescent substance abuse and its treatment have developed as important topics of inquiry in their own right, with more resources and high-quality research efforts being targeted on this persistent and pressing public health issue. These advances notwithstanding, few communities provide sufficient treatment services for adolescents who use alcohol, marijuana, nicotine, and other illicit drugs. Only about 10% of adolescents who need substance abuse treatment currently receive it (Substance Abuse and Mental Health Services Administration, [SAMHSA], 2002), and of those who receive treatment, only about one quarter receive the full range of services prescribed (Dennis & McGeary, 1999).

This chapter focuses on the nature of adolescent substance abuse and the services intended to treat it. For clarity, we use the term, *treatment services*, broadly to denote the full range of health and social services employed to contend with substance abuse disorders in adolescents. These

BEVERLY PRINGLE and JERRY FLANZER • National Institute on Drug Abuse, Bethesda, Maryland 20892.

*The views expressed in this chapter are those of the authors and not necessarily those of the National Institute on Drug Abuse.

may include medical, psychological, welfare, educational, employment, financial, and housing services, among others. We use the term, *therapy*, to denote specific talk, behavioral, and pharmacological strategies used to treat the symptoms of substance abuse. Substance abuse *treatments* and *treatment programs* for adolescents typically include one or more therapies plus other treatment services.

This chapter begins with a brief description of the nature of adolescent substance use and misuse, including the unique developmental issues of adolescence. We then review the small but growing set of substance abuse therapies showing the most promise for treating adolescents and describe the levels of care most commonly delivered to youth. The chapter concludes with a discussion of the key treatment service issues, including availability of services; breadth, integration, and targeting of services; staffing; financing; costs; and diffusion of research into practice.

SUBSTANCE USE AND ABUSE AMONG ADOLESCENTS: NATURE OF THE PROBLEM

Illicit substance use among adolescents has remained stable or decreased for 6 years in a row, according to 2002 data from *Monitoring the Future*, an annual study of youth drug trends funded by the National Institute on Drug Abuse (NIDA, 2003). The proportion of 8th and 10th graders reporting the use of any illicit drug during the prior year decreased significantly from 2001 to 2002 (20% to 18% for 8th graders, 37% to 35% for 10th graders). Adolescents reported specific declines in the use of marijuana, some club drugs, cigarettes, and alcohol. Nonetheless, a substantial proportion of adolescents report the use of substances each year, most commonly alcohol (39–72% past year use), marijuana (15–36% past year use), and nicotine (11–27% past 30-day use). The prevalence in use of other substances in 2002 trailed behind, ranging from a low of about 1% for past-year heroin use across the three grade levels, to a high of almost 8% for past-year use of tranquilizers among 12th graders and for past-year use of inhalants among 8th graders. The only statistically significant increases in adolescent substance use from 2001 to 2002 were 10th graders' past-year use of crack cocaine (1.8–2.3%) and 12th graders' past-year use of sedatives (5.9–7.0%) (NIDA, 2003).

Because the biology of adolescence is unique, the abuse—and even occasional use—of psychoactive substances during this period can have far-reaching harmful consequences. Important organ systems, including the reproductive, respiratory, skeletal, immune, and central nervous systems, mature during adolescence, which means that substances misused during this period can disrupt not only normal function, but also the natural maturational process. Adolescence is also marked by increased risk for infectious disease and accidental injury, making the additional effects of misused substances on the immune and central nervous systems especially harmful (Golub, 2000). Adolescents who use illicit substances are more likely to experience school truancy (Halfors et al., 2002); violence and delinquency (Dembo & Schmeidler, 2003); and other negative health consequences, such as unplanned pregnancy, sexually transmitted disease, trauma, accidents (Bonomo et al., 2001; Tapert, Aarons, Sedlar, & Brown, 2001; Taylor, Kreutzer, Demm, & Meade, 2003), and hepatitis C among injection drug users in particular (Gilvarry, 2000). High rates of comorbid psychiatric and behavioral problems—both internalizing disorders such as depression, anxiety, and traumatic distress and externalizing disorders such as hyperactivity, attentional deficits, violent conduct, and criminal behavior (Gilvarry, 2000; Greenbaum, Foster-Johnson, & Petrila, 1996; Rowe, Liddle, & Dakof, 2001)—are also prevalent among adolescent substance abusers. Taken together, these associated risks and characteristics make youth substance use a continuing and alarming public health concern.

For years, most adolescent substance abusers who received treatment did so in programs designed for adults (Kristiansen & Hubbard, 2001; White, 1998). Results were disappointing, and researchers determined that a firm understanding of youth development is critical for designing effective treatments for adolescents (Dennis, 2002). Researchers identified ways in which youth substance abusers differ from their adult counterparts and implications that these differences have for treatment (Winters, Stinchfield, Opland, Weller, & Latimer, 2000). For example, adolescents have shorter substance use histories than adults, but these histories often include a host of related troubles, such as conflicts with parents, difficulties with school performance and peer relationships, and legal problems (Etheridge, Smith, Rounds-Bryant, & Hubbard, 2001). Youth use more marijuana and alcohol than adults, and their patterns of substance use are different, involving more binge and opportunistic use (Dennis, 2002). Consequently, the alcohol detoxification clinics and systems that have been institutionalized for treating adult opiate addicts may have little value in treating adolescents. Moreover, adolescents' limited cognitive ability to recognize potential problems associated with risky behavior (including drug use and abuse) and to anticipate the negative, long-term consequences of their actions, renders inadequate many strategies used in motivating adults to seek and accept treatment. Fortunately, the recent spate of research on youth treatments has shown tailored services to be effective in achieving many behavioral and psychological improvements, including decreases in drug use, criminal activity, family problems, and other risky behaviors, plus increases in school and job functioning (Azrin et al., 2001; Hser et al., 2001; Jainchill, Hawke, De Leon, & Yagelka, 2000; Williams & Chang, 2000). These promising results have affirmed the value of recognizing and addressing the unique developmental needs of adolescents who use or abuse substances.

Although any use of illicit substances during adolescence may interfere with healthy development, not all youth who use substances will develop behaviors and symptoms severe enough to diagnose as abuse or dependence. However, for adolescents whose substance use escalates to abuse, the traditional "acute care" model of substance abuse treatment and recovery may no longer be adequate (McLellan, Lewis, O'Brien, & Kleber, 2000). Rather, researchers and clinicians describe a complex picture of recurring cycles involving substance use initiation, escalation to abuse, health services intervention, remission, lapse, and relapse (Dennis & Scott, 2002). Once adolescents are diagnosed with a substance abuse disorder, several full cycles spanning many years may be the norm for treatment rather than the exception. Emerging work on the nature and course of substance abuse, alone and in combination with other mental and physical health problems, has profound implications for revising current intervention paradigms, amending conceptualizations of treatment effectiveness, improving the organization and delivery of services, and developing better ways to finance services. A full understanding of how individual, social, and treatment factors interact to extend or curtail these drug use trajectories is important for developing and delivering optimally effective systems of intervention for adolescents at different developmental stages in their own maturation and in their substance use and treatment careers.

PROMISING TREATMENTS FOR ADOLESCENTS WITH SUBSTANCE USE PROBLEMS

Empirically tested, efficacious drug abuse therapies are the foundation for effective care. Different therapies are used alone and in combination within different treatment programs and modalities of care. Other health and social services often augment drug abuse therapies to increase treatment engagement, address psychosocial and health problems, and prevent or reduce relapse. The therapies most commonly used with adolescents include family-based and multisystemic therapies, cognitive-behavioral therapy, pharmacotherapy, 12-step treatments, and therapeutic communities. Review articles with details on the efficacy of these and other treatments include Crome (1999), Deas and Thomas (2001), Hser et al. (2001), Jainchill (2000), Muck, Zempolich, Titus, Fishman, Godley, & Schwebel, 2001, and Williams and Chang (2000).

Family-Based and Multisystemic Therapies

Of the therapies most commonly used to treat adolescent substance abuse, family-based therapies (Liddle et al., 2001; Robbins, Bacharach, & Szapocznik, 2002; Rowe & Liddle, 2003) and multisystemic therapy (Henggeler, Clingempeel, Brondino, & Pickrel, 2002) have received the most empirical research attention and are recognized as among the most promising (Cottrell & Boston, 2002; Winters, Latimer, & Stinchfield, 1999). The essential principle of these approaches is that adolescents' psychosocial environment, including their family and community, plays a role in establishing conditions related to the adolescents' drug use. Accordingly, treatment providers attempt to enlist these different social systems to help change the adolescents' psychosocial milieu to protect against risky behaviors such as drug abuse.

Cognitive-Behavioral Therapy

Cognitive-behavioral therapy (CBT) is widely employed for treating all kinds of behavioral problems in adolescents, including substance use and abuse (Crome, 1999). Theory underlying CBT posits that behavioral change can be influenced by a combination of the thoughts (e.g., anticipatory expectations, attributions, information processing) and emotions associated with particular behavioral events (Kendall, 1991). Thus, treatment providers use CBT to change undesirable behaviors such as drug use by modifying adolescents' maladaptive thoughts and coping skills through skills training in effective communication and social interaction, adaptive problem solving, anger management, constructive interpretation of emotions, and other strategies. Through CBT, adolescents learn how to avoid opportunities for use of drugs or alcohol, decline unwanted offers, tolerate and ease uncomfortable emotions, and reframe dysfunctional thoughts, all of which can assist adolescents in resisting temptations to use or abuse substances.

Pharmacotherapy

Pharmacological interventions for substance abuse typically are used to counteract intoxication and withdrawal symptoms or to prevent relapse. Less is known about pharmacological interventions—compared with psychosocial interventions—for treating adolescent substance abuse. This is due in part to difficulties in adequately assessing the safety and efficacy of pharmacological treatments in minority-age populations (Crome, 1999). However, in the case of alcohol, the most widely used substance among adolescents, it may also be due to the fact that only a small proportion of adolescents have yet developed alcohol dependence (Crome, 1997), and, consequently, do not require medication to manage withdrawal symptoms. Psychotropic medications to treat comorbid psychiatric disorders (e.g., depression) have been used more widely with adolescents than have medications to treat substance abuse *per se* (Deas & Thomas, 2001).

12-Step Programs

Twelve-step programs, such as Alcoholics Anonymous and Narcotics Anonymous, are ubiquitous in the substance abuse treatment community. These programs are based on 12 steps, developed by the founders of Alcoholics Anonymous (Alcoholics Anonymous, 1976), that comprise both a philosophy of and a process for recovery from alcohol abuse (Jainchill, 2000). Twelve-step programs conceive of addiction as a chronic illness involving denial and loss of self-control, and they emphasize spirituality as a key treatment component (Deas & Thomas, 2001). Recovering addicts often use 12-step group therapy sessions as social support to help in preventing relapse. The use of 12-step programs has received much more research attention with adults than with adolescents. Researchers and treatment providers have begun to suspect that some tenets of 12-step programs may not be developmentally appropriate for adolescents. This question has sparked several recent studies (i.e., Kelly, Myers, & Brown, 2000, 2002; Winters et al., 2000) to examine the efficacy of these approaches specific to adolescent populations.

Therapeutic Communities

As the name denotes, the therapeutic community focuses on the *community* as the salient therapeutic ingredient for facilitating change. The treatment, in essence, is full-time engagement with a community of peers and staff members through a variety of structured community activities, with the goals being abstinence from drugs and the development of personal insight, social responsibility, and commitment to specific therapeutic community values (Jainchill, 2000). Originally designed for adult addicts (see De Leon, 1997, 2000 for details), therapeutic communities have been modified for adolescents, including the use of smaller communities, shorter lengths of stay, greater family involvement, and less emphasis on confrontation (Etheridge et al., 2001; Jainchill, 2000). Therapeutic communities are, by definition, residential in nature. There is some variation in the treatment period for adolescents, but most therapeutic communities consider 6 to 12 months to be the recommended duration of treatment (Jainchill, 2000).

TREATMENT FACILITIES AND MODALITIES OF CARE FOR ADOLESCENTS

Approximately 37% of substance abuse treatment facilities in the United States (excluding those in criminal justice institutions) report offering special services for youth, according to data from the National Survey of Substance Abuse Treatment Services (Duffy, 2002). These facilities are similar to those without adolescent programs in that over half are private, nonprofit organizations; over three quarters provide drug or alcohol urine screening; and about one quarter of their clients are in treatment for alcohol problems only. Treatment facilities with special youth programs also differ from facilities without them. For example, facilities with special youth services tend to be somewhat larger than those without them (93 vs. 76 clients), and they are more prevalent in the Central and Western parts of the country (39% of substance abuse treatment facilities in those regions) than in the South (33%) and in the East (36%). The number of services provided in the facilities with adolescent programs and facilities without them is similar, but the mix of services differs. For example, family counseling and aftercare are more commonly provided in facilities with adolescent programs, whereas residential services and methadone or LAAM treatments are more commonly found in facilities without an adolescent program. Fewer facilities with adolescent services report substance abuse to be their main treatment focus (vs. mental health or other services), compared with adult service only facilities (Duffy, 2002).

Additional empirical information about community treatment services for youth, the youth who receive these services, and the modalities of care through which the services are delivered, comes from the Drug Abuse Treatment Outcome Studies for Adolescents (DATOS-A), 1993–1995, supported by NIDA. The DATOS-A program sample included 37 agencies in six cities (Pittsburgh, Minneapolis, Chicago, Portland, Miami, and New York), and the researchers assessed seven treatment services within three treatment modalities, or levels, of care. The treatment services were medical, psychological, family, legal, educational, vocational, and financial (Etheridge et al., 2001). The modalities of care were outpatient drug-free, short-term inpatient, and residential. Study results showed that the three modalities were distinguished by the location of service delivery, services provided, clientele served, and planned duration of treatment (Kristiansen & Hubbard, 2001; Rounds-Bryant, Kristiansen, & Hubbard, 1999).

Outpatient Care

Outpatient care for substance abuse typically connotes one or more treatment services delivered to adolescents who travel to one or more treatment facilities or by treatment providers who travel to the adolescents. In DATOS-A, outpatient drug-free programs included regular and intensive outpatient and day treatment programs, with planned durations of stay ranging from 1 month to 2 years (Kristiansen & Hubbard, 2001). The adolescent clientele tended to be somewhat younger than those receiving inpatient or residential care, reported lower rates of regular drug use and criminal activity, had the least drug treatment experience, and had higher chances of meeting diagnostic criteria for anxiety, depression, and attention deficit (Kristiansen & Hubbard, 2001; Rounds-Bryant et al., 1999). Delany, Broome, Flynn, and Fletcher (2001) found three groupings among the DATOS-A outpatient programs based on the services delivered: one group offered psychological, family, and aftercare services; a second group offered these three core services plus medical services; and a third group offered educational, vocational, and legal services—but not medical services—in addition to the core trio of psychological, family, and aftercare services. Program accreditation, greater diversity of client needs, and greater staff resources were all related to the provision of a broader range of services in these outpatient programs. The professional training of program directors, however, was not related to extent of service offerings in these programs, as it was in DATOS-A residential programs.

Inpatient Care

Inpatient care typically refers to the set of treatment services provided to adolescents during a hospital admission. In DATOS-A, short-term inpatient programs typically involved medical stabilization and various forms of psychological counseling (e.g., individual, group, family, 12-step), plus educational and aftercare services (Delany et al., 2001; Kristiansen & Hubbard, 2001). Although the planned length of stay ranged from only about 2 weeks to 1 month (Kristiansen & Hubbard, 2001), youth in these short-term programs received more medical, psychological, and family services than youth in the outpatient or residential programs. Thus, researchers concluded that despite the shorter treatment duration, the emphasis on provision of services appeared to be stronger (Etheridge et al., 2001). Adolescents in DATOS-A inpatient programs were more likely to be White, female, psychiatrically impaired, and to report far more criminal activity than their arrest rates indicated (Kristiansen & Hubbard, 2001).

Residential Care

As the term implies, *residential care* refers to the treatment services provided to adolescents while they are living in a treatment facility. In the DATOS-A study, residential care included a variety of therapeutic community programs (traditional, short-term, and modified), halfway houses, and shelter-based programs that provided traditional treatments plus services designed to help resocialize clients for reentry into society (Kristainsen & Hubbard, 2001). Overall, adolescents in DATOS-A residential programs were referred to treatment primarily through the juvenile or criminal justice systems, and, compared with youth receiving outpatient and inpatient care, they were more likely to use cocaine and heroin (Kristiansen & Hubbard, 2001; Rounds-Bryant et al., 1999). The planned length of stay in these residential programs ranged from about 3 months to 1 year, with a median planned stay of about 5 months (Delany et al., 2001; Kristainsen & Hubbard, 2001). Delany et al. (2001) found two major groupings of residential programs—one group that offered medical, psychological, educational, and family services, and a second group that offered those four services plus financial services and onsite aftercare. Programs in the latter group, which offered more services, tended to have smaller capacities, somewhat larger client-to-counselor ratios, a higher proportion of directors with terminal or professional degrees, and clients with fewer treatment needs. The professional training of program directors across the two residential program groupings was related to more extensive service offerings.

KEY SERVICE DELIVERY ISSUES

The extent to which adolescents who use and abuse substances do not obtain appropriate and adequate treatment services is alarming and raises questions about the availability of treatment services for youth; the breadth, integration, and targeting of those services; and the financing and costs of treatment services. Two additional service delivery issues that may be related to the undertreatment of adolescents are staffing and the transfer of efficacious treatment therapies and services into effective community interventions.

Availability of Treatment Services

Inadequacy of substance abuse treatment services for adolescents is widely reported, but the true scope of unaddressed needs in this population remains unclear (Delany et al., 2001). Based on a statewide study, Harrison and Fulkerson (1996, cited in Delany et al., 2001) estimated that three quarters of youth in the state of Minnesota who had a substance use disorder in 1995 did not receive treatment. Presumably, given the wide range of health and psychosocial problems associated with substance abuse during adolescence, ready availability of a broader range of treatment services than is currently available is critically needed.

Delany et al. (2001) analyzed data from DATOS-A to determine the association between organizational factors and availability of various services across the three treatment modalities studied: outpatient drug-free, short-term inpatient, and residential care. Results of these analyses showed that "three factors—program accreditation" (by, e.g., the Joint Commission on the Accreditation of Healthcare Organizations, the Commission on the Accreditation of Rehabilitation Facilities), "diversity of patient needs, and the staff/patient ratio—were found to be related to the range of on-site services available to patients, but these factors differed based on whether the program was providing care in a residential or an outpatient setting" (p. 600). For example, among outpatient programs, accreditation was related to the provision of a wider array of services, and those outpatient programs with more diverse patient needs and greater staff resources offered their patients a richer set of service options. In contrast, for the residential programs in DATOS-A, accreditation was related to fewer services and staff resources, and diversity of patient need did not have a significant effect on the range of services provided. The short-term inpatient programs were different still; they were relatively homogenous in terms of the services offered, generally including medical, psychological, educational, family, and aftercare services (Delany et al., 2001).

Breadth, Integration, and Targeting of Treatment Services

Effective treatment of adolescent drug abuse often requires the collective contributions of psychological, family, educational, vocational, employment, legal, recreational, and financial services in addition to specific drug abuse therapies (Williams & Chang, 2000). Program comprehensiveness is predictive of better treatment outcome in adolescents (Friedman & Glickman, 1986), as it is in adults (McLellan et al., 1994). Yet, *how* to deliver comprehensive and coordinated services to youth to simultaneously treat the symptoms of substance abuse, attenuate the varied and interrelated negative consequences, and minimize relapse is a persistent and perplexing dilemma.

Delivery of effective intervention services for clinically complicated youth is especially challenging. Given the high rates of comorbid psychiatric, medical, educational, family, legal, and other social problems in substance abusing youth, plus the fact that co-occurring disorders can interact in ways to support problem behaviors in one or more of these domains, treatment plans must encompass the full range of services needed to address these related problems in an integrated manner. The extent to which various services are fragmented or integrated may affect the degree to which they are both utilized and effective. Case management has a track record for promoting integration and continuity of care for individuals of all ages, especially among the dually diagnosed (e.g., Godley, Godley, Dennis, Funk, & Passetti, 2002; Ho et al., 1999; McLellan et al., 1999; Siegal et al., 1996). Ideally, case managers establish and maintain linkages across agencies to enlist services not provided by the drug treatment program, such as housing, medical care, child welfare, educational or vocational services, and legal help. Recently, researchers primarily studying treatment services utilization among adults are beginning to distinguish and study the differences between *on-site* and *off-site* case management (Friedmann, D'Aunno, Jin, & Alexander, 2000), which may have implications for delivery of services to youth and families as well.

Equally important is the targeting of appropriate services to the appropriate adolescents at the appropriate time in their drug use and treatment careers. Kendall and Kessler (2002) make the case for recognizing the developmental heterogeneity of youth in targeting interventions for psychopathology, substance abuse, or both: "Research attention must be paid to identifying the optimal match between the timing of the intervention and the level of the children's social, emotional, peer, and cognitive development" (p. 1305). For example, the design and delivery of aftercare or continuing care services—those support services that are provided after the intensive phase of substance abuse therapy has ended—is receiving increased research attention of late. Effective aftercare services for a 13-year-old with a short drug-use career and relatively few collateral problems, who has just completed her first treatment experience will likely be quite different from aftercare services for an 18-year-old youth with a long career of drug use and criminal involvement. Continuing care and recovery management services that support adolescents who have begun the recovery process have been especially underutilized and understudied.

Treatment Staff Working with Adolescents

The understanding that adolescents have problems and treatment needs unique from those of other drug-using populations raises questions about who should treat youth and what skills they should possess. Given the critical nature of the therapeutic alliance in efficacious psychotherapy (Horvath, 2001) and in retaining individuals in drug abuse treatment (Barber et al., 2001), knowledge about adolescent development and skill in relating to and counseling adolescents appears to be of consequence. Moreover, given the many different systems that influence the lives of drug abusing youth (e.g., family, education, mental health, medical, welfare, criminal justice), treatment practitioners need both knowledge of these interacting systems and to be adept at skill in navigating them.

Few studies have examined the adolescent treatment workforce (Pond, Aguirre-Molina, & Orleans, 2002). To address this knowledge gap, the Center for Substance Abuse Treatment and its Addiction Technology Transfer Centers (ATTCs) have gathered data on the characteristics and needs of the substance abuse treatment workforce. Early analyses of data for the northwestern United States indicate a growing disparity between demographic profiles of treatment providers and the adolescents they treat (Northwest Frontier Addiction Technology Transfer Center [NFATTC], 2000). For example, the workforce is predominantly White, female, and middle aged (47 years average age), whereas the adolescent treatment population is predominantly male, growing more racially and ethnically diverse, and initiating drug use at increasingly younger ages. Whether this demographic divide between clients and treatment providers matters is an issue of continuing debate among practitioners that calls for greater research attention.

The NFATTC survey also found that substance abuse treatment counselors serving adolescents often are former users themselves, not unlike the counselors treating adult substance abusers. Conventional wisdom has held that former users are among the most appropriate treatment providers for adults, but little empirical evidence supports this practice. Recently, some researchers have argued that former users may actually be harmful in the role of treatment providers for adolescents. Citing observations from her own research, Stevens (2003) has suggested that treatment delivered by young, healthy, gainfully employed, and recovering adults potentially can have iatrogenic effects by conveying to youth the impression that restoration of health after drug abuse during the teen years is easily attainable. Additional research can identify the knowledge, skills, and experiences that best equip counselors to work effectively with substance abusing youth.

Pollio's (2002) recent survey of state licensure boards regarding state certification requirements for substance abuse counselor revealed that no state in the United States currently offers provider certification specific to adolescents. Only five states stipulate that knowledge specific to the treatment of adolescents and youth is required for licensure. Two states include knowledge of human development in their licensing requirements, and two other states require knowledge of family counseling or family education. One additional state included knowledge of both human development and family issues. These findings raise questions about how adequately prepared are the practitioners currently treating youth drug abusers to do so.

Beyond licensing and training requirements, financing of treatment also influences the adolescent treatment workforce. The decrease in provider reimbursement rates that has resulted from transition to managed care has been credited with increased program instability and consequent workforce displacement (Pond et al., 2002). Pond et al. found poor compensation to be the most prevalent issue discussed in the literature on substance abuse treatment providers and in interviews with key informants about workforce issues. The NFATTC survey pointed to low pay as a barrier for individuals considering the field of substance abuse treatment.

Financing of Substance Abuse Treatment Services for Adolescents

Substance abuse treatment historically has been financed through public and private systems, but the clean delineation between these two systems has softened over the past decade (Cavanaugh, 2002), and the burden of financing has shifted from the private to the public sector (Dilonardo, Chalk, Mark, & Coffey, & the CSAT/CMHS Spending Estimates Team). It is clear, however, that financing—both public and private—of treatment services for substance abuse has not kept pace with the growing need (American Academy of Pediatrics, 2001). Moreover, the scant information available on financing substance abuse services for youth depicts a system based on the outdated view of substance abuse as an acute problem requiring acute care.

Two thirds of all children in the United States have private insurance, mainly through their parents' employers or through family-purchased plans (Kaiser Commission on Medicaid and the Uninsured, 2002). However, the health needs of adolescents are under-addressed, particularly in terms of coverage for ancillary and behavioral health services often indicated for treating substance abuse (Fox, McManus, & Reichman, 2002). A limited number of outpatient therapy visits for substance abuse are fully reimbursable in less than half of private plans and partially reimbursable in just over half. Residential care for substance abuse is especially rare and often limited to crisis intervention and detoxification services only. Reimbursable insurance coverage typically excludes family therapy (Cavanaugh, 2002), and the benefit limits and cost-sharing requirements for substance abuse services generally exceed those for general medical care (American Academy of Pediatrics, 2001).

Public funding for adolescent substance abuse presents a different set of issues. Many different sources of public funding support substance abuse treatment services for youth, including federal insurance and federal noninsurance-based financing, but these disparate funding streams are not well coordinated, and each has its own set of requirements and limitations (Cavanaugh, 2002; Solano, 1998). The results of a multistate case study of publicly supported substance abuse treatment for adolescents found that funding was both fragmented and insufficient to meet adolescents' treatment needs (Perry, 2002).

Two federal public insurance programs provide coverage for low-income youth: Medicaid and the Children's Health Insurance Program (CHIP). Medicaid covers about 20% of children in the United States, and CHIP covers an additional 3 million plus children (Kaiser Commission on Medicaid and the Uninsured, 2002). About 20% of low-income children remain uninsured. States administer Medicaid, with individual state policies governing how services are organized, financed, and delivered, creating discrepancies in financing and accessibility across states. Federal policy permits Medicaid funds to be used to cover emergency services for substance abuse and outpatient treatment services, but there is wide variation among the states in the type, amount, and intensity of adolescent substance abuse services provided under Medicaid at the state level (Geshan, 1999). Moreover, reimbursement rates and the supply of providers in some geographic areas are low.

Congress sought to broaden health care coverage for low-income children in 1997 [PL 105-33] by enacting the Children's Health Insurance Program, which targets low-income children who do not have other insurance coverage (Kaiser Commission on Medicaid and the Uninsured, 2002). States may use CHIP funds to expand Medicaid or to develop freestanding programs; again, practices vary by state. Freestanding CHIP programs tend to offer more limited benefits with more cost sharing requirements (General Accounting Office, 1999). All states but one cover some form of substance abuse treatment through CHIP, most commonly detoxification and limited outpatient treatment, but reimbursable services vary considerably (Howell, Roschwald, & Salake, 2000).

Federal noninsurance financing is the principal source of publicly funded substance abuse services for the uninsured and for those individuals who need additional treatment services to supplement those covered by insurance (Cavanaugh, 2002). Federal policies support services to treat adolescent substance abuse through block grants, categorical funding, and demonstration projects in six public policy domains: health, juvenile justice, family support and child welfare, education, housing, and labor (Cavanaugh, 2002). The type, amount, and intensity of services supported under these domains vary widely, and there is little coordination among them. In the health domain, the most important funding source is the Substance Abuse Prevention and Treatment Performance Partnership Block Grant (SAPTPPBG), administered by the Substance Abuse and Mental Health Services Administration. States support over half of all substance abuse treatment services with these dollars. In many states, however, SAPTPPBG funds for youth are spent primarily on prevention services, with little money targeted on youth treatment (Cavanaugh, 2002). Within the juvenile justice system, drug courts are a major recent initiative to address substance abuse, and the preliminary results are promising. Within the family and child welfare systems, adolescent substance abuse appears to be one among many needs competing for priority, and it rarely takes top billing. In the education domain, two major federal policies provide for the provision of adolescent drug abuse treatment services: the Vocational Rehabilitation Grants to States and the Individuals with Disabilities Act. The program for Safe and Drug Free Schools and Communities, funded with education dollars, focuses primarily on prevention efforts. In federal housing programs, adolescent drug abuse treatment services can be provided, but implementation is scarce. Finally, the Work Force Investment Act, administered by the Department of Labor, allows for substance abuse treatment services as a means for enabling successful employment of youth (Cavanaugh, 2002).

Costs of Treatment Services for Adolescents

Valid and reliable cost data on services used to treat youth substance abuse are surprisingly sparse. Such information is critical for making informed decisions about public health policy, budgeting, and optimal configurations of staffing and services required to produce the greatest treatment result per resources expended for various subpopulations of adolescent drug abusers. Economic data from the Fort Bragg Demonstration Project suggest, for example, that average treatment costs for adolescents with comorbid substance use and psychiatric disorders are more than twice as high as for adolescents with only one of these disorders (King, Gaines, Lambert, Summerfelt, & Bickman, 2000). Little work has been published on the comparative costs of treatment for this and other subpopulations of adolescents.

Early work in this area has emphasized the importance of evaluating the *full costs* of the delivery of treatment services (e.g., Anderson, Bowland, Cartwright, & Bassin, 1998; Cartwright, 1998; French, 1995)—above and beyond the personnel, supplies, and depreciation costs typically accounted for—to include "the value of all resources used in the treatment process including resources received either in kind or at below market rates (French et al., 2002, p. 85). Anderson et al. (1998) developed a method for estimating the full economic costs of delivering specific substance abuse treatment services and offered an example of how cost estimates might be produced for a best-practices treatment protocol. Of ultimate importance, is using cost and outcome data together to determine comparative cost-effectiveness and benefit-costs of treatment services provided (Anderson et al., 1998; Cartwright, 1998; Cohen, 1998; French et al., 2002).

French et al. (2002) applied another analytic method—the Drug Abuse Treatment Cost Analysis Program (French, 2001a, 2001b)—in the analysis of economic data from the Cannabis Youth Treatment (CYT) study. The CYT study, supported by the Center for Substance Abuse Treatment, examined different treatment approaches delivered to adolescents and their families (Dennis et al., 2002). Study goals included assessment of the effectiveness, full costs, and cost-effectiveness of the various treatment approaches. Researchers estimated the full costs of services delivery and reported economic cost estimates per total treatment episode ranging from $1,089 to $3,290 per adolescent; costs generally reflected intensity, duration, and number of services provided (for details, see French et al., 2002). The next steps will include combining these cost estimates with outcome data to conduct cost-effectiveness and cost–benefit analyses.

Diffusion of Research into Practice

Despite recent advances in treating adolescent drug abuse, far too little science-based treatment technology and knowledge makes its way into community treatment settings in a timely manner (Liddle et al., 2002; McLellan, 2002). Response to this perennial issue has progressed beyond simple exhortation of researchers to make studies more applied and findings more accessible to treatment providers. Efforts continue to package and deliver research findings to the field in easily digestible formats, including print media (e.g., Treatment Improvement Protocol Series, Technical Assistance Publication Series, both published by the Center for Substance Abuse Treatment, SAMHSA; NIDA Notes, published by NIDA), electronic media, conference presentations, hands-on workshops, and technical assistance. Researchers increasingly develop treatment manuals to assist practitioners in learning and adhering to specific evidence-based treatment practices. Along with this proliferation of treatment manuals, however, is the growing awareness that such manuals and other off-the-shelf products are useful but insufficient as stand-alone tools for accomplishing the technology transfer task (Godley, White, Diamond, Passetti, & Titus, 2001; Henggeler & Schoenwald, 2002). Fidelity to new treatment models—an important factor in the delivery of effective programs—is more complicated than following a manual.

Also important is what practitioners and community treatment agencies must do to efficiently capture and apply new knowledge and technologies in their organizations. As advances in treatment technology continue at an accelerating pace, practitioners and community service agencies need strategies for keeping abreast of the research and making informed selections from among the promising technologies available to them. This complicated process of continuous organizational change aimed at improvement is gaining attention in the field of drug abuse treatment (e.g., Lamb, Greenlick, & McCarty, 1998; Roman & Johnson, 2002). Simpson (2002), for example, integrated the organizational change literature and theory into a model for transferring research to practice in substance abuse treatment. The model involves four stages: *exposure* to new information, *adoption* or intention to try an innovation, *implementation* or trial use, and finally, *practice* or regular sustained use. Based on this model of technology transfer, Lehman, Greener, and Simpson (2002) developed an assessment tool for determining a treatment organization's readiness for change to assist researchers in studying change at the "receiving end" of the technology transfer process. The flow of research to practice is only a part of the system that needs to be developed, however. Greater and more effective inclusion of treatment providers in the research process is also called for—not simply as subjects of research, but as integral partners in research design, implementation, assessment, and technology transfer efforts (Brown & Flynn, 2002).

CONCLUSIONS

The world of substance abuse treatment for adolescents is changing rapidly. Efficacious therapies and other more comprehensive interventions are being developed at an accelerating pace. Nonetheless, challenges remain in delivering effective treatment services of adequate level, duration, intensity, and breadth to all youth who need them at the appropriate times in the youths' drug use and treatment careers. Meeting these challenges will require well-financed systems of care that recognize and accommodate drug abuse as the chronic relapsing condition that it is for many individuals. Much work needs to be done to establish an efficient system for both translating evidence-based treatments into practice and, conversely, using the treatment experiences and practical dilemmas of practitioners to inform new research. The time is right for a new generation of treatment services research to tackle these important public health issues by building on the recent and promising advances in the clinical treatment of adolescent drug abuse.

REFERENCES

Alcoholics Anonymous. (1976). *Alcoholics Anonymous: The story of how many thousands of men and women have recovered from alcoholism* (3rd ed.). New York: Alcoholics Anonymous World Services.

American Academy of Pediatrics. (2001). Improving substance abuse prevention, assessment, and treatment financing for children and adolescents. *Pediatrics, 108,* 1025–1029.

Anderson, D. W., Bowland, B. J., Cartwright, W. S., & Bassin, G. (1998). Service-level costing of drug abuse treatment. *Journal of Substance Abuse Treatment, 15,* 201–211.

Azrin, N. H, Donohue, B., Teichner, G. A., Crum, T., Howell, J., & DeCato, L. A. (2001). A controlled evaluation and description of individual-cognitive problem solving and family-behavior therapies in dually-diagnosed conduct-disordered and substance-dependent youth. *Journal of Child & Adolescent Substance Abuse, 11,* 1–43.

Barber, J. P., Luborsky, L., Gallop, R., Crits-Christoph, P., Frank, A., Weiss, R. D. et al. (2001). Therapeutic alliance as a predictor of outcome and retention in the National Institute on Drug Abuse Collaborative Cocaine Treatment Study. *Journal of Consulting and Clinical Psychology, 69,* 119–124.

Bonomo, Y., Coffey, C., Wolfe, R., Lynskey, M., Bowes, G., & Patton, G. (2001). Adverse outcomes of alcohol use in adolescents. *Addiction, 96,* 1485–1496.

Brown, B. S., & Flynn, P. M. (2002). The federal role in drug abuse technology transfer: A history and perspective. *Journal of Substance Abuse Treatment, 22*(4), 245–257.

Cartwright, W. S. (1998). Cost–benefit and cost-effectiveness analysis of drug abuse treatment services. *Evaluation Review, 22,* 609–636.

Cavanaugh, D. A. (2002). *Financing a system of care for adolescents with substance use disorders: Opportunities and challenges.* Paper prepared for the Robert Wood Johnson Foundation and presented for discussion at the Center for Substance Abuse Treatment's summit on adolescent systems of care (9/26–27/02).

Cohen, M. A. (1998). The monetary value of saving high-risk youth. *Journal of Quantitative Criminology, 14,* 5–33.

Cottrell, D., & Boston, P. (2002). Practitioner review: The effectiveness of family therapy for children and adolescents. *Journal of Child Psychology and Psychiatry, 43,* 573–586.

Crome, I. B. (1997). Editorial: Young people and substance problems—From image to imagination. *Drugs-Education Prevention and Policy, 4,* 107–116.

Crome, I. B. (1999). Treatment interventions—looking toward the millennium. *Drug and Alcohol Dependence, 55,* 247–263.

Deas, D., & Thomas, S. E. (2001). An overview of controlled studies of adolescent substance abuse treatment. *The American Journal on Addictions, 10,* 178–189.

Delany, P. J., Broome, K. M., Flynn, P. M., & Fletcher, B. W. (2001). Treatment service patterns and organizational structures: An analysis of programs in DATOS-A. *Journal of Adolescent Research, 16,* 590–607.

De Leon, G. (1997). Therapeutic communities: Is there an essential model? In G. De Leon (Ed.), *Community as method. Therapeutic communities for special populations and special settings* (pp. 3–18). Westport, CT: Praeger.

De Leon, G. (2000). *Therapeutic community—Theory, model, & method.* New York: Springer.

Dembo, R., & Schmeidler, J. (2003). Classification of high-risk youths. *Crime & Delinquency, 49,* 201–230.

Dennis, M. L. (2002). Treatment research on adolescent drug and alcohol abuse: Despite progress, many challenges remain. *Connection* (pp. 1–2, 7). Washington, DC: Academy-Health. http://www.academyhealth.org/publications/connection/may02.pdf

Dennis, M. L., & McGeary, K. A. (1999). Adolescent alcohol and marijuana treatment: Kids need it now. *TIE Communique* (pp. 10–12). Rockville, MD: Center for Substance Abuse Treatment.

Dennis, M. L., & Scott, C. K. (2002). Recovery management for chronic substance users: Preliminary evidence for a new paradigm. Presentation to the Division of Epidemiology, Services, and Prevention Research, NIDA, June 26, 2002, Rockville, MD.

Dennis, M. L., Titus, J. C., Diamond, G., Donaldson, J., Godley, S. H., Tims, F. et al. (2002). The Cannabis Youth Treatment (CYT) experiment: Rationale, study design and analysis plans. *Addiction, 97*(Suppl. 1), 16–34.

Dilonardo, J. D., Chalk, M., Mark, T. L., Coffey, R. M., & the CSAT/CMHS Spending Estimates Team. (2000). Recent trends in the financing of substance abuse treatment: Implications for the future. *Health Services Research, 35,* 60–71.

Duffy, S. Q. (2002). SAMHSA survey shows prevalence, characteristics of treatment facilities that offer programs for adolescents. *Connection* (pp. 3, 8). Washington, DC: Academy-Health.

Etheridge, R. M., Smith, J. C., Rounds-Bryant, J. L., & Hubbard, R. L. (2001). Drug treatment and comprehensive services for adolescents. *Journal of Adolescent Research, 16,* 563–589.

Fox, H. B., McManus, M. A., & Reichman, M. B. (2002). *Private health insurance for adolescents: Is it adequate?* Washington, DC: Maternal and Child Health Policy Research Center.

French, M. T. (1995). Economic evaluation of drug abuse treatment programs: Methodology and findings. *American Journal of Drug and Alcohol Abuse, 21,* 111–135.

French, M. T. (2001a). *Drug Abuse Treatment Cost Analysis Program (DATCAP): Program Version* (7th ed.). Coral Gables, FL: University of Miami. Available at http://www.DATCAP.com

French, M. T. (2001b). *Drug Abuse Treatment Cost Analysis Program (DATCAP): Program version user's manual* (7th ed.). Coral Gables, FL: University of Miami. Available at http://www.DATCAP.com

French, M. T., Roebuck, M. C., Dennis, M. L., Diamond, G., Godley, S. H., Tims, F. et al. (2002). The economic cost of outpatient marijuana treatment for adolescents: Findings from a multisite field experiment. *Addiction, 97*(Suppl. 1), 84–97.

Friedman, A. S., & Glickman, N. W. (1986). Program characteristics for successful treatment of adolescent drug abuse. *Journal of Nervous and Mental Disease, 174,* 669–679.

Friedmann, P. D., D'Aunno, T. A., Jin, L., & Alexander, J. A. (2000). Medical and psychosocial services in drug abuse treatment: Do stronger linkages promote client utilization? *Health Services Research, 35,* 443–465.

General Accounting Office. (1999). *Children's health insurance program: State implementation approaches are evolving.* Health, Education, and Human Services Division, GAO NO.: GAO/HEHS-99-65.

Geshan, S. (1999). Substance abuse benefits in state children's health insurance programs. *TIE Communique* (pp. 25–27). Rockville, MD: Center for Substance Abuse Treatment.

Gilvarry, E. (2000). Substance abuse in young people. *Journal of Child Psychology and Psychiatry and Allied Disciplines, 41,* 55–80.

Godley, M. D., Godley, S. H., Dennis, M. L., Funk, R., & Passetti, L. L. (2002). Preliminary outcomes from assertive continuing care experiment for adolescents discharged from residential treatment. *Journal of Substance Abuse Treatment, 23,* 21–32.

Godley, S. H., White, W. L., Diamond, G., Passetti, L., & Titus, J. C. (2001). Therapist reactions to manual-guided therapies for the treatment of adolescent marijuana use. *Clinical Psychology: Science and Practice, 8,* 405–417.

Golub, M. S. (2000). Adolescent health and the environment. *Environmental Health Perspectives, 108,* 355–362.

Greenbaum, P. E., Foster-Johnson, L., & Petrila, A. (1996). Co-occurring addictive and mental disorders among adolescents; Prevalence research and future directions. *American Journal of Orthopsychiatry, 66*, 52–60.

Halfors, D., Vevea, J. L., Iritani, B., Cho, H., Khatapoush, S., & Saxe, L. (2002). Truancy, grade point average, and sexual activity: A meta-analysis of risk indicators for youth substance use. *Journal of School Health, 72*, 205–211.

Harrison, P. A., & Fulkerson, J. (1996). *Minnesota student survey 1995: Prevalence of psychoactive substance use disorders.* St. Paul, MN: Department of Human Services.

Henggeler, S. W., Clingempeel, W. G., Brondino, M. J., & Pickrel, S. G. (2002). Four-year follow-up of multisystemic family therapy with substance-abusing and substance-dependent juvenile offenders. *Journal of American Academy of Adolescent Psychiatry, 41*, 868–874.

Henggeler, S. W., & Schoenwald, S. K. (2002). Treatment manuals: Necessary but far from sufficient. *Clinical Psychology: Science and Practice, 9*, 419–420.

Ho, A. P., Tsuang, J. W., Liberman, R. P., Wang, R., Wilkins, J. N., & Eckman, T. A. et al. (1999). Achieving effective treatment of patients with chronic psychotic illness and co-morbid substance dependence. *American Journal of Psychiatry, 156*, 1765–1770.

Horvath, A. O. (2001). The alliance. *Psychotherapy, 38*, 365–372.

Howell, E., Roschwald, S., & Salake, M. (2000). *Mental health and substance abuse services under the State Children's Health Insurance Program: Designing benefits and estimating costs.* Washington, DC: Mathematica Policy Research, Inc.

Hser, Y., Grella, C. E., Hubbard, R. L., Hsieh, S., Fletcher, B. W., Brown, B. S. et al. (2001). An evaluation of drug treatments for adolescents in 4 U.S. cities. *Archives of General Psychiatry, 58*, 689–695.

Jainchill, N. (2000). Substance dependency treatment for adolescents: Practice and research. *Substance Use and Misuse, 35*, 2031–2060.

Jainchill, N., Hawke, J., De Leon, G., & Yagelka, J. (2000). Adolescents in therapeutic communities: one-year posttreatment outcomes. *Journal of Psychoactive Drugs, 32*, 81–94.

Kaiser Commission on Medicaid and the Uninsured. (2002, May). *Health coverage for low-income children* (Fact Sheet). Retrieved May 7, 2003, from the World Wide Web. http://www.kff.org

Kelly, J. F., Myers, M. G., & Brown, S. A. (2000). A multivariate process model of adolescent 12-step attendance and substance abuse outcome following inpatient treatment. *Psychology of Addictive Behaviors, 14*, 376–389.

Kelly, J. F., Myers, M. G., & Brown, S. A. (2002). Do adolescents affiliate with 12-step groups? Multivariate process model of effects. *Journal of Studies on Alcohol, 63*, 293–304.

Kendall, P. C. (1991). *Child and adolescent therapy: Cognitive-behavioral procedures.* New York: Guilford.

Kendall, P. C., & Kessler, R. C. (2002). The impact of childhood psychopathology interventions on subsequent substance abuse: Policy implications, comments, and recommendations. *Journal of Consulting and Clinical Psychology, 70*, 1303–1306.

King, R. D., Gaines, L. S., Lambert, E. W., Summerfelt, W. T., & Bickman, L. (2000). The co-occurrence of psychiatric and substance use diagnoses in adolescents in different service systems: Frequency, recognition, cost, and outcomes. *Journal of Behavioral Health Services & Research, 27*, 417–430.

Kristiansen, P. L., & Hubbard, R. L. (2001). Methodological overview and research design for adolescents in the Drug Abuse Treatment Outcome Studies. *Journal of Adolescent Research, 16*, 545–562.

Lamb, S., Greenlick, M. R., & McCarty, D. (Eds.). (1998). *Bridging the gap between practice and research.* Washington, DC: National Academy Press.

Lehman, W. E., Greener, J. M., & Simpson, D. D. (2002). Assessing organizational readiness for change. *Journal of Substance Abuse Treatment, 22*(4), 197–209.

Liddle, H. A., Dakof, G. A., Parker, K., Diamond, G. S., Barrett, K., & Tejada, M. (2001). Multidimensional family therapy for adolescent drug abuse: Results of a randomized clinical trial. *American Journal of Drug and Alcohol Abuse, 27*, 651–688.

Liddle, H. A., Rowe, C. L., Quille, T. J., Dakof, G. A., Mills, D. S., Sakran, E. et al. (2002). Transporting an adolescent drug treatment into practice. *Journal of Substance Abuse Treatment, 22*, 231–243.

McLellan, A. T. (2002). Technology transfer and the treatment of addiction: What can research offer practice? *Journal of Substance Abuse Treatment, 22,* 169–170.

McLellan, A. T., Alterman, A. I., Metzger, D. S., Grissom, G. R., Woody, G. E., Luborsky, L. et al. (1994). Similarity of outcome predictors across opiate, cocaine, and alcohol treatment: Role of treatment services. *Journal of Consulting and Clinical Psychology, 62,* 1141–1158.

McLellan, A. T., Hagan, T. A., Levine, M., Meyers, K., Gould, F., Bencivengo, M. et al. (1999). Does clinical case management improve outpatient addiction treatment. *Drug and Alcohol Dependence, 55,* 91–103.

McLellan, A. T., Lewis, D. C., O'Brien, C. P., & Kleber, H. D. (2000). Drug dependence, a chronic medical illness: Implications for treatment, insurance, and outcome evaluation. *Journal of the American Medical Association, 284,* 1689–1695.

Muck, R., Zempolich, K. A., Titus, J. C., Fishman, M., Godley, M. D., & Schwebel, R. (2001). An overview of the effectiveness of adolescent substance abuse treatment models. *Youth & Society, 33,* 143–168.

National Institute on Drug Abuse. (2003, January 31). NIDA InfoFacts: Teen drug abuse—High school and youth trends. Retrieved May 7, 2003, from the World Wide Web. http://www.nida.nih.gov/Infofax/HSYouthtrends.html

Northwest Frontier Addiction Technology Transfer Center (NFATTC). (2000). *Advancing the current state of addiction treatment: A regional needs assessment of substance abuse treatment professionals in the pacific northwest.* Portland, OR: RMC Research Corp.

Perry, P. D. (2002). *Fragmented funding: Friend or foe? A multi-state case study of publicly supported adolescent alcohol and substance abuse treatment.* Paper presented at the CSAT/RWJF Adolescent Treatment Systems and Support Summit. Rockville, MD, September 26–27, 2002.

Pollio, D. E. (2002). States need to ensure expertise of adolescent providers through training and certification. *Connection.* Washington, DC: AcademyHealth.

Pond, A. S., Aguirre-Molina, M., & Orleans, J. (2002). *The adolescent substance abuse treatment workforce: Status, challenges, and strategies to address their particular needs.* Paper prepared for the RWJF and presented at the CSAT/RWJF Adolescent Treatment and Support Summit, Rockville, MD, September 26–27, 2002.

Robbins, M. S., Bacharach, K., & Szapocznik, J. (2002). Bridging the research-practice gap in adolescent substance abuse treatment: The case of brief strategic family therapy. *Journal of Substance Abuse Treatment, 23,* 123–132.

Roman, P. M., & Johnson, J. A. (2002). Adoption and implementation of new technologies in substance abuse treatment. *Journal of Substance Abuse Treatment, 22*(4), 211–218.

Rounds-Bryant, J. L., Kristiansen, P. L., & Hubbard, R. L. (1999). Drug abuse treatment outcome study of adolescents: A comparison of client characteristics and pretreatment behaviors in three treatment modalities. *American Journal of Drug and Alcohol Abuse, 25,* 573–591.

Rowe, C. L., & Liddle, H. A. (2003). Substance abuse. *Journal of Marital and Family Therapy, 29,* 97–120.

Rowe, C. L., Liddle, H. A., & Dakof, G. A. (2001). Classifying clinically referred adolescent substance abusers by level of externalizing and internalizing symptoms. *Journal of Child and Adolescent Substance Abuse, 11*(2), 41–65.

Siegal, H. A., Fisher, J. H., Rapp, R. C., Kelliher, C. W., Wagner, J. H., Obrien, W. F. et al. (1996). Enhancing substance abuse treatment with case management—Its impact on employment. *Journal of Substance Abuse Treatment, 13,* 93–98.

Simpson, D. D. (2002). A conceptual framework for transferring research to practice. *Journal of Substance Abuse Treatment, 22*(4), 171–182.

Solano, P. (1998, March). *Financing of drug treatment services: A review of the literature.* Task 2 Deliverable of Behavior and Health Research, Inc. Contract Number N01DA-5-6050.

Stevens, S. (2003). *Lessons from the field: Recruitment, retention and ethical considerations when working with substance involved women and adolescent girls.* Paper presented at "Recruitment and Retention of Participants in Drug Abuse Research: Incentives, Ethics, and Practical Considerations," as part of the conference. "Science Meets Reality: Recruitment and Retention of Women in Clinical Studies, and the Critical Role of Relevance," a symposium sponsored by the NIH, Office of Research on Women's Health, January 6–9, 2003, Washington, DC.

Substance Abuse and Mental Health Services Administration. (2002). *Results from the 2001 National Household Survey on Drug Abuse: Volume I. Summary of national findings.* Retrieved May 7, 2003, from the World Wide Web. http://www.samhsa.gov/oas/nhsda/ 2k1nhsda/vol1/toc.htm#v1

Tapert, S. F., Aarons, G. A., Sedlar, G. R., & Brown, S. A. (2001). Adolescent substance use and sexual risk-taking behavior. *Journal of Adolescent Health, 28,* 181–189.

Taylor, L. A., Kreutzer, J. S., Demm, S. R., & Meade, M. A. (2003). Traumatic brain injury and substance abuse: A review and analysis of the literature. *Neuropsychological Rehabilitation, 13,* 165–188 [Special Issue].

White, W. L. (1998). *Slaying the dragon: A history of addiction and recovery in America.* Bloomington, IL: Lighthouse Institute Publications.

Williams, R. J., & Chang, S. Y. (2000). A comprehensive and comparative review of adolescent substance abuse treatment outcome. *Clinical Psychology: Science and Practice, 7,* 138–166.

Winters, K. C., Latimer, W., & Stinchfield, R. (1999). Adolescent treatment. In P. J. Ott, R. E. Tarter, & R. T. Ammerman (Eds.), *Sourcebook on substance abuse: Etiology, epidemiology, assessment, and treatment* (pp. 350–361). Boston: Allyn and Bacon.

Winters, K. C., Stinchfield, R. D., Opland, E., Weller, C., & Latimer, W. W. (2000). The effectiveness of the Minnesota Model approach in the treatment of adolescent drug abusers. *Addiction, 95,* 601–612.

13

Targeted Prevention of Antisocial Behavior in Children

The Early Risers "Skills for Success" Program

MICHAEL L. BLOOMQUIST, GERALD J. AUGUST, SUSANNE S. LEE, BARRIE E. BERQUIST, and ROBIN MATHY

The onset of aggression and conduct problems during the early childhood years paves the way for the development of a pattern of serious antisocial behavior, including violence, substance abuse, and criminal offending during adolescence and young adulthood (Hinshaw & Lee, 2003). This developmental progression, however, is not inevitable. Indeed, the relative balance between risk and protective factors experienced along this pathway appears to determine whether these aggressive children ultimately experience deviant or healthy outcomes (Tolan, Guerra, & Kendall, 1995).

Risk factors for antisocial behavior emerge across multiple levels. Child risk factors typically pertain to individual characteristics such as difficult temperament, deficient emotional regulation, learning delays, and deficiencies or distortions in social information processing. Parental risk factors include depression, substance abuse, negative attributions, and unrealistic expectations. Familial risk factors center on economic hardship, social isolation, and marital discord. These factors become manifest in coercive

MICHAEL L. BLOOMQUIST, GERALD J. AUGUST, SUSANNE S. LEE, BARRIE E. BERQUIST, and ROBIN MATHY • Department of Psychiatry, University of Minnesota Medical School, Minneapolis, Minnesota 55454.

parent–child relationships, family violence, and instability. Peer rejection, school failure, and affiliation with deviant friends are risk factors that can emerge during the middle childhood years. Social contexts characterized by depraved neighborhoods, substandard schools, and unsupervised recreational facilities can also constitute significant risk factors for children growing up in economically disadvantaged communities (see Hinshaw & Lee, 2003, for a review).

Protective factors insulate children from risks associated with the development of antisocial behavior. They promote a more normative or resilient developmental pathway related to positive developmental outcomes despite the existence of risks. Children's protective factors include academic success, positive social skills, prosocial peer relations, and positive attitudes toward school. Protective factors within a child's environment include having caregivers who employ supportive and authoritative parenting, teachers who encourage children to become connected to their school, and community institutions that provide opportunities and resources for children to develop prosocial skills and positive friendships (see Masten & Coatsworth, 1998, for a review).

The goals of early intervention and prevention programs for aggressive children who are at risk of developing antisocial behavior are to reduce the impact of risk factors and enhance the influence of protective factors. If these goals are accomplished, children are expected to develop more healthy outcomes as they mature into adolescence (Yoshikawa, 1994). Increasingly, a "developmental-ecological and multisystemic" framework has guided intervention and prevention of antisocial behavior (Bloomquist & Schnell, 2002; Henggeler, Schoenwald, Borduin, Rowland, & Cunningham, 1998; Tolan et al., 1995). The goal of this framework is to modify cumulative risk over the developmental age periods and across multiple intersecting systemic domains, including child, parent and family, school, peer, and community contexts. Intervention designs informed by this approach are thus multifaceted with components for the child (e.g., academic enrichment, social competence training), parents (e.g., support, behavioral skills training), and school (e.g., classroom-wide behavioral management systems, life skills curriculum) (see Bloomquist & Schnell, 2002, for a review).

Targeted prevention incorporates both selective and indicated prevention approaches (Gordon, 1983). Selective preventive interventions focus on individuals who are not yet showing any symptoms of developing problems despite being at heightened risk. The risk ranges from imminent to lifetime based on family history, exposure to adverse life events, or living in unhealthy environments. Indicated preventive interventions are directed at high-risk individuals who already display early symptoms of developing a problem.

The most promising targeted prevention programs designed to date are for children at risk for antisocial behavior. These include the Montreal Prevention Experiment (Vitaro, Brendgen, Pagani, Tremblay, & McDuff, 1999); The Fast Track Program (Conduct Problems Prevention Research Group, 2002); the Metropolitan Area Child Study (Metropolitan Area Child Study Research Group, 2002); the Incredible Years: Parents, Teachers, and

Children Training Series (Webster-Stratton & Reid, 2003); and the First Steps to Success Program (Walker et al., 1998). Collectively, findings from controlled studies have demonstrated the beneficial effect of these programs in modifying proximal variables such as children's social skills and parents' behavior management skills. Research evaluating the impact of these programs on distal outcomes, such as reductions in the prevalence of conduct disorders, school dropout, and drug abuse in adolescence and adulthood is currently underway.

The Early Risers "Skills for Success" Program is another example of a targeted prevention program. Early Risers has been developed and evaluated by this chapter's authors.[1] The remainder of this chapter describes the organizational structure, operational structure, and program structure of the Early Risers model. Within each component, evidence-based "best practices" that inform the Early Risers Program are presented. We briefly discuss training, supervision, and fidelity procedures. We conclude this chapter with an overview of research evaluation as well as future plans for wide-scale dissemination of the Early Risers Program.

THE EARLY RISERS MODEL OF TARGETED PREVENTION

The Early Risers model is a targeted prevention program for children who screen positive for the presence of aggression in the early elementary grades, and who often live within a poverty context. Comprehensive and coordinated intervention services are delivered for 2 or 3 years to qualifying children and their families in home or community settings. Child- and family-focused intervention components, known as "CHILD" and "FAMILY," respectively, are provided (see Table 1). The overarching goals of the Early Risers Program are to enhance children's functioning in self-regulation, social, and academic developmental domains, while facilitating family functioning and parenting skills. As a result, it is hypothesized that children's social, behavioral, affective, and academic developmental competencies are enhanced (August, Anderson, & Bloomquist, 1992), and bonds between the child, parents, prosocial peers, and the school institution are strengthened (Catalano & Hawkins, 1996), thereby preventing later antisocial behavior.

Organizational Structure

The Early Risers Program is modeled after a "community systems of care" approach (Burns & Goldman, 1999), and as such, it features comprehensive and coordinated services designed to help the child and family experience a seamless array of education, training, advocacy, support, and specialized health services. Its administrative design includes a partnership of collaborators who represent community schools, community health

---

[1]Other colleagues who have been part of the program development and evaluation are George Realmuto, M.D., Elizabeth Eagan, Ph.D., and Joel Hektner, Ph.D. at the University of Minnesota.

Table 1. Overview of Early Risers "Skills For Success" Program Interventions Components

---

CHILD component
1. Summer Program—Children attend a 6- to 8-week summer program focusing on social skills, reading enrichment or tutoring, and recreation.
2. "Circles of Friends" Program—Children attend weekly groups focusing on social skills, reading enrichment or tutoring, and recreation during the school year.
3. Monitoring and Mentoring School Support Program—Each child's academic functioning and school adjustment is systematically monitored and school-based interventions are provided according to each child's level of need throughout the school year. Interventions include goal setting or attainment strategies, reading enrichment, tutoring, consultation with teachers, and facilitating involvement of parents around school issues.

FAMILY component
1. Family Skills Program—A needs-adjusted parent-focused intervention is provided during the school year to enhance parent's knowledge of child development, and parenting skills, and to improve broader family interactions.
2. Family Support Program—Each family's functioning is systematically monitored throughout the duration of the Early Risers Program, and home-based interventions are provided according to each family's level of need. Interventions include goal setting or goal attainment strategies, and assisting families in accessing community services.

Note: These intervention components are delivered over 2 or 3 years, and modified thereafter for booster follow-up services.

or social services agencies, and university-based prevention specialists. Usually one service provider assumes primary responsibility for delivering Early Risers, but community partners contribute resources (e.g., financial, office space, personnel, etc.), or coordinate in service provision. These partners are also jointly involved in ongoing oversight of the Early Risers Program.

Operational Structure

Staffing and Logistics

The program can be delivered within a variety of community sites such as faith centers, neighborhood service centers, YMCAS, and YWCAS. However, schools appear to provide the optimal milieu. Program staff is typically recruited from within the ranks of one of the collaborating community agencies or from the schools. The primary service provider for the program is the community prevention specialist, more commonly referred to as the program's "family advocate." The typical family advocate has a bachelor's degree and several years of professional experience working with children and families in education or human service settings. A full-time family advocate can serve a caseload of up to 25 children and their families. "Child assistants" (i.e., paraprofessionals) help the family advocates deliver the CHILD programs. In a large-scale implementation where more than one family advocate is employed, a program manager is necessary to coordinate program activities, provide onsite supervision of the family advocates, and maintain oversight of program fidelity. In a more recent expansion of the program, a part-time licensed master's-level mental health professional was added to the program staff. This person is involved primarily with the FAMILY component serving as a consultant for the family advocate, or as a direct provider to those families who are experiencing more serious mental health problems. Whenever possible, consultants from various community agencies are identified to assist family advocates in locating and utilizing appropriate community resources and services for their families.

Child Screening and Recruitment Procedures

In a large-scale implementation of a targeted program, screening is necessary to efficiently identify at-risk children (August, Realmuto, Crosby, & MacDonald, 1995). Population-based screening of at-risk children is a sensitive issue as selection errors are to be expected (e.g., false-positive or false-negative errors). Problems related to labeling, stigma, and iatrogenic effects need to be given careful consideration in designing a screening devise. The Early Risers' Program employs a population-based procedure to identify children in early elementary school (e.g., K, 1st, and 2nd grades) who appear to be at elevated risk for developing antisocial behavior. Screening is typically performed by classroom teachers who are asked to complete a standardized behavior rating scale (e.g., Child Behavior Checklist–Teacher Rating Form) on all eligible students in their classes (eligibility criteria include consent to screen from parents). Children who are qualified for participation in the prevention intervention include those who receive scores on keyed aggressive and disruptive items that place them above a specified threshold. The specified threshold can vary from 10% to 30% of the student enrollment, depending on the community site of the program, perceived need of the program in the community, and available resources.

Children who qualify for participation are subsequently recruited. The family advocate conducts recruitment during a home visit. The family advocate describes the screening results and explains the goals and intended outcomes of the Early Risers Program. Parents are given a brochure that provides details on all program activities and names of staff to contact if questions arise.

Program Structure

CHILD Component

CHILD is offered continuously throughout the year. The recommended sequence begins with the 6-week Summer Program, followed by the "Circle of Friends" Program, and then the Monitoring and Mentoring School Support Program during the regular school year.

Summer Program. Research shows that over the summer months many high-risk children lose ground in academics and social skills (Cooper, Nye, Charlton, & Lindsay, 1996). Hence, a summer program provides opportunities to deliver intensive and focused programming to children who need them most.

The Early Risers Summer Program is adapted from the Pelham and Hoza (1996) summer treatment program for elementary-aged children with attention-deficit/hyperactivity disorder or oppositional defiant disorder. Children in the Pelham and Hoza program receive intensive behavioral, social, milieu, recreational, and education-focused interventions. These interventions are delivered 5 days per week over 8 weeks during the summer. Pelham and Hoza found that children who attended their summer treatment program exhibited significant improvements on ratings by parents, program counselors, teachers, and self-reports in the areas of behavior, social skill development, and improved self-esteem.

Program modifications were made to the Early Risers Summer Program from Pelham and Hoza (1996) to accommodate the slightly younger age group it serves as well as to facilitate its prevention focus. The program takes place Monday through Friday for 6–8 weeks (typically mid-June to mid-August). Previously, the Early Risers Summer Program has been conducted in both full- and half-day formats. The half-day format typically offers social skills training (1 hour), reading enrichment (1 hour), and cultural and creative arts activities (1 hour). The full-day format typically provides an additional 3-hour academic component, as well. Ten to 15 children are organized into a "track" with 2 or 3 staff (i.e., family and child assistants). In previous applications of the program, peer mentors were recruited to serve as positive role models and to provide opportunities for the at-risk children to develop friendships with prosocial children.

"Circle of Friends" Program. Each child is invited to attend the "Circle of Friends" Program during the academic year. The children attend a 90–120 minute group held one afternoon or evening per week. The group focuses on social competence training, which is augmented with reading skills enhancement, homework assistance, and recreational activities. Some children also attend a regularly scheduled after-school program offered by the school or community center on alternative weekdays. One evening per month, family members attend a parent–child activity consisting of food, recognition ceremonies, entertainment, and games.

Monitoring and Mentoring School Support Program. This program is based on an adaptation of Christenson and colleagues' "Check and Connect" model of school-based services for elementary through high-school-aged children (Christenson, Sinclair, Lehr, & Hurley, 2000). In Check and Connect, practitioners engage in systematic monitoring of each child's behavior and academic status at school, and provide advocacy, direct services, and service coordination. The overall goal is to promote coordination among the child, family, and school. In Check and Connect, all students receive "basic interventions" that include monitoring and problem solving about specific issues that emerge in the context of school. Children who are at higher risk receive "intensive services." Services include practical interventions, facilitating home–school collaboration, and assisting the child and family in accessing school-based services. Christenson et al. reported that the Check and Connect program reduced school absences and tardiness in elementary through high school populations. It also improved children's overall school adjustment, and reduced the likelihood that they would drop out.

In Early Risers, the Monitoring and Mentoring School Support Program is delivered as a needs-adjusted intervention with monitoring of all program children and mentoring tailored to the assessed needs of each child. The monitoring component is implemented in the form of three annual monitoring assessments (fall, winter, spring) conducted in collaboration with the child's teacher. Indicators of child adjustment that are assessed over time include (1) absenteeism per month, (2) behavioral classroom management concerns, (3) academic difficulties, (4) bus incidents or behavioral referrals, and (5) level of parental involvement regarding child problems. Children are then classified into three levels of need, including Level 1 (low need), Level 2 (moderate need), and Level 3 (high need). Subsequent delivery of services corresponds to these levels of need.

Of the approximately 25 children on a family advocate caseload, all qualify for some monitoring, but typically only 5–15 children who are in greatest need require individualized mentoring services. All children enrolled in Early Risers receive the Level 1 monitoring portion of the intervention. The monitoring involves systematic collection and evaluation of pertinent school adjustment information (as discussed above). If a problem is discovered through Level 1 monitoring, children are then eligible for two levels of mentoring services. Level 2 or "basic" mentoring services are provided to children with moderate needs or problems. Level 2 services include at least biweekly visits with the child and episodic consultation with teachers as indicated. Child-centered activities include encouragement of academic achievement, contracting for improved behavior in the school, and individualized training of social skills and problem-solving skills. Level 3 or "intensive" mentoring services include child-focused academic tutoring, intensive individualized social skills training, or referrals for additional school- or community-based services. Early Risers' parents are almost always involved in some fashion with Level 3 mentoring. Often there is a need to coordinate one or more parent–teacher meetings to synchronize home and school. Parents are encouraged to attend school functions and conferences, to communicate with teachers, to assist with homework, to encourage their child's reading, and to share information with the teacher.

FAMILY Component

FAMILY is modeled in part, after the Triple P—Positive Parenting Program (Sanders, Turner, & Markie-Dadds, 2002). Triple P is a multilevel system of parent and family education and support. The Early Risers' FAMILY component includes the Family Skills Program and the Family Support Program. Both programs are organized around a predetermined level of family need. This level of need is determined by either an informal family assessment or a formal interview-based assessment. Family advocates organize available information including their observations, expressed family concerns, and results from standardized questionnaires to determine (1) the child's functioning, (2) the parents' personal functioning, and (3) whether or not the family's basic physical and emotional needs are being fulfilled. Each family's need is designated on a continuum ranging from Level 1 (low need) to Level 2 (moderate need) to Level 3 (high need).

Family Skills Program. The Early Risers Family Skills Program provides information and specific skills training to enhance a parent's child management and personal coping skills, and broader family interactions. To accomplish this, the interventions utilized in the Family Skills Program include (1) training parents in child management procedures, (2) facilitating the parent–child relationship through play and bonding strategies, (3) teaching personal coping strategies, and (4) improving familial interaction skills. In Early Risers, the Family Skills Program is offered according to the levels of need described earlier. Levels 1, 2, and 3 provide increasingly intensive services.

All parents in the Early Risers Program are offered Level 1 programming. Participating families receive one to two, 60–90-minute sessions delivered in the home. Sessions focus on global parenting and normal child development. Families receive information about normal stages of child development addressing social, emotional, and academic domains, and associated parenting challenges. During the initial in-home session(s), parents are invited to a "Parents Excited About Kids (PEAK)" parent group. The PEAK group is offered at the school or community center. This program is information-oriented and delivered over eight, 90–120-minute sessions. Four of these sessions are based on the Triple P "Tips Sheets" concept (Sanders et al., 2002). The tip sheets give parents ideas to manage common child problems such as self-esteem, homework, behavior at school, chores, bedtime, tantrums, and so on. The final four sessions is based on parent-generated topics that can be delivered by the family advocate with the assistance of outside speakers. If parents are unable or unwilling to attend the PEAK group, an attempt is made to deliver an abbreviated version of this intervention during the in-home Family Support Program visits (described in the next section).

The program manager or mental health professional delivers Level 2 groups known as PEAK-2. This intervention typically involves approximately 15–25% of the families. Parents are encouraged to attend the PEAK-1 group prior to participating in the PEAK-2 group. Parents are invited to attend the PEAK-2 groups if their child is displaying moderate-to-severe behavior problems and the family is judged to be functional. PEAK-2 consists of eight, 60-minute sessions and focuses on behavioral strategies targeting specific problematic behaviors (e.g., aggression, oppositional behavior, and stealing). Topics or areas of focus are selected from a menu to meet the apparent unique needs of the attending families in a particular group. The areas of focus might include promoting children's social and educational development, observing and tracking child behavior, child-directed interaction and play, shaping positive behavior, ignoring mild negative behavior, defusing power struggles, deescalating parent–child conflict, time out or removal of privileges for noncompliance, standing or house rules, and monitoring or supervising children. Again, if parents do not attend the PEAK-2 group, elements of it are offered during Family Support Program home visits.

Level 3 is an in-home intervention delivered by a mental health professional. The focus is on severe child, parent, or family problems. Approximately 5–10% of families need this level of service. Ideally parents or families are referred to this service after they have completed Level 1 and Level 2 interventions. Level 3 is an individually tailored intervention of about eight to twelve, 60-minute sessions. The focus is on behavioral strategies to change targeted child behavior (e.g., aggression, defiance, and stealing), and also on parent or family problems (e.g., parent depression, stress, and relationship problems). Areas of focus are individualized for each family. They might include some child-focused strategies provided in Level 2, as well as use of a token system, specific interventions for stealing, parent stress management, cognitive restructuring of parent thoughts, or family-wide interaction skills such as problem solving, communication, and conflict resolution. In addition, referrals to other more intensive community-based services are also part of this intervention.

The Family Skills Program is provided over 2 years. The first year calls for delivery of the sessions as described above. Year 2 is basically for maintenance and reinforcement of previously learned skills. This takes place as family advocates interact with the families during in-home Family Support Program meetings. During the second year, the PEAK-1 and PEAK-2 groups described for year 1 can also be offered to families who did not previously participate or who may have changed levels over the year. If a third year of family skills programming is offered, it tends to be more informal, activity-based, and centered around topics and activities that are of specific interest to the children and families. The goal of the third year is to maintain previous gains by providing periodic contact with the family members.

Family Support Program. Our approach to family support is modeled after the Family-Centered Intensive Case Management program (Evans, Armstrong, & Kuppinger, 1996). In this program, case managers assess the needs of each family, develop a service plan for each family, link each family to needed services, coordinate meetings between the family and service providers, and monitor each family's ongoing needs and outcomes. Essentially, the case manager provides direct interventions, assists families in developing informal support systems, and functions as an advocate for the family within the community and at school. Evans et al. found that Family-Centered Intensive Case Management resulted in improvements in child and family functioning for children aged 5–12 years who had a wide range of adjustment problems.

Similarly, the Early Risers Family Support Program is a tailored case management-anchored delivery system, composed of three key elements. These core elements include (1) determining a family's level of need by assessing family functioning (discussed earlier), (2) setting strategic goals to achieve family, parent, and child stability, and (3) linking families to community resources and services in order to assist them in meeting the goals for their child or family. Family support services are delivered primarily within the context of a home visitation model. Thus, family advocates typically drive to the home of the family for face-to-face visits or contacts. If needed, however, the family support interventions can be delivered in a community center, a local restaurant, a child's school, or some other agreed-upon location. Families are assigned a set number of visits or contacts determined by their level of need. They are prescribed a minimum of 4, 6, and 12 visits at Levels 1, 2, and 3, respectively. The exact number of contacts can be adjusted if necessary. The success of the Family Support Program is dependent upon the quality of the relationship between the family advocate and the family, and the ability of the family advocate to assist the family in accessing the community resources it needs.

Of the approximately 25 families on a family advocate caseload, typically only 5–10 families require high-level services at any one point in time. Family advocates work with family members to set and achieve personal and child-centered goals. Progress toward achieving goals is determined via a goal attainment scaling methodology. A menu of brief interventions and service options are made available to the family. These include assisting families in advocating for their child at school, accessing community-based therapeutic services, accessing social or human services, and other such options.

Training, Supervision, and Fidelity

The Early Risers training, supervision, and fidelity protocol is guided by the Multisystemic Therapy Program example (Henggeler et al., 1998). Training for all staff is conducted by university prevention specialists in a standardized fashion. Each staff member is given a detailed Early Risers Program Manual that describes all intervention components and provides many useful forms to assist with screening, recruitment, intervention provision, documentation, and fidelity monitoring. The initial Early Risers training protocol involves a 4-day training seminar. All staff is required to demonstrate mastery over all aspects of service delivery and be "checked out" by training staff before completing training. Thereafter, training staff remains available to intervention staff for ongoing consultation on an as-needed basis.

The program manager provides ongoing supervision of intervention staff in a group format. This format allows opportunities for family advocates to collaborate on program issues, permits staff to brainstorm resolutions to problems or access resources, and furnishes ample opportunities for role play, modeling, and rehearsal. Periodic individual supervision with each family advocate helps provide feedback and correction of intervention sessions and also serves as an opportunity to review case management notes. The program manager and community consultant assist the family advocates in determining the level of child and family need, intervention planning, family goal setting, action plans, intervention options, and assist family advocates in locating resources.

The fidelity of program delivery is monitored throughout. Information is systematically collected and reviewed by the university prevention specialist and the program manager. This includes examination of child and parent attendance, documentation of services provided, direct observation of intervention provision, and consumer satisfaction data. Adjustments in programming, staffing, and training are made based on fidelity monitoring.

TRANSFERRING EARLY RISERS FROM RESEARCH TO PRACTICE

Early Risers was developed with the ultimate goal of utilization in "real world" practice settings. Efficacy and small-scale effectiveness studies were conducted prior to exporting it to broader practice settings. First, an Early Risers' efficacy study was conducted in schools located in four semirural communities in Minnesota. Across these communities, 20 elementary schools were matched for relevant SES variables and randomly assigned to program or control conditions. Kindergarten children in the 20 schools were screened by their classroom teachers for aggressive behavior. Those who met high-risk criteria were enrolled in the study (124 program, 121 control). The prevention trial began in the summer following the kindergarten year and ran continuously for 5 years. Three of the 5 years included intensive intervention, followed by 2 years of "booster" intervention at which time participants had completed the fifth grade. An evaluation conducted following the first 2 years of intervention indicated that program children made significantly greater gains in academic achievement and classroom behaviors than the controls. Only the most severely aggressive children, however, showed reductions in behavioral problems (e.g., aggression, hyperactivity, and impulsivity) (August, Realmuto, Hektner, & Bloomquist, 2001). These effects were maintained following a third program year and complemented by gains in social skills and adaptability (August, Hektner, Egan, Realmuto, & Bloomquist, 2002). At a 4-year evaluation, evidence for generalization of program effects via peer assessments in the natural school setting was found. Relative to controls, program children were viewed by their peers as higher in leadership and social etiquette, and they chose friends who were lower in aggression (August, Egan, Realmuto, & Hektner, 2003).

With validation of the program established, the next step was to transport the program to a community setting and determine if program effects could be sustained when delivered by community practitioners in a natural practice setting. The Early Risers effectiveness study was conducted in an urban, economically disadvantaged community with mostly African American families. Pillsbury United Communities in Minneapolis was the primary service delivery agency adopting the program. Pillsbury United Communities is a nonprofit agency that offers a network of neighborhood family centers strategically located in high-risk neighborhoods throughout the city. The overall strategy of this effectiveness trial was to provide a program support infrastructure to the agency (e.g., manuals, preprogram training, ongoing supervision and technical assistance, and regular monitoring of intervention fidelity with feedback and correction). However, the host agency was allowed to make program implementation adaptations in response to constraints faced by the agency. Kindergarten and 1st-grade children enrolled in 10 Minneapolis public schools were screened for aggressive behavior, randomized into program and control conditions, and recruited for the study. The program was implemented over a 2-year period. It included a baseline assessment followed by annual evaluations thereafter. In comparison to the efficacy study, low rates of client participation plagued this effectiveness study. Only half of the child participants attended at least half of the child sessions. Despite these problems, outcome analyses showed program-related benefits. Similar to the results of the efficacy study, the children who participated in the Early Risers Program made significant gains in social competence and school adjustment with only the most severely aggressive children showing reductions in externalizing behavior problems (August, Lee, Bloomquist, Realmuto, & Hektner, 2003). Academic achievement gains found in the efficacy study were not replicated in the effectiveness research.

The next step is to turn the program completely over to community provider systems and determine whether the program can be successfully implemented with minimum program support services provided by the program developers. A pilot practice initiative is currently under way in Hennepin County, Minnesota. In this effort, the same intervention components and administrative units as the Early Risers effectiveness study are being utilized. The Hennepin County Children, Families, and Adult Services Department will provide contractual oversight of the program and pay for the standardized CHILD—Summer, CHILD—Circle of Friends, and FAMILY—Family Skills Programs by unit of service delivered. Medical Assistance Targeted Child Welfare Case Management will be billed by unit of service delivered for the case management-orientated CHILD—Monitoring and Mentoring School Support and FAMILY—Family Support Programs. Maximum effort will be expended to improve attendance of participants in the program by emphasizing school-based and in-home delivery practices. A program evaluation study is planned to determine the level of engagement (feasibility) and pre-to–post-changes (impact).

SUMMARY

In this chapter we presented a comprehensive preventive intervention, the Early Risers "Skills for Success" Program. Early Risers is an example of a targeted prevention intervention designed to alter the developmental pathway leading to antisocial behavior in at-risk children as indexed by the presence of early-onset aggressive behavior. The CHILD and FAMILY components have been designed to reduce risk factors and promote protective factors over time across child, family, peer group, school and community systems. Randomized controlled studies provided evidence for the program's positive effect on child's proximal outcome variables such as reduced aggressive behavior and enhanced social skills. There is also evidence that the Early Risers Program can be successfully implemented by community practitioners in community settings. The Early Risers

Program's effectiveness in preventing the onset and continuation of antisocial behavior as these high-risk children enter adolescence will be determined through ongoing longitudinal research.

REFERENCES

August, G. J., Anderson, D., & Bloomquist, M. L. (1992). Competence enhancement training for children: An integrated child, parent, and school approach. In S. Christenson & J. C. Conoley (Eds.), *Home-school collaboration: Enhancing children's academic and social competence* (pp. 175–213). Silver Springs, MD: National Association of School Psychologists.

August, G. J., Egan, B. A., Realmuto, G. R., & Hektner, J. M. (2003). Parceling component effects of a comprehensive prevention program for disruptive elementary school children: Testing predictors of participation and outcome across individual intervention components. *Journal of Abnormal Child Psychology, 31*, 515–527.

August, G. J., Hektner, J. M., Egan, B. A., Realmuto, G. M., & Bloomquist. M. L. (2002). The Early Risers longitudinal prevention trial: Examination of 3-year outcomes in aggressive children with intent-to-treat and as-intended analyses. *Psychology of Addictive Behaviors 16*, (Suppl. 4), 27–39.

August, G. J., Lee, S. S., Bloomquist, M. L., Realmuto, G. M., & Hektner, J. M. (2003). Dissemination of an evidence-based prevention innovation for aggressive children living in culturally diverse, urban neighborhoods: The Early Risers effectiveness study. *Prevention Science, 4*, 271–286.

August, G. J., Realmuto, G. M., Crosby, R. D., & MacDonald, A. W., III (1995). Community-based multiple-gate screening of children at risk for conduct disorder. *Journal of Abnormal Child Psychology, 23*, 521–543.

August, G. J., Realmuto, G. M., Hektner, J. M., & Bloomquist, M. L. (2001). An integrated components preventive intervention for aggressive elementary school children: The "Early Risers" program. *Journal of Consulting and Clinical Psychology, 69*, 614–626.

Bloomquist, M. L., & Schnell, S. V. (2002). *Helping children with aggression and conduct problems: Best practices for intervention.* New York: Guilford.

Burns, B. J., & Goldman, S. K. (Eds.). (1999). *Systems of care: Promising practices in Children's Mental Health, 1998 Series, Volume IV: Promising practices in wraparound for children with serious emotional disturbance and their families.* Washington, DC: Center for Effective Collaboration and Practice, American Institute for Research.

Catalano, R. R., & Hawkins, J. D. (1996). The social development model: A theory of antisocial behavior. In J. D. Hawkins (Ed.), *Delinquency and crime: Current theories.* New York: Springer-Verlag.

Christenson, S. L., Sinclair, M. F., Lehr, C. A., & Hurley, C. M. (2000). Promoting successful school completion. In D. Minke & G. Bear (Eds.), *Preventing school problems-promoting school success: Strategies and programs that work* (pp. 224–240). Bethesda, MD: National Association of School Psychologists.

Conduct Problems Prevention Research Group. (2002). Evaluation of the first 3 years of the Fast Track prevention trial with children at high risk for adolescent conduct problems. *Journal of Abnormal Child Psychology, 30*, 19–35.

Cooper, H., Nye, B., Charlton, K., & Lindsay, J. (1996). The effects of summer vacation on achievement test scores: A narrative and meta-analytic review. *Review of Educational Research, 66*, 227–268.

Evans, M. E., Armstrong, M .I., & Kuppinger, A. D. (1996). Family-Centered Intensive Case Management: A step toward understanding individualized care. *Journal of Child and Family Studies, 5*, 55–65.

Gordon, R. S. (1983). An operational classification of disease prevention. *Public Health Reports, 98*, 107–109.

Henggeler, S. W., Schoenwald, S. K., Borduin, C. M., Rowland, M. D., & Cunningham, P. B. (1998). *Multisystemic treatment of antisocial behavior in children and adolescents.* New York: Guilford Press.

Hinshaw, S. P., & Lee, S. S. (2003). Conduct and oppositional defiant disorders. In E. J. Mash & R. A. Barkley (Eds.), *Child psychopathology* (2nd ed., pp. 144–198). New York: Guilford.

Masten, A. S., & Coatsworth, J. D. (1998). The development of competence in favorable and unfavorable environments: Lessons from research on successful children. *American Psychologist, 53,* 205–220.

Metropolitan Area Child Study Research Group. (2002). A cognitive-ecological approach to preventing aggression in urban settings: Initial outcomes for high-risk children. *Journal of Consulting and Clinical Psychology, 70,* 179–194.

Pelham, W., & Hoza, B. (1996). Intensive treatment: Summer treatment program for children with ADHD. In E. D. Hibbs & P. S. Jenson (Eds.), *Psychosocial treatment for child and adolescent disorders: Empirically based strategies for clinical practice* (pp. 311–340). Washington, DC: American Psychological Association.

Sanders, M. R., Turner, K. M. T., & Markie-Dadds, C. (2002). The development and dissemination of the Triple P-Positive Parenting Program: A multilevel, evidence-based system of parenting and family support. *Prevention Science, 3,* 173–189.

Tolan, P. H., Guerra, N. G., & Kendall, P. (1995). A developmental-ecological perspective on antisocial behavior in children and adolescents. *Journal of Consulting and Clinical Psychology, 63,* 579–584.

Vitaro, F., Brendgen, M., Pagani, L., Tremblay, R. E., & McDuff, P. (1999). Disruptive behavior, peer association, and conduct disorder: Testing the developmental links through early intervention. *Development and Psychopathology, 11,* 287–304.

Walker, H. M., Kavanagh, K., Stiller, B., Golly, A., Severson, H. H., & Feil, E. G. (1998). First step to success: An early intervention approach for preventing school antisocial behavior. *Journal of Emotional and Behavioral Disorders, 6,* 66–80.

Webster-Stratton, C., & Reid, M. J. (2003). The incredible years parents, teachers, and children training series: A multifaceted treatment approach for young children with conduct problems. In A. E. Kazdin & J. R. Weisz (Eds.), *Evidence-based psychotherapies for children and adolescents.* (pp. 224–240). New York: Guilford.

Yoshikawa, H. (1994). Prevention as cumulative protection: Effects of early family support and education on chronic delinquency and its risks. *Psychological Bulletin, 115,* 28–54.

14

Implementing Effective Youth Violence Prevention Programs in Community Settings

PATRICIA A. GRACZYK and PATRICK H. TOLAN*

The past decade has seen remarkable growth in the field of youth violence prevention. There is an increased understanding of the biological and contextual factors that place youth at risk for violence, enhanced awareness of the importance of identifying protective factors, and a proliferation of rigorously designed empirical studies that has allowed for the categorization of many prevention efforts as efficacious, promising, or ineffective. As society's view of youth violence shifts from one that perceives youth violence solely as a juvenile justice issue to a broader perspective that recognizes youth violence as a public health issue, greater attention is being focused on: clarifying the nature of youth violence and patterns in its occurrence and prevalence; using epidemiological methodologies to identify putative causal, risk, and protective factors; developing and evaluating the effectiveness and generalizability of interventions; and widespread dissemination of effective interventions (U.S. Department of Health and Human Services (USDHHS), 2001). All these factors combine to set the stage in the coming decade for even greater progress in understanding the roots of youth violence and finding ways to prevent and treat it.

A major challenge that remains to be addressed by researchers, practitioners, and policy makers alike is to find ways to facilitate the utilization

PATRICIA A. GRACZYK and PATRICK H. TOLAN • Institute for Juvenile Research, Department of Psychiatry, University of Illinois at Chicago, Chicago, Illinois 60612.

*A Faculty Scholar award from the University of Illinois provided support for Dr. Tolan.

of quality youth prevention programs by community organizations. Efforts to prevent youth violence can be significantly compromised when organizations adopt programs that are ineffective or of unknown effectiveness. In the landmark report on youth violence, the Surgeon General concluded that, in spite of the variety of intervention programs available with demonstrated effectiveness in preventing and reducing youth violence, community organizations (e.g., schools) continue to use interventions of questionable quality (USDHHS, 2001). Mendel (2000) proposed that violence and other delinquent acts could be reduced substantially by the simple act of funneling monies from ineffective programs to programs that work. However, the utilization of programs that are ineffective or of unknown effectiveness is but one challenge to efforts to diffuse effective violence prevention practices. When effective programs are adopted by community organizations, frequently they are so poorly implemented that positive effects are compromised (Gottfredson et al., 2000; USDHHS, 2001). To summarize, many violence prevention initiatives currently being implemented within this country fall short of addressing the serious problems facing young people and society that these initiatives are intended to address.

What can be done to help organizations deliver high-quality violence prevention programs? Although the answer to this question is complex and multifaceted, we propose that a major advance would involve a more systematic and carefully defined focus on organizational and service delivery characteristics that affect program delivery.

We start this chapter by presenting a brief overview of current knowledge about youth violence and effective violence prevention interventions. Youth violence refers to physical acts by young people that can result in injury or death to another individual (USDHHS, 2001). As youth violence prevention programs move from well-controlled efficacy trial conditions to less-controlled community settings, organizational and service delivery characteristics assume increasing importance. Therefore, we then focus our discussion on organizational and service delivery issues from the perspective of violence prevention and broader organizational literatures. Our review of these literatures is intended to be selective and descriptive, and highlights three processes we believe are of particular relevance to the successful implementation of violence prevention programs in community organizations. These processes are (1) program adoption, (2) staff training, and (3) efforts to strike an optimal balance between fidelity to a program's design and adaptation to the local context.

CURRENT KNOWLEDGE ABOUT YOUTH VIOLENCE PREVENTION

Prevalence of Youth Violence

In the United States, homicide rates among youth aged 15–19 years began declining in 1994, after reaching record rates in the latter half of the

1980s. Nonetheless, the rates of homicide continue to be among the highest recorded for this age group, and the United States continues to be extreme among the world's countries in the rate of youth homicides. Homicide is the second leading cause of death among young people aged 15–24 years overall, and African American youth are five times more likely to be victims of homicide than are Whites (Snyder & Sickmund, 1999). In contrast to the decline in homicide rates, the incidence of nonlethal youth violence (i.e., aggravated and simple assaults) has remained relatively stable over the past two decades. Rates of nonlethal violence have been averaging 34–44 per 1000 youth aged 12–17 years overall, with Native Americans having the highest rates of victimization for violent crimes compared to persons of other ethnic or racial backgrounds (Snyder & Sickmund, 1999). The rates for nonlethal violence in the United States are still elevated compared with other industrialized Western nations; however, they do not stand out as distinctively as homicide rates.

Youth self-reported behavior contributing to violence also has declined since 1993. According to the 2001 National Youth Risk Behavior Survey (Centers for Disease Control and Prevention, 2002), 33.2% of high school students reported they were involved in physical fights in the previous year (compared to 42.5% in 1993), 17% carried a weapon the previous month (compared to 26.1% in 1993), 12.5% participated in physical fights on school property (compared to 16.2% in 1993), and 6.4% brought a weapon to school (compared to 11.8% in 1993). Contrary to this downward trend in the prevalence of violent-related behavior is the upward trend in young people who fear for their safety. In 2001, 6.6% of students surveyed reported that they felt unsafe going to school compared to 4.0% of students in 1997. In summary, although youth violence and behaviors contributing to violence had decreased from 1993 to 2001, more young people feel less safe in school or going to and from school.

Types of Adolescent Violence

All youth violence is not the same. Distinguishing among the various types of adolescent violence may be helpful in understanding differing contributing risk factors, needed responses, and targeting of violence prevention efforts. Within the general category of violence, there are important variations in motives, apparent causes, populations most at risk and, we suggest, the types of interventions needed. Four types of violence have been proposed by Tolan and Guerra (1994) and are briefly described below.

Situational Violence

Over half the violent acts committed by youth involve situational violence that is not well explained by individual characteristics or prior behavior (e.g., a fight at a sporting event; Tolan, 2001). Police records, emergency room surveys, and other archival sources show increases in violence during extreme heat, on weekends, and during times of social stress (Rotton & Frey, 1985). Similarly, an increase in aggression can occur if pursued goals are blocked or unforeseen impediments to plans occur (Averill, 1983). Living in poverty, particularly impoverished inner-city communities, is linked to frequent but unpredictable stressful events (Tolan & Gorman-Smith, 1997). In addition to these intrusive events, minority youth in these neighborhoods grow up facing ongoing discrimination and social disparities (Gibbs, 1989; Prothrow-Stith, 1992). Apart from the particular situational factors bearing down on inner-city youth, research has identified two other social catalysts for youth violence: firearm access and substance use, particularly alcohol (Cook, 1991; Rosenberg, 1991). When there is access to firearms or alcohol has been consumed, the risk of violence increases, separate from any risk explainable by individual characteristics (Rosenberg, 1991).

Relationship Violence

Approximately 25% of youth violence involves interpersonal disputes between persons within ongoing relationships (Tolan, 2001). Thus, relationship violence or violence among friends and family members is a common form of adolescent violence. Dating violence, for example, occurs at disturbing rates. Bergman (1992) found that 15.7% of adolescent females and 7.8% of males reported being physically victimized on dates. Notably, most victims continued to date after the violence (e.g., 79.2% of female victims), and over half of the victims were assaulted more than once by the perpetrator. In some cases, relationship violence erupts as an unusual incident, whereas in other cases it occurs periodically. In many cases, it appears that relationship violence is a familial habit; violence among parents often extends to and among children (Steinmetz, 1986; Straus & Gelles, 1986). In any case, violence as part of a longstanding relationship is a critical consideration in intervention planning, and seems to be related to a mixture of social and psychological characteristics (Tracy, Wolfgang, & Figlio, 1990).

Predatory Violence

Predatory violence is defined as that perpetrated intentionally, usually as part of some criminal act. Muggings, robbery, and gang assaults are common forms of this type of violence. Most estimates indicate that about 20% of adolescents commit such acts (Tracy et al., 1990), but only a small portion of this group (5–8% of males and 3–6% of females) is responsible for most of the predatory violence. Predatory violence is the type most studied and is the target of almost all the adolescent violence prevention programs. There is considerable research on the development of this type of violence, at least as part of a pattern of ongoing antisocial behavior (Huesmann, Eron, Lefkowitz, & Walder, 1984; Moffitt, 1993; Tolan & Loeber, 1993). This type of behavior seems to be predictable, develops slowly over time with onset by early adolescence, lasts long after adolescence, is dependent on multiple risk factors, and seems to require intensive and early prevention and treatment intervention methods (Huesmann et al., 1984, Moffitt, 1993; 1984; Tolan & Loeber, 1993). The age of first offense is a particularly critical predictor of risk for predatory violent behavior, as opposed to prediction of aggression, general antisocial behavior, or any violence (Tolan & Gorman-Smith, 1997).

Psychopathological Violence

Psychopathological violence refers to violent acts committed by individuals with psychotic symptoms, and accounts for approximately 5% of homicides (Tolan, 2001). Of the four types, this form represents the clearest example of individual pathology, although environmental precipitants may be necessary for its occurrence (Cornell, Benedek, & Benedek, 1987; Mungas, 1983). Research, although scant, suggests that such behavior is related to the neural system and severe psychological trauma and is not merely a byproduct of the learning situations and contributors to other types of violence (Lewis, Shanock, Pincus, & Glaser, 1980). Psychopharmacological and other management methods targeted at carefully identified individuals seem warranted here, whereas these techniques are less effective when used as interventions for other types of violence (Tolan & Guerra, 1994).

What Can Work with Youth Violence

In the past 5 years, major national reviews have identified many efficacious, promising, ineffective, and even harmful preventive interventions that target violence or risk and protective factors associated with violence. There are multiple reviews that can be consulted (e.g., Catalano, Arthur, Hawkins, Berglund, & Olson, 1998; Lipsey & Wilson, 1998; Sherman et al., 1997; Tolan & Guerra, 1994). Each emphasizes somewhat different criteria but also have remarkable similarities in findings. Also, all identify efficacious programs, that is, programs that seem to have reliably determined benefits for reducing youth violence. Perhaps the most authoritative review is found in the Surgeon General's report on Youth Violence (USDHHS, 2001) and the related Blueprints for Violence Prevention project at the University of Colorado, Center for Prevention of Violence, conducted by the Center for the Study and Prevention of Violence (Elliott & Tolan, 1998). Readers are referred to these reviews for information about specific youth violence prevention interventions.

Rather than repeating the content of these reviews here, we summarize the findings and implications for these for what can work in reducing youth violence:

- There are many empirically supported avenues for treating and preventing youth violence that range from individual, to family, to school setting, and community focus (Elliott & Tolan, 1998; USDHHS, 2001).
- It appears that multicomponent programs are necessary to reach high-risk youth and affect risk that is distributed across the

general population and concentrated among high-risk youth (Tolan & Guerra, 1994).

- Focus on the family as at least one component of a violence prevention initiative seems necessary. For high-risk youth, a family focus appears necessary and perhaps central in preventive efforts (Henggeler, Melton, Brondino, Scherer, & Hanley, 1997).
- There is evidence that programs that affect social problem-solving and related cognitive attitudes about use of violence and bonding to school reduce rates of violence in the general population (Hawkins, Farrington, & Catalano, 1999). However, the effects for high-risk children remain unproven (Conduct Problems Prevention Research Group, 1999; Metropolitan Area Child Study Group & Gorman-Smith, 2003).
- To affect the overall prevalence of violence, the most promising approach is to combine universal or primary prevention efforts that attempt to dissuade acceptance of violence in peer groups, classrooms, homes, and the community with indicated prevention or secondary prevention efforts targeting youth showing behavioral risk. These indicated prevention initiatives must be multicomponent, substantial in length, and coordinate and address home (family), school, and community functioning of targeted at-risk youth (Tolan, 1998).
- The scant evaluation research on policy impact consistently supports prevention over rehabilitation, therapeutic or enhancement, and support of youth over punitive or penal approaches, and community-based efforts over institutional efforts (Tolan & Gorman-Smith, 1997).
- The viability of interventions and policies depends heavily on the acceptance and support of the approaches by those organizations and individuals charged with delivering them.
- The impact of a given program depends greatly on the organization of its delivery, including the provision of appropriate training and support to implementers. The effects of sound organization may be as great as that of the actual intervention activities (Lipsey & Derzon, 1998).

WHAT IS IMPORTANT TO MAKE "WHAT *CAN* WORK" BE USEFUL AND EFFECTIVE

The last two points in the previous list echo those expressed in the Surgeon General's report (USDHHS, 2001) about the critical gap between what is understood about how to prevent youth violence and what it takes to have that occur at a scale that would have significant impact. These observations underscore the kinds of issues now surfacing with greater frequency and intensity than ever before as efficacious prevention initiatives are being disseminated to a wide variety of community-based settings around the country. These settings differ extensively in structure, mission, resources, population served, and the repertoire of implementer knowledge, skills, and attitudes required for the effective delivery of violence prevention interventions. Thus, greater attention to what is important in getting effective interventions that can be effectively done in a way that promotes their effectiveness is needed. Central to accomplishing that goal is recognizing the importance of the interface between efficacious violence prevention interventions, organizational factors that can facilitate or impede their implementation, and the types of training local implementers will need to insure that interventions are delivered with sufficient fidelity. It is to these issues we now turn.

Program Adoption

Planning decisions made prior to program implementation can have a significant effect on the success of a youth violence prevention intervention. When an organization is considering the adoption of an intervention, it is important that a primary adoption criterion is to select an empirically validated program. In addition, organizational and target population characteristics should be considered. To assist in this process, organizations can conduct what Stufflebeam refers to as *context and input evaluations* (Stufflebeam & Shrinkfield, 1985). Context evaluations include an accurate assessment of the target population and its needs as well as a subsequent determination of the program's capability to address those needs. In schools, such information is often obtained from student records. Information can also be obtained through other means such as surveys, focus groups, and interviews (Perry, 1999). Organizational structure and resources are the issues addressed in input evaluations. Input evaluations encourage organizations to analyze their infrastructure to determine if it is sufficient to handle programmatic needs. At this stage, analyses consider such factors as available and needed personnel and material resources, budgeting issues, and feasibility. In short, it is important that community organizations assess the fit of the program with the organization and the needs of the youth to be served prior to implementing the program.

The Incredible Years Series (IYS; Webster-Stratton et al., 2001) provides a good example of a program that assists organizations in determining the fit of the program to the organization. IYS is an empirically supported violence prevention program designated as a Blueprints model program and a promising intervention in the Surgeon General's report (USDHHS, 2001). The program provides a comprehensive questionnaire on its Website (www.incredibleyears.com) to help organizations determine their readiness for using the IYS program. Readiness questions cover such issues as target population characteristics and needs; organizational goals and philosophy; organizational commitment of time, material, and human resources to training and program delivery; characteristics of candidate implementers; and participant recruitment. Along with questions, this survey also provides a rationale for including questions and related program requirements, such as the need for both administrators and service providers to be motivated and interested in the delivery of the program. This tool and others like it provide organizations with critical pieces of information that allow them to systematically evaluate the likelihood that candidate programs can be implemented successfully within their organizations to serve the needs of their communities.

Implementer Training

Once a program has been chosen for adoption, the training provided to implementers gains in importance and is a critical prerequisite for effective program delivery. When using the term training in this chapter, we are referring to preimplementation training activities as well as ongoing technical assistance and support provided during the initial phases of implementation. Developers of violence prevention interventions use a variety of training models and, at this time, there is limited empirical evidence within the violence prevention field or broader prevention field that either identifies characteristics of effective training models or organizational factors that are associated with positive training outcomes. To provide some guidance on this issue, we summarize information from the broader training literature and discuss its relevance to violence prevention.

Organizational support for training activities can take many forms and can influence training results by influencing implementers' motivation to learn, actual learning and retention, and their willingness to transfer newly trained knowledge and skills to their work environment. Prior to training, Baldwin and Magjuka (1991) found that trainees distinguished between management "permission" and management "support," with the latter requiring a time commitment on the part of the manager either during the training or in follow-up activities afterward. Trainees who at the start of the training activity believed that their managers supported the activity and expected supervisory follow-up after training also reported stronger intentions to transfer trained knowledge and skills to the job.

The importance of principal support in school-based prevention work has received initial support from recent studies and our own experiences in implementing the *Metropolitan Area Child Study* (MACS; Metropolitan Area Child Study Group, 2002) in schools serving disadvantaged communities. Findings from a large national survey of school-based delinquency prevention efforts revealed that principal support predicted usage of best practices and high-quality methods (Gottfredson et al., 2000; Gottfredson & Gottfredson, 2002). Results from Greenberg and colleagues' (Kam, Greenberg, & Walls, 2003) effectiveness study revealed that principal support was associated with enhanced outcomes for inner-city students who participated in the *PATHS Curriculum* (Promoting Alternative Thinking Strategies; Greenberg, Kusche, & Mihalic, 1998), a program designated as a model Blueprints program and a promising universal program in the Surgeon General's report (USDHHS, 2001). Specifically, they found that a combination of principal support and high-quality implementation resulted in significant increases in student emotional competence and significant decreases in student behavioral dysregulation and aggression compared to students in schools with low principal support.

When undertaking teacher training for MACS, we worked to gain strong support from central administration at the district level, engaged principals in a meeting to explain the approach, to address their concerns, and to gain their support, and then met with teachers to undertake the same processes. This process helped to build the expectation that MACS was helpful to the teachers, and that their efforts to learn and implement the program would be supported by the organization.

In addition, post-training supervisory support and peer support have been found to be important in determining whether trainees use what they learned (e.g., Seyler, Holton, Bates, Burnett, & Carvalho, 1998). In community organizations, supervisors and peers can respond positively or negatively when newly trained implementers of violence prevention programs attempt to implement the intervention. Colleagues may provide support by encouraging implementers to use what they have learned; however, peers may also resist change and actively discourage implementers from introducing any new activities into the school or agency setting that might ultimately impact other members of the group. Similarly, supervisors can encourage implementers' efforts to use the intervention by establishing posttraining goals for the implementers, allocating needed resources, or by providing recognition for transfer efforts. There is also some evidence to suggest that negative responses by supervisors may have more influence on transfer efforts than positive responses (Bates, Holton, Seyler, & Carvalho, 2000).

Finally, implementers of violence prevention programs will enter training activities with preconceived notions about the relevance of the training activities to them and their organization. Implementers who view delivering a violence prevention program as a digression from their primary role or of minor relevance to the mission of their organization may be less inclined to implement the program or to implement it with sufficient integrity. This issue may be particularly relevant to classroom-based or school-based violence prevention programs. The mission of schools is often narrowly defined to focus solely on academic achievement and the role of teachers limited to enhancing the academic achievement of their students. With the added pressure of high-stakes testing, schools may marginalize violence and other prevention efforts in deference to the intense demands of academic accountability (Adelman & Taylor, 2003). In the example of the MACS intervention teacher training, it was important to recognize that teachers actively evaluate the training requirements, the program utility, and the competing responsibilities when engaging (or not) in training of a program meant to aid with violence prevention. This will affect not only skill acquisition, but also fidelity to procedures, program maintenance and adaptation, and likelihood of implementation in a manner that can have similar effects to those found in efficacy trials.

Unfortunately, the field of youth violence prevention has not undertaken much systematic study of how these factors affect implementation and ultimately participant outcomes. Although some studies are underway, their ability to direct on these matters is still uncertain. What is clear is that such work will be critical for advancing from what can work to what will work in actual implementation.

Balancing Fidelity and Adaptation

A third significant issue facing community organizations adopting evidence-based youth violence prevention interventions is to determine how to implement them with sufficient fidelity while at the same time, adapting them to local circumstances in a way that maximizes positive outcomes for targeted participants. Thus, issues involving treatment fidelity or implementation quality and adaptation have come to the forefront and warrant attention in a more comprehensive and systematic fashion than they have generally received in the past.

Treatment fidelity refers to the degree to which an intervention is conducted as it was originally intended (Durlak, 1998) and historically has referred to the discrepancy between the intervention as designed and the intervention as delivered. Recently, we proposed an expanded definition of treatment fidelity for school-based prevention efforts (Graczyk, Domitrovich, & Zins, 2003; Greenberg, Domitrovich, Graczyk, & Zins, in press) that is based on Chen's (1990, 1998) original model of implementation quality. According to the model, treatment fidelity is a function of the extent to which the intervention was implemented as designed as well as the extent to which the recommended implementation support system (e.g., training, ongoing technical assistance) was used. Thus, organizations need to consider both the intervention and the recommended supports to delivery in their efforts to insure adequate treatment fidelity and ultimately positive intervention effects.

Within the youth violence prevention and related prevention fields, factors that influence effective program implementation have been identified and there are several references available that discuss these factors (e.g., Gottfredson et al., 2000; Graczyk et al., 2003; Greenberg et al., in press; Lipsey & Derzon, 1998; Lipsey & Wilson, 1998). Identified factors can be grouped according to the characteristics of the program itself, the training and technical support provided to the implementers, and the environmental conditions. In our expanded model (Graczyk et al., 2003; Greenberg et al., in press), characteristics of intervention include such things as the program's essential components or "active ingredients," the dosage or amount of the intervention delivered to the target population, the quality of materials, and participant responsiveness. The training and technical support components include training content and training methods, model of supervision used, and implementer characteristics. Examples of environmental conditions that might impact the implementation of a school-based prevention intervention include classroom climate, administrative support, the interface between the program and district goals, and the quality of school–community collaborations. Preliminary support for this model is found in the Gottfredson et al. (2000) study of school-based delinquency prevention programs. Higher-quality implementation was associated with more standardized materials and methods, extensive and high-quality training and supervision, principal support, and integration of the program into normal school operations. It is clear that the extent to which a youth violence prevention initiative is delivered well is predicated on a set of factors that extend beyond attributes of the program itself.

Nonetheless, variations in program implementation are to be expected as community-based organizations attempt to deliver an evidence-based youth violence prevention intervention due to the inherent differences between real-world settings and the controlled circumstances in which programs were originally evaluated. Program developers can assist organizations in addressing the fidelity–adaptation conundrum in several ways. First, program developers can specify the active ingredients of an intervention. Active ingredients are typically based in the program's causal theory and are critical to the intervention's potential for generating positive outcomes. Implementers should be advised to make every effort to deliver these critical components to the target population. Aspects of the intervention that are not included in this category are those that could be modified to fit the setting without compromising program effects. For example, in the MACS program the social-cognitive intervention is focused on modifying child beliefs about the acceptability of aggression, the utility of aggression in solving problems, their responsibility to others in controlling anger and aggression, and formulating plans for conflict management that are more thoughtful and prosocial. These principles and the primary activities used to orient the students and help them undertake the needed behavioral practice are prescribed. It is believed that one cannot add on or leave out components and still have the same intervention and the same confidence in likely benefits. However, the examples used can and should be locally developed and relevant. Moreover, there is more emphasis on community-based violence in higher-risk communities than there might be in less-threatening neighborhoods where violent incidents stand out more in contrast to typical life. Along with suggestions for adaptations based on environmental considerations, program developers can provide guidelines for adaptations based on other considerations such as characteristics of the target population. As an example, developers of the *Incredible Years Series* (Webster-Stratton et al., 2001) provide specific guidelines for adapting their program depending on participant risk status and ethnicity.

Regrettably, there is currently little empirically derived information available to guide community organizations in their adaptation efforts. What information is available suggests that the more organizations digress from a program or preventive strategy as it was designed and evaluated, the greater the risk that program effects will be compromised (e.g., Botvin, Baker, Dusenbury, Botvin, & Diaz, 1995; Botvin, Baker, Dusenbury, Tortu, & Botvin, 1990; Connell, Turner, & Mason, 1985; Gottfredson, Gottfredson, & Hybl, 1993). Therefore, to insure optimal outcomes, organizations are advised at this time to follow a program's protocol to the greatest extent possible and to seek advice from the program's developers or technical assistance staff before initiating any adaptations in their settings.

CONCLUSIONS

The first goal of this chapter was to highlight the body of knowledge that has accumulated within the field of youth violence prevention over the past decade, as it has the potential to expand and strengthen the services that are currently being provided by community-based organizations. In our discussion of the four types of youth violence—situational, interpersonal, predatory, and psychopathological—we noted that, although most youth violence is of the situational or interpersonal type, most research and preventive interventions have targeted predatory violence. Clearly, a greater emphasis on developing and implementing effective preventive efforts to decrease the two most frequent forms of youth violence is warranted.

As high-quality violence prevention initiatives become the focus of widespread dissemination efforts, processes contributing to their successful implementation by community organizations become increasingly more significant. Such processes include program adoption, implementer training, and treatment fidelity. Thus, discussion of these three processes within community organizations served as the second goal of this chapter.

One way to clarify the role of organizational factors to a program's success is to incorporate them into the program's theory, specifically into the theory's implementation support system. According to Chen (1998), there are two major components of a comprehensive program theory. The first is the causative or causal theory, which specifies how the program produces its intended outcomes. The second is the prescriptive theory, which provides guidelines for delivering the interventions and describes the context that is necessary for the successful implementation of the intervention, and includes consideration of the implementation support system. Both the causal and prescriptive theories of an intervention need to be considered. The causal theory can assist practitioners in screening and in identifying the appropriate intervention to be used when a particular outcome is targeted. The prescriptive theory is equally important because it guides the daily activities of the program and identifies the environmental supports needed to ensure high-quality programming. Inclusion of organizational factors in a program's theory will allow researchers to test for organizational effects in their research designs, which will in turn provide a greater understanding of the role of organizational issues in achieving program outcomes.

We also recommend that more attention be paid to training issues in the violence prevention area, both scientifically and practically. More specifically, we propose that: (1) successful transfer of training be a major consideration when youth violence prevention initiatives are disseminated to community organizations; (2) organizational and individual factors be included in statistical models that test the effectiveness of training activities in promoting successful transfer, and (3) research be conducted that compares different training models for the same violence prevention initiative.

Effective transfer of training is a function of successful adaptation (Ford & Weissbein, 1997). Stated simply, the question is not "if" community-based practitioners will adapt programs to their unique settings, but "how" they will adapt it. As mentioned earlier, program developers can provide guidance to organizations by specifying the active ingredients of an intervention and providing specific guidelines for adaptation. Furthermore, program developers can include content in their training activities that goes beyond coverage of the violence prevention intervention itself and includes information and skills to help implementers adapt the intervention to their settings.

Administrators and supervisors in community organizations can increase their return on investment in staff training activities and support high-quality program implementation by fostering a positive implementation climate. Such support should include opportunities and resources that allow program implementers time to practice, improve, learn from their mistakes, support one another in their implementation efforts, and effectively adapt what they learned to their daily work situations.

We hope that by devoting greater attention to organizational and service delivery issues in the future, community organizations will be better able to attain a high degree of success in their usage of evidence-based youth violence prevention approaches. We propose that greater consideration of these issues will help advance violence prevention from a field of great promise to one of great effect.

REFERENCES

Adelman, H. S., & Taylor, L. (2003). Toward a comprehensive policy vision for mental health in schools. In M. D. Weist, S. W. Evans, & N. A. Lever (Eds.), *Handbook of school mental health: Advancing practice and research* (pp. 23–43). New York: Kluwer.

Averill, J. R. (1983). Studies on anger and aggression: Implications for theories of emotion. *American Psychologist, 38*, 1145–1160.

Baldwin, T. T., & Magjuka, R. J. (1991). Organizational training and signals of importance: Linking pretraining perceptions to intentions to transfer. *Human Resource Development Quarterly, 2*, 25–36.

Bates, R. A., Holton, E. F., Seyler, D. L., & Carvalho, M. A. (2000). The role of interpersonal factors in the application of computer-based training in an industrial setting. *Human Resource Development International, 3*(1), 19–42.

Bergman, L. (1992). Dating violence among high school students. *Social Work, 37*, 21–27.

Botvin, G. J., Baker, E., Dusenbury, L., Botvin, E. M., & Diaz, T. (1995). Long-term follow-up results of a randomized drug abuse prevention trial in a white middle-class population. *Journal of the American Medical Association, 273*, 1106–1112.

Botvin, G. J., Baker, E., Dusenbury, L., Tortu, S., & Botvin, E. M. (1990). Preventing adolescent drug abuse through a multi-modal cognitive-behavioral approach: Results of a 3-year study. *Journal of Consulting and Clinical Psychology, 58*, 437–446.

Catalano, R. F., Arthur, M. W., Hawkins, J. D., Berglund, L., & Olson, J. J. (1998). Comprehensive community- and school-based interventions to prevent antisocial behavior. In R. Loeber & D. Farrington (Eds.), *Serious and violent juvenile offenders: Risk factors and successful interventions* (pp. 248–283). Thousand Oaks, CA: Sage.

Centers for Disease Control and Prevention. (2002). *Surveillance summaries*, June 28, 2002. MMWR 2002:51 (No. SS-4).

Chen, H. T. (1990). *Theory-driven evaluations.* Newbury Park, CA: Sage.

Chen, H. T. (1998). Theory-driven evaluations. *Advances in Educational Productivity, 7*, 15–34.

Conduct Problems Prevention Research Group. (1999). Initial impact of the fast track prevention trial for conduct problems: I. The high risk sample. *Journal of Consulting and Clinical
Psychology, 67,* 631–647.

Connell, D. B., Turner, R. R., & Mason, E. F. (1985). Summary of the findings of the School
Health Education Evaluation: Health promotion effectiveness, implementation, and costs.
Journal of School Health, 55, 316–323.

Cook, P. J. (1991). The technology of personal violence. In M. Tonry (Ed.),*Crime and justice: An annual review of research. Vol. 14* (pp. 1–71). Chicago: University of Chicago
Press.

Cornell, D. G., Benedek, E. P., & Benedek, D. M. (1987). Characteristics of adolescents
charged with homicide: Review of 72 cases. *Behavioral Sciences and the Law, 5,* 11–23.

Durlak, J. A. (1998). Why program implementation is important. *Journal of Prevention and
Intervention in the Community, 17,* 5–18.

Elliott, D. S., & Tolan, P. H. (1998). Youth violence, prevention, intervention and social policy:
An overview. In D. Flannery & R. Hoff (Eds.), *Youth violence: A volume in the psychiatric
clinics of North America* (pp. 3–46). Washington, DC: American Psychiatric Association.

Ford, J. K., & Weissbein, D. A. (1997). Transfer of training: An updated review and analysis.
Performance Improvement Quality, 10(2), 22–41.

Gibbs, J. T. (1989). Black adolescents and youth: An update on an endangered species. In
R. L. Jones (Ed.), *Black adolescents* (pp. 3–27). Berkeley, CA: Cobb & Henry.

Gottfredson, D. C., & Gottfredson, G. D. (2002). Quality of school-based prevention programs:
Results from a national survey. *Journal of Research in Crime and Delinquency, 39*(1), 3–35.

Gottfredson, G. D., Gottfredson, D. C., Czeh, E. R., Cantor, D., Crosse, S. B., & Hantman, I.
(2000). *National Study of Delinquency Prevention in Schools.* Ellicott City, MD: Gottfredson
Associates, Inc.

Gottfredson, D. C., Gottfredson, G. D., & Hybl, L. G. (1993). Managing adolescent behavior:
A multiyear, multischool study. *American Educational Research Journal, 30,* 179–216.

Graczyk, P. A., Domitrovich, C. E., & Zins, J. E. (2003). Facilitating the implementation of
evidence-based prevention and mental health promotion efforts in schools. In M. D. Weist,
S. W. Evans, & N. A. Lever (Eds.), *Handbook of school mental health: Advancing practice
and research* (pp. 301–308). New York: Kluwer Academic/Plenum.

Greenberg, M. T., Domitrovich, C. E., Graczyk, P. A., & Zins, J. E. (in press). *The study of imple-
mentation in school-based prevention research: Theory, research, and practice.* Rockville,
MD: Center for Mental Health Services, Substance Abuse and Mental Health Services
Agency, Department of Health and Human Resources.

Greenberg, M. T., Kusche, C., & Mihalic, S. (1998). Promoting alternative thinking strategies
(PATHS). In D. S. Elliott (Series Ed.), *Blueprints for violence prevention.* Boulder, CO: Center for the Study and Prevention of Violence, Institute of Behavioral Science, University
of Colorado at Boulder.

Hawkins, J. D., Farrington, D. P., & Catalano, R. F. (1999). Reducing violence through the
schools. In D. S. Elliott, B. A. Hamburg, & K. R. Williams (Eds.), *Youth violence: New
perspectives for schools and communities.* Cambridge: Cambridge University Press.

Henggeler, S. W., Melton, G. B., Brondino, M. J., Scherer, D. G., & Hanley, J. H. (1997).
Multisystemic therapy with violent and chronic juvenile offenders and their families: The
role of treatment fidelity in successful dissemination. *Journal of Consulting and Clinical
Psychology, 65,* 821–833.

Huesmann, L. R., Eron, L. D., Lefkowitz, M. M., & Walder, L. O. (1984). Stability of aggression
over time and generations. *Developmental Psychology, 20,* 1120–1134.

Kam, C., Greenberg, M. T., & Walls, C. T. (2003). Examining the role of implementation quality
in school-based prevention using the PATHS curriculum. *Prevention Science, 4*(1), 55–63.

Lewis, D. O., Shanock, S. S., Pincus, J. H., & Glaser, G. H. (1980). Violent juvenile delinquents: Psychiatric, neurological, psychological, and abuse factors. *Annual Progress in
Child Psychiatry & Child Development, 1,* 591–603.

Lipsey, M., & Derzon, J. (1998). Predictors of violent or serious delinquency in adolescence
and early adulthood: A synthesis of longitudinal research. In R. Loeber & D. Farrington (Eds.), *Serious & violent juvenile offenders: Risk factors and successful interventions*
(pp. 86–105). Thousand Oaks, CA: Sage.

Lipsey, M., & Wilson, D. B. (1998). Effective intervention for serious juvenile offenders. A synthesis of research. In R. Loeber and D. Farrington (Eds.), *Serious & violent juvenile offenders: Risk factors and successful interventions* (pp. 313–345). Thousand Oaks, CA: Sage.

Mendel, R. A. (2000). *Less hype, more help: Reducing juvenile crime, what works and what doesn't.* Washington, DC: American Youth Policy Forum.

Metropolitan Area Child Study Group. (2002). A cognitive-ecological approach to preventing aggression in urban settings: Initial outcomes for high-risk children. *Journal of Consulting and Clinical Psychology, 70,* 179–194.

Metropolitan Area Child Study Research Group, & Gorman-Smith, D. (2003). Effects of teacher training and consultation on teacher behavior toward students at high risk for aggression. *Behavior Therapy, 34,* 437–452.

Moffitt, T. E. (1993). Adolescence-limited and life-course-persistent antisocial behavior: A developmental taxonomy. *Psychological Review,100,* 674–701.

Mungas, D. (1983). An empirical analysis of specific syndromes of violent behavior. *Journal of Nervous and Mental Disease, 171,* 354–361.

Perry, C. L. (1999). *Creating health behavior change: How to develop community-wide programs for youth.* Thousand Oaks, CA: Sage.

Prothrow-Stith, D. (1992, June). Can physicians help curb adolescent violence? *Hospital Practice,* 193–207.

Rosenberg, M. L. (1991). *Violence in America.* New York: Oxford University Press.

Rotton, J., & Frey, J. (1985). Air pollution, weather, and violent crimes: Concomitant time-series analysis of archival data. *Journal of Personality and Social Psychology, 49,* 1207–1220.

Seyler, D. L., Holton, E. F., Bates, R. A., Burnett, M. F., & Carvalho, M. A. (1998). Factors affecting motivation to transfer training. *International Journal of Training and Development, 2*(1), 2–16.

Sherman, L., Gottfredson, D., MacKenzie, D., Eck, J., Reuter, P, & Bushway, S. (1997). *Preventing crime: What works, what doesn't, what's promising: A report to the United States Congress.* College Park: University of Maryland.

Snyder, H. N., & Sickmund, M. (1999). *Juvenile offenders and victims: 1999 national report.* Washington, DC: U.S. Department of Justice, Office of Juvenile Justice and Delinquency Prevention.

Steinmetz, S. K. (1986). The violent family. In M. Lystad (Ed.), *Violence in the home: Interdisciplinary perspectives* (pp. 51–70). New York: Brunner/Mazel.

Straus, M. A., & Gelles, R. J. (1986). Societal changes in family violence from 1975 to 1985 as revealed by two national surveys. *Journal of Marriage and Family, 48,* 465–479.

Stufflebeam, D. L., & Shrinkfield, A. J. (1985). *Systematic evaluation.* Boston: Kluwer-Nijhoff.

Tolan, P. H. (1998). Community and prevention research. In P. Kendall, J. Butcher, & G. Holmbeck (Eds.), *Handbook of research methods in clinical psychology* (2nd ed., pp. 403–418). New York: Wiley.

Tolan, P. H. (2001). Youth violence and its prevention in the United States: An overview of current knowledge. *Injury Control and Safety Promotion, 8,* 1–12.

Tolan, P. H., & Gorman-Smith, D. (1997). Treatment of juvenile delinquency: Between therapy and punishment. In D. Stoff, J. Brieling, & J. Maser (Eds.), *Handbook of antisocial behavior* (pp. 405–415). New York: Wiley.

Tolan, P. H., & Guerra, N. G. (1994). *What works in reducing adolescent violence: An empirical review of the field.* Monograph prepared for the Center for the Study and Prevention of Youth Violence. Boulder: University of Colorado.

Tolan, P. H., & Loeber, R. L. (1993). Antisocial behavior. In P. H. Tolan & B. J. Cohler (Eds.), *Handbook of clinical research and practice with adolescents* (pp. 307–331). New York: Wiley.

Tracy, P. E., Wolfgang, M. E., & Figlio, R. M. (1990). *Delinquency careers in two birth cohorts.* New York: Plenum.

U.S. Department of Health and Human Services. (2001). *Youth violence: A report of the Surgeon General.* Rockville, MD: U.S. Department of Health and Human Services, Centers for Disease Control and Prevention, National Center for Injury Prevention and Control;

Substance Abuse and Mental Health Services, Administration, Center for Mental Health Services; and National Institutes of Health, National Institute of Mental Health. (available at http://www.surgeongeneral.gov/library/youthviolence/)

Webster-Stratton, C., Mihalic, C., Fagan, A., Arnold, D., Taylor, T., & Tingley, C. (2001). *Blueprints for violence prevention, book eleven: The Incredible Years: Parent, teacher, and child training series.* Boulder, CO: Center for the Study and Prevention of Violence.

15

Adolescent Sex Offender Programs

WILLIAM D. MURPHY, JACQUELINE PAGE,
and REBECCA ETTELSON

The management of adolescent sex offenders involves the coordination of
a variety of systems, primarily the mental health system, juvenile justice
system, and the child protective system (CPS). The focus of this chapter
is on delivery systems for adolescent sex offenders. However, to understand current approaches, we will first describe some basic literature on
the (1) scope of the problem, (2) characteristics and classification system for
this group, and (3) assessment and risk assessment approaches. Throughout this chapter, it is noted that anyone considering delivery systems for
adolescent sex offenders should give thought to how these systems will
interact and work together.

SCOPE OF THE PROBLEM

Early studies of adolescent sex offenders tended to dismiss concerns
about this population (Markey, 1950). However, beginning in the 1980s,
evidence gathered from a number of sources suggested adolescent sex offenders accounted for 30–50% of offenses against children and 15–20%
of rapes (Barbaree, Hudson, & Seto, 1993) with more recent reviews presenting similar findings (Righthand & Welch, 2001; Weinrott, 1996). In
addition, data from the National Incident Data Reporting Systems (Snyder,
2000) on offenses reported to the police show a very similar pattern. The
age of offenders committing the greatest number of sexual assaults is 14,
although this varies with the age of the victim. For those victims between

WILLIAM D. MURPHY, JACQUELINE PAGE, and REBECCA ETTELSON • Department of
Psychiatry, University of Tennessee Health Science Center, Memphis, Tennessee, 38105.

the ages 6 to 11, the greatest number of offenses is committed by 13–14-year-olds. For 12–17-year-old victims, the most frequent age of the offender is 17 years, and for those over 18 years, the most frequent age of the offender is in their mid-20s. Also, an early study by Abel and Rouleau (1990) reported that a significant number of adult offenders, especially those offenders against children, begin their offending during adolescence. These data are part of the impetus for the application of adult models to adolescent sex offenders. There was a tendency to view all adolescent sex offenders as having a chronic disorder that would require extensive treatment and lifelong management. It was also assumed that all adolescent offenders were at relatively high risk for future offending and therefore needed significant restrictions to manage their offending risk.

Although there have been few randomized controlled studies of adolescent sex offender treatment, there have been numerous reports of recidivism rates of identified adolescent sex offenders. Reviews by Righthand and Welch (2001) and Weinrott (1996) indicated across a number of studies that official recidivism rates tend to be in the 10–12% range for sexual reoffenses but two to three times higher for nonsexual offenses. It should be noted, however, that there are reports of higher recidivism rates (Långström, 2002) suggesting that there are probably subgroups who are higher risk. The rate of 10–12% is much lower than many had originally assumed, and it should be noted that reconviction rates for adult offenders are not as high as the general population assumes (Hanson et al., 2002). It also should be noted that although rates are low, it does appear that adolescent sex offenders are more likely to recidivate sexually than general delinquents (Hagan, Gust-Brey, Cho, & Dow, 2001; Sipe, Jenson, & Everett, 1998). For example, Hagan et al. found in an 8-year follow-up study that the sex offender reoffense rate for a combined group of rapists and child molesters was 18% versus 10% for a group of nonsexual offenders.

Although generally sexual recidivism for this population is low, there still is a great deal of variability across studies. The significant recidivism for nonsexual offenses in adolescents does not differ from adult populations (Hanson et al., 2002). This variability in recidivism rates has led Becker and Kaplan (1988) to postulate that there may be different trajectories for adolescent sex offenders similar to Moffitt's (1993) work on adolescent limited and life course persistent antisocial or delinquent behavior in adolescents. Becker and Kaplan suggested three trajectories: the Dead-End Path with no further sexual or nonsexual recidivism, the Delinquency Path where the offender may commit more sexual offenses but as part of a general antisocial pattern, and the Sexual Interest Path where the offender develops specific paraphilic interest. Early research and theorizing tended to assume only the latter.

CHARACTERISTICS AND CLASSIFICATION

In designing treatment programs and intervention systems, an important factor is the treatment needs of the population. Research has attempted to determine sex offender-specific characteristics of this population that might relate to etiology and treatment needs. These studies have been descriptive studies of offenders and comparisons of adolescent sex offenders to other groups such as violent non-sex offenders and nonviolent, non-sex offenders with only a few studies comparing these groups to nonoffenders. Major reviews of the literature (Righthand & Welch, 2001; Veneziano & Veneziano, 2002; Weinrott, 1996) all come to the same conclusion: Adolescent sex offenders are extremely heterogeneous and across studies they tend to have more similarities to other delinquent populations than differences. These adolescents vary across most of the dimensions of adolescent functioning, including degree of social competence, delinquency, impulsivity, sexual preoccupation or deviation, academic functioning, intellectual functioning, exposure to trauma, and family psychopathology.

Because of this heterogeneity, there have been a number of attempts to develop classification systems that might rationally or empirically define groups with specific treatment needs (Butler & Seto, 2002; Hunter, Figueredo, Malamuth, & Becker, 2003; Knight & Prentky, 1993; Worling, 2001). It is not the purpose of this chapter to try to describe in detail each of these systems, but if one looks across them, there are similarities in terms of dimensions in which the classifications are based. Two major dimensions include delinquency or impulsivity and sexual deviation or preoccupation. Other dimensions include factors such as degree of social competence, emotional management, and family functioning.

ASSESSING RISK AND NEED

In terms of programming for this population, the principles of risk, need, and responsivity from the general correctional rehabilitation literature (Andrews & Bonta, 1998) provide a framework for assessing risk and treatment needs and determining the level of service delivery. In this framework, *risk* refers to risk of reoffending, both generally and sexually, and is usually based on static (i.e., unchangeable) factors. *Need* (sometimes referred to as dynamic risk factors) includes those factors that, if changed, would lead to a reduction in risk. Finally, *responsivity* is the delivery of treatment in "a style and mode that is consistent with the ability and learning style of the offender" (Andrews & Bonta, 1998, p. 245). Such factors include intellectual and academic functioning, cultural factors, and possibly comorbid psychiatric disorders.

Clinicians and policy makers who are designing delivery systems still face a number of significant decisions. Many times there has to be a determination of (1) level of care, (2) the components of treatment programs, and (3) the extent of external monitoring needed to maintain community safety. Studies on the characteristics of offenders and attempts at developing typologies have identified potentially important dimensions, some which have more empirical support than others.

In the general area of delinquent and adolescent violent behavior, there is a rather large meta-analytic literature that has established empirically validated static and dynamic risk factors (Lipsey & Derzon, 1998). These include such well-known factors as early childhood aggression, school problems, previous offenses, substance abuse, abusive parents or exposure to violence, antisocial parent, association with antisocial peers, and lack of parental supervision among others. Although not always developed into actuarial scales, there are empirically established static and dynamic factors that can guide decision making in terms of degree of risk and treatment needs for the general area of violent and serious delinquency.

For adolescent sex offenders a number of risk or need instruments are currently undergoing validation and include the Juvenile Sex Offender Assessment Protocol-II (Prentky, Harris, Frizzell, & Righthand, 2000, available at www.csom.org), the Estimate of Risk of Adolescent Sex Offender Recidivism (Worling & Curwen, 2001), and the Protective Factor Scale (Bremer, 2001). Each of these scales rate offenders on slightly different variables but have similar general broad areas, which include sexual deviation or preoccupation, impulsivity or delinquency, attitudes supportive of offending, emotional management or social competence, family functioning, and general community stability. Current standards of practice would suggest that as one is designing programs, these scales and specific items on the scales can serve as a guide to the level of care needed, the types of interventions needed, and the level of external controls; with appropriate recognition of their limitations (Caldwell, 2002).

TREATMENT DELIVERY

As the above discussion suggests, the first step in programming for the adolescent sex offender is an adequate assessment that focuses on the offender's risk, needs, and factors that would affect responsivity. There are a variety of approaches to assessment of adolescent sex offenders (Colorado Sex Offender Management Board, 2002; Murphy & Page, 1999; Utah Network on Juveniles Offending Sexually, 1996). Regardless of the assessment methodology, the purpose is to identify those factors identified in the previous section that relate to risk, treatment need, and reponsivity.

The Utah Network on Juveniles Offending Sexually (1996) describes a triage model of assessing sex offenders. This model recognizes that not all offenders are high risk and describes four levels of assessment. The Level A assessment is provided by a line worker, such as a Juvenile Court intake probation officer or a CPS investigator with appropriate training. This evaluation would focus on the review of police statements, victim or witness statements, interviews of the parents and juvenile, an assessment of supervision by the parents, and an interview with any collateral contacts. For low-risk offenders, no further assessment may be required. The Level B assessment would be performed by a clinician who specializes in juvenile sex offender assessments and would occur where the line worker assesses that there is higher risk or need for higher supervision. At this level, more detailed structured interviews are conducted and there may be administration of formal risk assessment instruments. For those youth who again appear to be at high risk but also may have other mental health or correctional problems, referrals would be made for Level C evaluations. This third level of assessment would include detailed interviewing, use of risk assessment instruments, and the use of formal psychological measures or procedures and plethysmographic assessment (i.e., physiological measure of sexual arousal). The final level referred in their guidelines as Level D would be similar to Level C evaluation but would occur in an inpatient or residential facility rather than in an outpatient setting. Youth referred for these types of evaluations would be those who present significant concerns to the community, where there is little information known and those who may have more acute mental health disorders requiring both assessment and stabilization. At all levels of assessment, the assessment is designed to determine risk level, potential to reoffend, appropriate level of clinical interventions needed and appropriate level of supervision needed. This model of assessment recognizes that not all offenders are at high risk, all may not need extensive psychosexual evaluations and is a model that if appropriately implemented with appropriately trained professionals can be cost effective.

After the initial assessment, there are basically three decisions to be made. These decisions include determining (1) the type of treatment (or treatment program) that is needed, (2) what level of intensity and level of structure are indicated, and (3) the degree of external monitoring that is needed. On one level these decisions are similar to those that general mental health practitioners make in that the needs of the youth and family are taken into consideration. However, when working with adolescent sex offenders, the clinician also has a responsibility to community safety, which often complicates the decision-making process.

TYPE OF TREATMENT

Before discussing issues related to determining the type of treatment and treatment program that is needed, we will briefly summarize what is generally meant by sex offender-specific treatment. Adolescent sex offender treatment tends to be cognitive-behavioral in nature within a relapse prevention framework (Murphy & Page, 2000). Treatment focuses on (1) reducing denial; (2) correcting attitudes that support offending and thinking patterns used to justify offending; (3) identifying factors that trigger or place the offender at risk; (4) developing coping skills and strategies to manage risk; (5) increasing motivation by assisting the offender to understand the consequences of their offending to themselves, their families, and hopefully the victim; (6) where appropriate, teaching skills to manage urges and decrease deviant arousal; and (7) increasing the youth's ability to form appropriate relationships and develop a more healthy approach to sexuality. Treatment tends to be delivered in groups with family therapy being an adjunct to the group. Families may be seen in traditional family therapy, in multifamily groups, or family education groups. However, to re-state, there are many offenders who need interventions in other areas and programs must be able to address concomitant problems, either within the program or by coordinating with other providers.

The type of treatment program should be determined by the specific treatment need. Treatment needs can be viewed as varying across three major dimensions: sex offending, general delinquency or violence, and general mental health needs. Each dimension is viewed as a continuum with family functioning cutting across all three. Any one youth can be at different points on each of the dimensions (Chaffin, 2003). It is important that there is an attempt to assess each dimension independently; however, it should also be recognized that factors such as impulsivity or social competency, may impact each identified area.

Systems for intervening in mental health needs or generalized antisocial and violent behavior are covered in other chapters of this book. However, some general comments about the interaction of sex offender treatment and treatment of general antisocial behavior are warranted. For offenders high on the dimension of general antisocial or violent behavior and low on sex offender risk and need, empirically valid treatment for juvenile delinquency such as multisystemic therapy (MST; Henggeler, Mihalic, Rone, Thomas, & Tibbons-Mitchell, 1998) or functional family therapy (Alexander et al., 1998) with more limited sex offender-specific treatment might be warranted (Chaffin, 2003). It should also be noted that there is some preliminary evidence that MST may in itself reduce sex offender risk (Borduin, Henggeler, Blaske, & Stein, 1990; Borduin & Schaeffer, 2001). Sex offender treatment is generally delivered in a group format and clinicians need to be concerned about possible iatrogenic effects of placing highly delinquent adolescents in groups with other antisocial peers (Dishion, McCord, & Poulin, 1999). However, there is no evidence at this time that participation in group therapy increases sex offender risk specifically. Those youth who are high on both the sex offending dimension and the general antisocial or violent behavior dimension will require interventions that take into account both of these treatment needs.

LEVEL OF CARE

Once the level of risk and treatment needs have been identified, the decision-making process involves determining the level of care that the youth needs. The guiding principle for level of care determination in the general mental health area is placement in the least restrictive environment. However, when working with adolescent sex offenders, community safety also becomes a critical component of the decision. Whereas the least restrictive environment principle continues to be taken into consideration, the clinician also must consider safety issues and risk. It is clear that in the past there has been a tendency to place many adolescent sex offenders in restrictive residential care when some of these adolescents could have been managed in a less restrictive environment. However, there are those youth who will require structured or secure placements although this number is probably fewer that we previously believed. At times placement in a more restrictive level of care has occurred because of the lack of alternatives. It is agreed that delivery systems for the management of sex offenders should be able to match risk and this is best accomplished in systems with continua of care as presented (Bengis, 1997; Chaffin, 2003; Colorado Sex Offender Management Board, 2002; Utah Network on Juvenile Offending Sexually, 1996). Components of such a continuum might include outpatient programs, intensive outpatient programs, day treatment programs, specialized therapeutic foster care, group homes, independent living programs, staff secure residential programs, and locked secure residential programs.

The majority of adolescent sex offenders can probably be managed in outpatient programs. Participants in an outpatient program would generally have lower or moderate risk on most of the dimensions and in addition have adequate community support. Outpatient programs typically involve a group therapy session once a week, which is supplemented by family therapy and individual psychotherapy if needed. For those offenders who have more moderate risk but have support systems that can provide adequate monitoring, more intensive outpatient programs might be used.

Traditional intensive outpatient programs see the individual 3–4 hours a day 2–3 days a week, whereas day treatment programs may have the youth 6–8 hours a day for 5 days a week, although these vary across settings. Unfortunately, in many jurisdictions it is difficult to have enough adolescents in sex offender-specific traditional intensive outpatient programs or day treatment programs for the service to be cost effective. However, specific aspects of these programs that assist in meeting the youth's needs can sometimes be provided in an adapted format. This can involve increasing the number of groups per week or increasing individual or family therapy.

Another type of intensive outpatient program is the use of in-home services, school and community liaison, and linking the youth with more prosocial community activities. Although not inexpensive, these programs may be more feasible for smaller programs and smaller jurisdictions and can be targeted to only those offenders who are of higher risk. These types of interventions are especially useful to those offenders who are at moderate-to-high risk in the delinquency area.

Structured or therapeutic foster homes and group homes can serve as an alternative placement for youth who are at moderate risk and cannot remain in the home. The youth's inability to remain in the home may be due to possible victims in the home or significant family issues or dysfunction that suggests they would not be adequately monitored if left in the home. These types of less restrictive placements can also be utilized as a step-down placement for youth who have been in a more structured or secure setting. The placement can be combined with outpatient services that may vary in intensity depending on the youth's needs and level of risk.

Independent living programs provide for the needs of older youth and may be especially beneficial to those who have been in restrictive environments for a significant period of time. These programs focus on assisting the youth in working toward independence. Youth who have spent lengthy periods of time in residential settings often need this type of assistance to successfully reintegrate into the community as a young adult. Structure within independent living programs may vary from staff supervised to the young adult living in his own apartment. Youth involved in independent living programs would also be involved in an outpatient program with the focus of treatment depending on their individualized needs.

The highest level of care is residential or correctional-based treatment. Residential programs include staff-secure settings and locked-secure settings. Locked-secure residential programs may operate as a mental health program or within a juvenile correctional facility. Programs within juvenile correctional facilities are typically the most secure by the nature of the setting. These programs may be referred to as locked-secure residential programs or as correctional-based programs and vary in nature with some being quite similar to mental health-based programs whereas others are more rooted in a correctional philosophy.

Staff-secure facilities are appropriate for those youth who are high risk on the sex offending variable or exhibit a moderate level of emotional or behavioral problems that necessitate a more structured environment, but are not at high risk for escape or violence against other youth or staff. Locked-secure facilities are more appropriate for the groups that are both high on sex offending risk and generally high on antisocial behavior. Youth who have severe behavioral and emotional problems or are high on the antisocial behavior dimension may also be treated in locked-secure facilities. In many jurisdictions, the most violent offenders will be found in juvenile correctional facilities. However, because decisions to send a youth to a juvenile correctional facility are often made by judges, at times lower-risk offenders are unfortunately placed in such facilities, which may have unwanted iatrogenic effects.

In summary, decisions regarding treatment needs and level of care of adolescent sex offenders should be based on an adequate assessment process that focuses on factors that are specific to reducing the risk for sex offending and general criminal behavior. Unfortunately, these factors are not all empirically established, but there is a literature that at least provides clinicians with guidelines. The most effective delivery systems will have a continuum of care which, in the end, is more cost-effective than having only options of outpatient versus residential. In addition, programs must be able to address needs across a variety of dimensions and must recognize that for some adolescent sex offenders, sex offender treatment may not need to be intensive, and other areas, such as adolescent antisocial behavior or mental health problems, may be of more importance.

A NEED FOR COORDINATED SYSTEMS

No matter what the level of care, effective sex offender management requires the involvement of a number of systems with appropriate external supervision (Center for Sex Offender Management [CSOM], 1999; National Adolescent Perpetrator Network [NAPN], 1993). This range of services can include child protective services, especially when there is a victim in the home, but frequently also involves juvenile or family court and juvenile probation officers. Adolescent sex offender programs need to establish working relationships with these systems and states such as Colorado (Colorado Sex Offender Management Board, 2002) and Utah (Utah Network on Juveniles Offending Sexually, 1996) have detailed programs that address interagency cooperation. Coordination of efforts between the different agencies can be extremely beneficial to the treatment process in addition to ensuring that other agencies involved are aware of the program rules and guidelines for supervision. Agencies such as probation, the juvenile court, and child protective services provide important external monitoring to ensure that treatment program rules and supervision guidelines are followed. Gaining interagency cooperation may require significant time in developing protocols, educating other agencies, and being educated regarding other agencies' functioning. However, in our experience such time will improve the clinician's ability to provide services to this population.

GUIDELINES AND RESOURCES

There is a variety of guidelines and program models for this population on the national, state, and local levels. Many of these also include descriptions of staff qualifications. On the national level, there are two primary organizations, the Association for the Treatment of Sexual Abusers (ATSA; www.atsa.com) and the National Adolescent Perpetrator Network through the Kemp Center at the University of Colorado Health Science Center. ATSA has both a Code of Ethics and Standards and Guidelines for Practice (available at www.atsa.com). The ATSA Standards provide a general overview of currently accepted assessment and treatment practices, although it should be noted that these were originally developed for work with adult offenders and as the ATSA Standards note, there needs to be some caution in applying some of the standards to adolescents. The National Adolescent Perpetrator Network published a report (National Task Force on Juvenile Sexual Offending, 1993) that presents assumptions regarding issues on reporting, investigation, prosecution and intervention. The 1993 report is, at this point, somewhat out of date and NAPN is currently in the process of revising it.

The National Crimes Victims Research and Treatment Center at the Medical University of South Carolina has also published child physical and sexual abuse guidelines (available at www.musc.edu; Saunders, Berliner, & Hanson, 2003). This report describes treatment protocols for interventions in a number of areas of child abuse and rates the interventions in terms of how well they are empirically supported. A brief description is given of current components of adolescent sex offender treatment which is similar to that described earlier in this chapter. In terms of the evaluation of empirical support, adolescent sex offender treatment is rated as a "supported and acceptable treatment" but not as empirically established. For those working in residential facilities, there are published standards of treatment for youth in sex offender-specific residential programs. These standards were developed by an expert panel and cover the major issues one has to be concerned with in running adolescent programs (Bengis et al., 1999). It covers areas such as residents' rights, staff qualifications, safety standards, and intervention standards.

On the national level, there are two federally supported projects, the Center for Sex Offender Management (www.csom.org), sponsored by the Office of Justice Programs and the U.S. Department of Justice, and the National Center on Sexual Behavior in Youth, sponsored by the Office of Juvenile Justice and Delinquency Prevention through the Center on Child Abuse of Neglect at the University of Oklahoma Health Sciences Center (www.ncsby.org). The Center for Sex Offender Management was established in 1996 and provides information exchange, training, technical assistance, and analyzes the accomplishment of 19 multidisciplinary programs nationwide that have displayed promising practices with sex offenders. The CSOM's website provides information on both adult and adolescent offenders and has a number of publications and training resources. The National Center on Sexual Behavior in Youth was more recently established as a national training and technical assistance center. The National Center provides a number of training resources and treatment guidelines for both adolescent offenders and children with sexual behavior problems.

As earlier noted, there are also statewide models such as the previously cited programs in Utah and Colorado. For programs looking for statewide implementation models, the resources of these two groups provide extensive protocols for interagency cooperation, outline specific assessment approaches and treatment requirements, and provide detailed information on provider qualifications.

Finally, there are descriptions of innovative local programs (Hunter, Gilbertson, Vedros, & Morton, in press) that describe two programs, Wraparound Milwaukee and the Norfolk Juvenile Sex Offender Program. The Wraparound Milwaukee program was developed for high-risk youth including adolescent sex offenders and is a "community-based, family centered, culturally competent, multiple system and strength based alternative to institutional and deficit based care" (Hunter et al., in press). The program uses offense-specific assessment, multisystem collaboration and a variety of services from foster care to group homes and a variety of outpatient programs including in-home programs. The program has proven effective in increasing outpatient participation and decreasing the need for residential care. The Norfolk program has many similar features and uses interagency involvement including the court system, probation service, district attorneys, offender providers, victim treatment providers,the public school system, and representatives from the defense bar. The program model uses both socio-ecological approaches and sex offender-specific interventions. This program involves sex offender treatment groups, in-home services, groups for parents and caretakers, and community monitoring.

Both of these programs appear to include program features that are thought to be effective, but to date these programs are still undergoing evaluation and have not been empirically validated.

CONCLUSION

There have been advances in the field's understanding of adolescent sex offenders and their assessment and treatment, but there are several limitations to the current approaches to services for this population. On the positive side, not all adolescent offenders are viewed as being at high risk and in need of intensive interventions and life-long monitoring. Instead, the need for more individualization and flexibility in treatment programming for this population is recognized. There are also a number of risk and need instruments under development. In addition there are descriptions of promising treatment approaches and delivery systems that are also being researched. However, the major limitation at this time is that none of these are fully validated and empirically established. The field also is lacking with regard to primary prevention programs, which ultimately should be the main goal. As the field moves forward, it is hoped that clinicians will have better empirical data to guide decision making and interventions with this specialized population. Enhancing and improving the delivery of services will require the combined efforts of researchers, treatment providers, state agencies, juvenile court systems, and other relevant agencies including those who govern funding for programs within the treatment continuum.

REFERENCES

Abel, G. G., & Rouleau, J. L. (1990). The nature and extent of sexual abuse. In W. L. Marshall, D. R. Laws, & H. E. Barbaree (Eds.), *Handbook of sexual assault: Issues, theories, and treatment of the offender* (pp. 9–21). New York: Plenum.

Alexander, J., Barton, C., Gordon, D., Grotpeter, J., Hansson, K., Harrison, R. et al. (1998). *Blueprints for violence prevention, Book Three: Functional family therapy.* Boulder, CO: Center for the Study and Prevention of Violence.

Andrews, D. A., & Bonta, J. (1998). *The psychology of criminal conduct* (2nd ed.). Cincinnati, OH: Anderson.

Barbaree, H. E., Hudson, S. M., & Seto, M. C. (1993). Sexual assault in society: The role of the juvenile offender. In H. E. Barbaree, W. L. Marshall, & S. M. Hudson (Eds.), *The juvenile sex offender* (pp. 1–24). New York: Guilford.

Becker, J. V., & Kaplan, M. S. (1988). The assessment of adolescent sexual offenders. *Advances in Behavioral Assessment of Children and Families, 4,* 97–118.

Bengis, S. (1997). Comprehensive service delivery with a continuum of care. In G. Ryan & S. Lane (Eds.), *Juvenile sexual offending: Causes, consequences, and correction* (pp. 211–218). San Francisco, CA: Jossey-Bass.

Bengis, S., Brown, A., III, Freeman-Longo, R., Matsuda, B., Ross, J., & Thomas, J. (1999). *Standards of care for youth in sex offense-specific residential programs.* Holyoke, MA: NEARI Press.

Borduin, C. M., Henggeler, S. W., Blaske, D. M., & Stein, R. J. (1990). Multisystemic treatment of adolescent sexual offenders. *International Journal of Offender Treatment and Comparative Criminology, 34,* 105–113.

Borduin, C. M., & Schaeffer, C. M. (2001). Multisystemic treatment of juvenile sexual offenders: A progress report. *Journal of Psychology and Human Sexuality, 13,* 25–42.

Bremer, J. F. (2001). *The Protective Factors Scale.* St. Paul, MN: Project Pathfinder, Inc.

Butler, S. M., & Seto, M. C. (2002). Distinguishing two types of adolescent sex offenders. *Journal of the American Academy of Child and Adolescent Psychiatry, 41,* 83–90.

Caldwell, M. F. (2002). What we do not know about juvenile sexual reoffense risk. *Child Maltreatment, 7,* 291–302.

Center for Sex Offender Management. (1999). *Understanding juvenile sexual offending behavior: Emerging research, treatment approaches and management practices.* Silver Spring, MD: Author.

Chaffin, M. (2003). *Triage decision making guidelines for adolescent sex offenders.* Oklahoma City, OK: National Center on the Sexual Behavior of Youth.

Colorado Sex Offender Management Board. (2002). *Standards and guidelines for the evaluation, assessment, treatment and supervision of juveniles who have committed sexual offenses.* Denver, CO: Author.

Dishion, T. J., McCord, J., & Poulin, F. (1999). When interventions harm: Peer groups and problem behavior. *American Psychologist, 54,* 755–764.

Hagan, M. P., Gust-Brey, K. L., Cho, M. E., & Dow, E. (2001). Eight-year comparative analyses of adolescent rapists, adolescent child molesters, other adolescent delinquents, and the general population. *International Journal of Offender Therapy and Comparative Criminology, 45,* 314–324.

Hanson, R. K., Gordon, A., Harris, A. J. R., Marques, J. K., Murphy, W. D., Quinsey, V. L. et al. (2002). First report of the collaborative outcome data project on the effectiveness of treatment for sex offenders. *Sexual Abuse: A Journal of Research and Treatment, 14,* 169–194.

Henggeler, S. W., Mihalic, S. F., Rone, L., Thomas, C., & Tibbons-Mitchell, J. (1998). *Blueprints for violence prevention, Book Six: Multisystemic therapy.* Boulder, CO: Center for the Study and Prevention of Violence.

Hunter, J. A., Figueredo, A. J., Malamuth, N. M., & Becker, J. V. (2003). Juvenile sex offenders: Toward the development of a typology. *Sexual Abuse: A Journal of Research and Treatment, 15,* 27–48.

Hunter, J. A., Gilbertson, S. A., Vedros, D., & Morton, M. (2004). Strengthening community-based programming for juvenile sexual offenders: Key concepts and paradigm shifts. *Child Maltreatment, 9,* 177–189.

Knight, R. A., & Prentky, R. A. (1993). Exploring characteristics for classifying juvenile sex offenders. In H. E. Barbaree, W. L. Marshall, & S. M. Hudson (Eds.), *The juvenile sex offender* (pp. 1–24). New York: Guilford.

Långström, N. (2002). Long-term follow-up of criminal recidivism in young sex offenders: Temporal patterns and risk factors. *Psychology, Crime, and Law, 8,* 41–48.

Lipsey, M. W., & Derzon, J. H. (1998). Predictors of violent or serious delinquency in adolescence and early adulthood: A synthesis of longitudinal research. In R. Loeber & D. P. Farrington (Eds.), *Serious and violent juvenile offenders: Risk factors and successful interventions* (pp. 86–105). Thousand Oaks, CA: Sage.

Markey, O. B. (1950). A study of aggressive sex misbehavior in adolescents brought to Juvenile Court. *American Journal of Orthopsychiatry, 20,* 719–731.

Moffitt, T. E. (1993). Adolescence-limited and life-course-persistent antisocial behavior: A developmental taxonomy. *Psychological Review, 100,* 674–701.

Murphy, W. M., & Page, I. J. (1999). Adolescent perpetrators of sexual abuse. In R. T. Ammerman & M. Hersen (Eds.), *Assessment of family violence: A clinical and legal sourcebook* (2nd ed, pp. 367–389). New York: Wiley.

Murphy, W. M., & Page, I. J. (2000). Relapse prevention with adolescent sex offenders. In D. R. Laws, S. M. Hudson, & T. Ward (Eds.), *Remaking relapse prevention with sex offenders: A sourcebook* (pp. 353–368). Thousand Oaks, CA: Sage.

National Task Force on Juvenile Sexual Offending. (1993). The Revised report from the National Task Force on Juvenile Sexual Offending, 1993 of the National Adolescent Perpetrator Network, *Juvenile and Family Court Journal, 44,* 1–121.

Prentky, R., Harris, B., Frizzell, K., & Righthand, S. (2000). An actuarial procedure for assessing risk with juvenile sex offenders. *Sexual Abuse: A Journal of Research and Treatment, 12*, 71–93.

Righthand, S., & Welch, C. (2001). *Juveniles who have sexually offended: A review of the professional literature.* Washington, DC: Office of Juvenile Justice and Delinquency Prevention.

Saunders, B. E., Berliner, L., & Hanson, R. F. (Eds.). (2003). *Child physical and sexual abuse: Guidelines for treatment* (Final Report: January 15, 2003). Charleston, SC: National Crime Victims Research and Treatment Center.

Sipe, R., Jensen, E. L., & Everett, R. S. (1998). Adolescent sexual offenders grown up: Recidivism in young adulthood. *Criminal Justice and Behavior, 25*, 109–124.

Snyder, H. N. (2000). *Sexual assault of young children as reported to law enforcement: Victim, incident, and offender characteristics.* Washington, DC: National Center for Juvenile Justice.

Utah Network on Juveniles Offending Sexually. (1996). *Juvenile sex offender specific protocols and standards manual* (3rd ed.). Price, UT: Author.

Veneziano, C., & Veneziano, L. (2002). Adolescent sex offenders: A review of the literature. *Trauma, Violence, and Abuse, 3*, 247–260.

Weinrott, M. R. (1996). *Juvenile sexual aggression: A critical review.* Boulder, CO: Center for the Study and Prevention of Violence.

Worling, J. R. (2001). Personality-based typology of adolescent male sexual offenders: Differences in recidivism, rates, victim-selection, characteristics, and personal victimization histories. *Sexual Abuse: A Journal of Research and Treatment, 13*, 149–166.

Worling, J. R., & Curwen, T. (2001). Estimate of risk of adolescent sexual recidivism (Version 2.0: The "ERASOR"). In M. C. Calder (Ed.), *Juveniles and children who sexually abuse: Frameworks for assessment* (pp. 372–397). Lyme Regis, Dorset, UK: Russell.

16

Rural Mental Health Services

DAVID L. FENELL and ALAN J. HOVESTADT

Providing affordable and comprehensive metal health services for those who need these services is a tremendous challenge for the helping professions. The demand for services across the nation exceeds the ability of the mental health community to provide them. This is especially true for rural communities. DeLeon (2000) reported that even though 25% of the citizens of the United States live in rural areas, as many as two thirds of rural counties do not have basic mental health programs or adequately trained providers to meet the needs in those areas. Benson (2003a) supported this assertion and reported that much of rural America is underserved by mental health professionals. Her research suggested that approximately 60% of rural areas lack adequate mental health services. These statistics demonstrate that the challenges involved in providing mental health services for children, adolescents, and families in rural communities are formidable. To provide a comprehensive array of services, Rural Mental Health Centers (RMHC) must be efficiently organized, staffed, and allocated adequate resources to support the programs and services needed in the rural community. Even efficiently organized centers will not be successful in providing services without visionary leadership, highly skilled service providers, and technically competent support staff members who are accepted by and able to work well with citizens of rural areas (Fenell, Hovestadt, & Cochran, 1987; Hovestadt, Fenell, & Canfield, 2002).

Rural areas are difficult to define. However, most scholars agree that they consist of small communities that are distant from large metropolitan areas. Cities in rural areas are small, composed of fewer than 50,000

DAVID L. FENELL • Counseling and Human Services Program, University of Colorado at Colorado Springs, Colorado Springs, Colorado, 80933.   **ALAN J. HOVESTADT** • Counselor Education and Counseling Psychology, Western Michigan University, Kalamazoo, Michigan, 49008.

individuals, surrounded by open countryside, and removed from settled suburbs of larger cities (Murray & Keller, 1991). Rural areas have certain common characteristics that distinguish them from urban areas including lower population density; less access to goods and services; greater familiarity among the members of the community; less affluence; less access to education; and more health and mental health problems (Campbell, 2003).

Murray and Keller (1991) surveyed demographic research that revealed most mental health professionals choose to practice in urban areas and university towns. Many mental health professionals avoid rural practice because they believe that they may be professionally isolated, removed from cultural stimulation, unable to obtain quality education for their children, and may not be able to adapt to rural values. Nonetheless, quality mental health services are desperately needed in rural areas. Campbell (2003) reported that depression is almost twice as high among rural adolescents compared to the national norm and suicide rates in certain rural areas are three times higher than expected. Further, rural adolescents engage in binge drinking, drug abuse, and drive under the influence of alcohol more often than urban adolescents. The need for quality mental health services in rural communities is clearly present. However, meeting the need is as much a challenge for the helping professions today as it was a decade ago (Benson, 2003a).

The purpose of this chapter is to describe rural mental health service delivery. To accomplish this goal we will first describe the organization and delivery of mental health services developed to respond to the myriad of problems experienced by children, adolescents, and families in rural communities. Then we will describe the unique characteristics needed by rural mental health administrators and service providers to be successful working in rural areas. Highly skilled mental health professionals and administrators who are accepted by the citizens of the rural community in which they work are needed to organize and deliver services. Without these uniquely qualified professionals, rural mental health centers are unlikely to operate at their full potential (Fenell et al., 1987; Hovestadt et al., 2002).

RURAL MENTAL HEALTH CENTER ORGANIZATION

The organization of rural mental health centers is not significantly different from the organization of urban centers. However, the way in which services are provided may differ considerably because rural mental health professionals are often responsible for large, geographically remote service areas. Thus, rural providers may spend a large portion of their time traveling to satellite centers to provide services to clients who live at considerable distance from the RMHC (Murray & Keller, 1991). Effective RMHCs are led by visionary, down-to-earth administrators. These leaders are able to organize services, work well with local citizens, and hire and retain quality professional staff that respect community values and are able to relate well with community members.

Like their urban counterparts, most RMHC executive directors are appointed by and report to a governing board composed of influential community members who provide oversight and general direction for the center. In large RMHCS, the executive director's responsibilities are similar to those of an urban director. The director is responsible for hiring and supervising staff, determining mental health needs of the community, developing service delivery programs, evaluating program effectiveness, conducting research, administering the budget, fund raising, establishing linkages with other community service and health organizations, community relations and responding to other center administrative requirements (Fenell et al., 1987).

Small RMHCS require flexible organizational structures. The smallest centers might be staffed by a single mental health service provider who must "do it all." This individual would be both administrator and service provider, alternating jobs as the situation required (Kersting, 2003a). Other small centers may be staffed by two or three professionals who must establish collaborative working relationships with allied helping professionals to meet all community needs. One of the problems identified by rural mental health professionals, especially those working in small centers is professional burnout, which may result from high demands for services and the multiple roles these individuals perform (Dittmann, 2003).

Mental health professionals in small centers must be able to provide generalist mental health services and work in an administrative capacity as required by the circumstances. The staff of small centers must quickly identify and develop linkages with physicians, dentists, clergy, and other service organizations in the community to identify those citizens in need of mental health services and identify the most frequently reported mental health issues. To adequately respond to the demand for services, small centers must develop training programs to prepare paraprofessionals from the community to assist the professional staff in meeting certain community mental health needs such as delivering psychoeducational programs covering a variety of preventive mental health topics (Kinney, 1985). Finally, it must be remembered that establishing an effective RMHC organization will not be sufficient if the staff members are not able to develop and maintain cordial relationships with community members. An aloof doctor–patient relationship does not work well in rural America (Hovestadt et al., 2002).

SERVICES DELIVERED BY RURAL MENTAL HEALTH CENTERS

Human and Wasem (1991) identified a framework for the delivery of mental health services in rural areas. First, services must be *available*. There must be an agency or center to provide mental health service and appropriate personnel to staff the agency. DeLeon (2000), Benson (2003a), and Murray and Keller (1991) have described the shortage of qualified mental health personnel in rural communities. Thus, availability of services is not a given in all rural areas. The second element of the framework is *accessibility.* Even if services are available, are clients able to make use of them? Rural mental health service delivery areas vary from the smallest at 5,000 square miles to the largest at 60,000 square miles with accessibility problems increasing with the size of the area served. Accessibility of services may be affected by several factors including the distance between the client and the provider, lack of public transportation, lack of finances to pay for services, and lack of RMHC satellite offices strategically positioned throughout the service area to meet community mental health needs. The third element of the framework is *acceptability* of mental health service. Human and Wasem believe that for services to be acceptable, they must be provided in a way that is congruent with the values of the rural community.

Are there clearly distinguishable differences between rural mental health service delivery and service delivery provided by urban centers? The research on this subject is contradictory (Jones, Robbins, & Wagenfeld, 1974; York, Denton, & Moran, 1989). Weigel and Lloyd (2002) recently completed a study comparing rural and urban mental health counseling practices and found that there are certain significant differences between rural and urban mental health practices. The differences reported in this study were contextual issues pertaining to the requirements to meet the needs in extended service delivery areas of the rural settings compared to the urban settings. Even though some research suggested that rural communities experience proportionately more mental health problems than urban areas (Campbell, 2003), the specific mental health services provided by each type of center are not appreciably different. Other research suggested that rural mental health needs are similar in kind, but different in emphasis than in urban areas (Benson, 2003a). In the following section we will describe key services that a fully staffed RMHC might provide. The literature reviewed for this chapter is unanimous in recognizing that most rural areas do not have sufficient mental health services to meet the needs of the rural population (Benson, 2003a; DeLeon, 2000; Murray & Keller, 1991). Thus, only the most affluent and well-supported rural communities will have centers with all the services described.

Needs Assessment, Program Development, and Outcome Research

The primary mission of RMHCs is to meet the mental health needs of the rural communities they serve. But how are these needs to be identified? Once identified, how are the needs to be met? Finally, how can the RMHC be sure that the programs provided are meeting their goals (Lund, 1978)? To accomplish these tasks the RMHC needs a designated section tasked with needs assessment, program development, and outcome research (Fenell et al., 1987; Nettekoven & Sundberg, 1985). The major difficulty experienced by the RMHCs that attempt to develop an effective assessment and research section is that the urgent demands of the clientele for direct service are so great that time is not available for planning programs that meet other important community needs. In these situations, an expedient needs assessment may be accomplished by simply identifying the types of problems that present at the center and then developing programs to respond to them. Even so, RMHC staff members must strive to make time to conduct needs analyses to ensure they are addressing the most urgent community needs in addition to evaluating other ways they may serve the community.

Basic Mental Health Services

Benson (2003a) reported that rural, urban, and suburban communities experience similar types and rates of mental health problems whereas Campbell (2003) and Murray and Keller (1991) have noted differences between rural and urban mental health needs. In either case, RMHCs need to be prepared to provide important and frequently utilized services such as individual and group counseling. Because of the high demand for services in rural areas, group counseling sessions can extend the ability of mental health professionals to make direct contact with more clients (Corey, 2000).

Individual and group counseling services are especially important in the treatment of depression and the feelings of hopelessness that may lead to suicidal ideation. Foxhall (2000) reported that depression among rural adolescents is nearly twice the national average. Campbell (2003) reported that suicide rates in the rural west are three times higher than the national average. Once depression develops in rural clients it tends to persist (Linn & Husani, 1985), perhaps because the relatively stable characteristics of rural communities reinforce the symptoms. Basic crisis intervention services are necessary to provide quick response to problems such as depression and suicidal threats and to prevent them from exacerbating. A telephonic, 24-hour on-call system is frequently implemented to respond to the crises that occur during the hours that the RMHC is closed.

Substance Abuse Treatment

Rural adolescents are more likely to use tobacco products, drink to excess, abuse drugs, and drive when impaired than adolescents from urban communities (Campbell, 2003). Adults in rural areas experience problems with alcohol and drugs as well. The personal and social costs of substance abuse and related behaviors are high. Thus, RMHCs frequently provide substance abuse prevention and treatment programs as part of the service delivery system (Wagenfeld, 1991). Locally recruited paraprofessionals who have experience in resolving their own substance abuse problems often augment the RMHC staff. These paraprofessionals, under professional staff supervision, may work individually with clients and conduct psychoeducational groups (Kinney, 1985).

Marital and Family Therapy and Parent Education

Members of rural communities frequently hold traditional values, and this is often manifested in that they place great importance on family, church, and community. When psychological problems develop, often the first line of defense is to seek family, church, and community support (Human & Wasem, 1991). Stoller and Lee (1994) reported that rural marriages tend to be more stable than urban marriages. This may be true because of the traditional rural value system that views marriage as sanctioned by God and divorce as wrong. Despite the lower divorce level, rural couples do experience significant marital difficulties. Thus, RMHCS offer services for couples seeking to improve their relationships. In addition, family therapy is provided to help families deal with the problems of child rearing, adolescent depressions, substance abuse, and other family-related issues. Mental health providers trained in a systemic orientation are often most effective in providing marital and family services (Hovestadt et al., 2002). However, professionals who do not have systems training may also be effective helping rural families (Fenell & Weinhold, 2003). Parent education programs may be offered to help parents manage the normal, but often distressing, developmental problems experienced by most families. Additionally, many RMHCS provide domestic violence prevention and treatment programs. The farm crisis that emerged in the 1980s put tremendous economic and social stressors on families. Marriages were stressed, relationships deteriorated, and domestic violence issues sometimes emerged (Murray & Keller, 1991). RMHCS were called upon to institute programs to respond to this crisis. Benson (2003a) reported that families that sought professional help were able to respond more effectively to the crisis than families that did not seek help.

Other Services

The services described above are those most frequently provided. However, other important services that receive that less attention in the literature are often provided. Some RMHCS offer services for the severely mentally ill including those with schizophrenic, bipolar, and other chronic mental health conditions (Wagenfeld, 1982). Close coordination with medical personnel who prescribe and monitor medications is necessary in providing this service. Services are sometimes offered for the developmentally disabled and the elderly with dementia problems (Crawford, 2003). Because rural mental health professionals are typically generalists (Hovestadt et al., 2002), the staff may not be trained to treat the severely mentally ill, the elderly, and those with developmental disabilities. Therefore, many RMHCS have developed *Telehealth* capabilities (Benson, 2003c). Telehealth is a technology-based system that links providers who are separated by distance and allows rural mental health practitioners to access experts in the field on the treatment of a variety of complex mental health problems (Maheu, 2001). It allows rural providers who may not have specialized knowledge in some areas to consult with experts to help devise treatment for or referral of patients with problems outside the scope of the RMHC's ability to provide services. A more detailed discussion of telehealth services is provided by Liss elsewhere in this volume.

Another service provided by RMHCS is consultation to community organizations. When a community organization experiences interpersonal conflicts among its members, RMHC professionals can intervene with conflict resolution assistance. Additionally, RMHC staff may provide consultation or supervision for teachers, counselors, and administrators of local schools concerning appropriate interventions for children with school-related problems (Kennedy, 2003).

All the services described above would rarely be provided by a single RMHC. Qualified staff and funding simply are not available in most communities to provide a comprehensive array of services. Thus, those who elect to serve as mental health providers in rural communities must become generalists and must be prepared to consult regularly with specialists to implement services that the staff may not be equipped to deliver. But no matter how comprehensive the array of services may be, those residing in the rural community will not make use of them unless they trust the administrator and service providers of the RMHC. Mental health professionals who are successful in rural communities have certain qualities that make it more likely that they will be accepted into the community and thus be able to effectively deliver mental health services. We will discuss those qualities in the remainder of this chapter.

CHARACTERISTICS OF EFFECTIVE RURAL MENTAL HEALTH DIRECTORS AND SERVICE PROVIDERS

Fenell et al. (1987) conducted research to identify most important characteristics of RMHC senior administrators. Hovestadt et al. (2002) identified the characteristics of effective rural mental health service providers. They identified several characteristics essential to organizing, leading, and working as mental health professionals in successful rural mental health centers that are capable of providing mental health services to children, adolescents, and families. The most important characteristics identified in this research are described below along with their implication for the effective organization and delivery of mental health services to the rural community. These characteristics can help potential candidates for RMHC positions assess their qualifications and readiness for rural mental health center work as well as serving as a guide for governing boards as they evaluate applicants for staff positions in their centers.

Leadership Ability

A fundamental characteristic of the effective RMHC director according to Fenell et al. (1987) is *leadership ability*. This characteristic is not unique to rural mental health centers, as directors of urban and suburban centers need this ability as well (Weigel & Lloyd, 2002). This characteristic is also important for RMHC staff members who are responsible for program delivery and supervision of other staff members. Leadership includes the ability to make decisions, set priorities, delegate responsibilities, and teach and motivate staff. These skills make it possible to resolve the myriad of problems that can occur in the administration of a RMHC (Cedar & Salasin, 1979). Rural communities experience the full spectrum of mental health problems. The idyllic pastoral setting often associated with the rural lifestyle is rapidly disappearing as many of the problems of urban America have reached the rural communities.

Political Savvy

Another critical skill needed by rural mental health personnel is *political savvy*. It is widely understood that rural communities tend to be close knit with formal and informal communication and leadership systems. Miller and Ostendorf (1982) reported that an effective RMHC director and staff must have the ability to understand and interface with formal and informal community organizations with diverse constituencies and multiple concerns. To be able to do this, knowledge of systems theory is helpful (Fenell & Weinhold, 2003) as is the ability to understand and accommodate the power structure within the community. Successful professionals are able to identify with and accommodate the influential systems and organizations within the community and involve the members of these organizations in the programs of the RMHC. Political savvy is also important as the RMHC staff lobbies local governance groups, county and state legislators to provide funding and other types of support for the RMHC.

Ability to Manage Budgets and Obtain Resources

Effective rural mental health center directors and program managers are charged with budget management. Depending on the size of the organization budgets can amount to as much as several million dollars per year for comprehensive organizations or as little as $100,000 for a one-person center. The RMHC director is ultimately responsible for the center's budget even though some larger centers hire a staff person to manage the budget and some budget management may be delegated to program managers. Whether the center is a large or a small one, careful stewardship of available resources is an essential skill. In virtually all cases, RMHC funding is not sufficient to meet all needs. Therefore, it is important to be able to identify and apply for sources of external funding (Miller & Ostendorf, 1982). The ability to obtain external funding through grant writing is needed if innovative programs are to be added to the basic programs supported by the annual budget.

Ability to Select and Retain RMHC Personnel

Another important characteristic of effective rural mental health center directors and program managers is the ability to identify, hire, and guide the careers of mental health center professional and administrative staff. No organization can respond to the demands of its constituencies without well-trained and competent personnel who desire to remain with the organization (Fenell et al., 1987). Thus, this characteristic might be the most important of all. Because of the isolated nature of rural centers, it is imperative that staff get along well and work together collaboratively. The director takes the lead in maintaining staff harmony through the use of effective personnel management techniques. More importantly, however, is the genuine caring demonstrated through the personal interest the director takes in each staff member.

In addition to these skills the effective RMHC director must identify and hire competent staff that has the requisite personality, background, values, and skills set that will facilitate their ability to serve well in rural America. The majority of graduate students in the mental health disciplines are from urban and suburban areas. They have little knowledge of rural mental health career opportunities. Even when students are made aware of rural opportunities, they may avoid these positions because of the negative stigma associated with rural communities (Lichtenstein, Nettekoven, & Sundberg, 1986). Mental health professionals are stereotypically liberal, progressive, inclusive, and not highly religious. They tend to have flexible value systems and are supportive of opportunities for groups that have been historically discriminated against including many minority groups, women, and gays and lesbians. They may perceive the rural community as holding rigid conservative values, tied to the past, highly religious, an insular closed system, and not recognizing the need to accommodate groups who have suffered past discrimination (Campbell, 2003). Thus many mental health professionals are concerned that they will not be a good fit in rural mental health because of this potential clash of values, beliefs, and behaviors (Piercy, Hovestadt, Fenell, Franklin, & McKeon, 1982). Because these attitudes toward rural mental health work are so prevalent, the RMHC director often finds it difficult to identify, hire, and retain competent staff who will find the rural environment a good fit.

There are several desirable characteristics of rural mental health professionals, including the executive director of the center. To obtain the best staff possible, the RMHC center director will assess potential applicants for the qualities identified and described in the following sections.

An Appropriate Mental Health Specialization

Rural communities have the same types of psychological problems as other settings. Thus, to best meet the range of needs of community members it is important to hire staff with a variety of differing specializations. Important specialization areas include marriage, family therapy (Hovestadt et al., 2002), responding to the needs of the rural elderly (Chalifoux, Neese, Buckwalter, Litwak, & Abraham, 1996), child therapy (Kennedy, 2003), and treating affective disorders, and drug and alcohol abuse treatment (Campbell, 2003). A staff with a variety of specialties can increase the scope of services provided by the center as professionals cross-train each other and train paraprofessionals to supplement the professional staff by providing appropriate services (Hovestadt et al., 2002).

Ability to Function as a Generalist

This quality seems to contradict the previous one. However, both qualities, possessing a needed specialization *and* being able to function as a generalist, can and do coexist in rural mental health practice. Being a generalist is especially critical in small rural mental health centers with only a few professional staff members (Murray & Keller, 1981). In small centers the staff must treat each problem that comes through the door. The therapist may not be trained to treat clients with certain presenting problems. Therefore, it is ethically important for rural mental health professionals to have access to a variety of referral sources to treat these clients. A growing number of centers with limited access to specialized mental health care have implemented *distance counseling* through the use of interactive video technology. This technology holds great promise for small, isolated rural communities where mental health specialization is not available (Benson, 2003c).

Rural Community Appreciation and Understanding

This characteristic is one of the most important for both RMHC administrators and staff members. The literature on rural mental health is replete with references to the importance of this characteristic (Fenell et al., 1987; Hovestadt, Fenell, & Piercy, 1983; Murray & Keller 1991). The rural system is a highly complex organization, composed of numerous interrelated subsystems, and with clearly defined overt and covert rules of behavior. For the RMHC to organize to provide effective services to the rural clientele, it must hire a staff that is aware of these factors and can interact effectively with all elements of the rural organization. Moreover, to increase the odds of acceptance in the rural community, RMHC staff members need to live, work, and play in the community. Those who work in rural areas by day and retreat to urban centers by night often take longer in establishing effective working relationships with their clientele.

Individuals raised in rural communities are frequently self-reliant and often unwilling to seek help. Moreover, they stereotypically hold traditional values; are politically and fiscally conservative, and may hold strong fundamentalist religious beliefs (Fenell et al., 1987; Hovestadt et al., 2002). As in all treatment settings, the therapist must be successful in establishing therapeutic relationships with clients (Rogers, 1957). In addition, rural therapists must be able to establish rapport with influential individuals and subsystems within the community. Rural communities tend to be "close-knit." If key members of the community believe that RMHC personnel do not understand the organization of the community, appreciate the community, and accept the values of the people within the community, then it is unlikely that the members of the community will feel comfortable seeking services from the center (Weigel & Lloyd, 2002). On the other hand, when the community members observe the RMHC staff living in the community, participating in community activities and establishing local friendships, trust builds and the utilization of services often increases.

Personality Attributes Relevant to Rural Life

A good fit between person and environment is important for successful rural mental health practice (Miller & Ostendorf, 1982). Certain personality traits seem to contribute to this success including flexibility, dependability, trustworthiness, maturity, self-awareness, empathy, and an ability to tolerate isolation. In addition, a good sense of humor and an easy-going relationship style facilitate successful practice. Professionals who possess these characteristics seem to get along with the community members well, enjoy their work, and are less likely to terminate employment prematurely (Hovestadt et al., 2002).

Relevant Professional Background and Training

To best organize for effective service delivery in rural settings, the RMHC director and staff should have *relevant professional background and training*. While this is the ideal, most mental health professionals come to the RMHC with little or no understanding of the requirements for successful practice in the rural setting (Murray & Keller, 1991). Only a few training programs exist that were specifically designed to prepare mental health professionals for work in rural settings (Hargrove, 1991; Kersting, 2003b). Most training programs prepare their graduates for work in urban settings and provide their students with the clinical skills and ethical knowledge necessary for success in urban practice. Many of the graduates who opt for work in rural communities do so initially because of the National Health Service Corps program that repays the educational debts of health professionals who agree to practice in underserved rural areas (Chamberlin, 2003).

Hovestadt et al. (1983) developed a rural training program for students preparing for work in rural settings. The program was designed to prepare the students for the realities of rural practice. One of the student activities required in this rural east Texas program was eating breakfast at the "Chat and Chew Café" early in the morning when the farmers, ranchers, and local business owners were present and discussing the events of the community. Another event was to attend the local African American Baptist church and meet the pastor and congregation members. A third event was to attend a local high school football game and interact with other folks in attendance. A final activity was to meet and interview local mental health personnel and identify the joys and sorrows of rural practice. Through completion of these activities the students began to develop an appreciation of the members of that rural community and an understanding that would equip them to be successful in rural practice.

Other rural mental health training programs are located at the University of Florida, Idaho State University, and Nebraska. Programs specifically focused on services for Native Americans are located at the University of North Dakota, Oklahoma State University, the University of Montana, and the University of Colorado (Benson, 2003b). These programs attempt to teach their students to be self-sufficient and resourceful in the rural environment; develop the necessary skills to become culturally compatible with the rural environment and its people; develop a wide range of generalist skills to provide help to a variety of mental health concerns and develop financial skills to manage the RMHC and to meet personal financial obligations (Kersting, 2003a). It is projected that as more academic programs add rural mental health training, the number of underserved rural areas will decline. However, this projection will need to be confirmed through comprehensive program evaluations and follow-up studies.

Stressors in Rural Mental Health

Working as a mental health service provider in rural areas can be a pleasant experience for those who enjoy the rural lifestyle, interacting with their clients and families in informal settings and a slower pace of life. Another advantage of rural practice is that the cost of living is often less than in urban settings; homes are more affordable and in some communities many of the social problems of the cities are absent. Additionally, those professionals who enjoy outdoor activities like hunting, fishing, hiking, and camping often enjoy working in a rural environment.

There are also significant drawbacks to rural practice. Therapists who work in rural areas often report that they feel professional isolation from colleagues and may not be able to get supervision when needed. They are often isolated from urban social activities such as the theater, art galleries, museums, and concerts. Although the cost of living may be low in rural areas, salaries are usually low as well and annual raises are modest. Professionals have reported that living in a rural community makes them feel like they are on call all the time. Some therapists enjoy the out of office contact with clients whereas others find it difficult to manage (Dittmann, 2003). Thus, burnout can occur if the provider does not take concrete measures to prevent it. Additionally, rural practice provides ethical challenges to some professionals. Dual relationships, for example, are almost unavoidable as your client might also be your car mechanic (Dittmann, 2003). Finally, therapists may struggle with the lack of personal privacy for themselves and their family that can occur in rural settings (Weigel & Lloyd, 2002).

CONCLUSION

This chapter has described the organization and delivery of rural mental health services and has identified essential characteristics that professional staff members must possess to be successful in the rural environment. The information in this chapter highlights the significant issues of rural mental health service delivery. Further, it may serve as a guide for professionals considering employment in rural mental health. The topics covered in this chapter may suggest areas of curriculum development for academic programs designed to prepare professionals for rural mental health work. Finally, the information here may serve as a guide for the selection of rural mental health center directors and professional staff members who will bear the responsibility of providing competent and comprehensive mental health services to this traditionally underserved population.

REFERENCES

Benson, E. (2003a). Beyond "urbancentrism". *Monitor on Psychology, 34*(6), 54–55.

Benson, E. (2003b). Psychology in Indian country. *Monitor on Psychology, 34*(6), 56–57.

Benson, E. (2003c). Telehealth gets back to basics. *Monitor on Psychology, 34*(6), 58–59.

Campbell, C. D. (2003). Rurality as a form of diversity: Preparing for rural practice. *The Family Psychologist, 19*(3), 13–14.

Cedar, T., & Salasin, J. (1979). *Research directions for rural mental health.* McLean, VA: Mitre Corp.

Chalifoux, Z., Neese, J. B., Buckwalter, K. C., Litwak, E., & Abraham, I. L. (1996). Mental health services for the rural elderly: Innovative service strategies. *Community Mental Health Journal, 32,* 497–503.

Chamberlin, J. (2003). Slot offers loan repayment and other rewards. *Monitor on Psychology, 34*(6), 61.

Corey, G. (2000). *Theory and practice of group counseling* (5th ed.). Pacific Grove, CA: Brooks/Cole.

Crawford, N. (2003). Knocking down access barriers. *Monitor on Psychology, 34*(6), 64–65.

DeLeon, P. H. (2000). Rural America: Our diamond in the rough. *Monitor on Psychology, 31*(7), 5.

Dittmann, M. (2003). Maintaining ethics in a rural setting. *Monitor on Psychology, 34*(6), 66.

Fenell, D. L., Hovestadt, A. H., & Cochran, S. W. (1987). Characteristics of effective administrators of rural mental health centers. *Journal of Rural Community Psychology, 8*(1), 23–35.

Fenell, D. L., & Weinhold, B. K. (2003). *Counseling families: An introduction to marriage and family therapy.* Denver: Love Publishing.

Foxhall, K. (2000). Rural life holds particular stressors for women. *Monitor on Psychology, 31*(1), 30–32.

Hargrove, D. S. (1991). Training Ph.D. psychologists for rural service: A report from Nebraska. *Community Mental Health Journal, 27,* 293–298.

Hovestadt, A. H., Fenell, D. L., & Canfield, B. S. (2002). Characteristics of effective providers of marital and family therapy in rural mental health settings. *Journal of Marital and Family Therapy, 28,* 225–231.

Hovestadt, A. H., Fenell, D. L., & Piercy, F. P. (1983). Integrating marriage and family therapy within counselor education: A three level model. In B. F. Okun & S. T. Gladding (Eds.), *Issues in training marriage and family therapists.* Ann Arbor, MI: ERIC Clearinghouse No. ED237839.

Human, J., & Wasem, C. (1991). Rural mental health in America. *American Psychologist, 46,* 232–239.

Jones, J. D., Robins, S. S., & Wagenfeld, M. O. (1974). Rural mental health centers: Are they different? *International Journal of Mental Health, 3,* 77–92.

Kennedy, J. (2003). Man of many roles. *Monitor on Psychology, 34*(6), 67.

Kersting, K. (2003a). Professional pioneering on the frontier. *Monitor on Psychology, 34*(6), 68.

Kersting, K. (2003b). Teaching self-sufficiency in rural practice. *Monitor on Psychology, 34*(6), 60–62.

Kinney, H. (1985). Utilization of psychoeducational interventions in rural mental health programs. *Journal of Rural community Psychology, 6*(2), 45–51.

Lichtenstein, E., Nettekoven, L., & Sundberg, N. (1986). Training for mental health promotion in rural settings. *Journal of Rural community Psychology, 1*, 31–40.

Linn, J. G., & Husani, B. A. (1985). Chronic medical problems, coping resources and depression: A longitudinal study of rural Tennesseans. *American Journal of Community Psychology, 13*, 733–742.

Lund, D. A. (1978). Mental health program evaluation: Where do you start? *Evaluation and Program Planning, 1*, 31–40.

Maheu, M. (2001). *E-health, telehealth and telemedicine*. San Francisco: Jossey-Bass.

Miller, M., & Ostendorf, D. G. (1982). Administrative, economic and political considerations in the development of rural mental health services. In P. A. Keller & J. D. Murray (Eds.), *Handbook of rural community mental health*. New York: Human Sciences Press.

Murray, J. D., & Keller, P. A. (1991). Psychology in rural America: Current status and future directions. *American Psychologist, 46*, 220–231.

Nettekoven, L., & Sundberg, N. (1985). Community assessment methods in rural mental health promotion. *Journal of Rural Community Psychology, 6*(2), 21–43.

Piercy, F. P., Hovestadt, A. J., Fenell, D. L., Franklin, E., & McKeon, D. (1982). A comprehensive training model for therapists serving rural populations. *Family Therapy, 9*, 239–249.

Rogers, C. R. (1957). The necessary and sufficient conditions of therapeutic personality change. *Journal of Consulting Psychology, 21*, 95–103.

Stoller, E. P., & Lee, G. R. (1994). Informal care of rural elders. In R. T. Coward, C. N. Bull, G. Kulkulka, & J. M. Galliher (Eds.), *Health services for rural elders*. New York: Springer.

Wagenfeld, M. O. (1982). Psychopathology in rural areas: Issues and evidence. In P. A. Keller & J. D. Murray (Eds.), *Handbook of rural community mental health*. New York: Human Sciences Press.

Wagenfeld, M. O. (1991). Mental health in rural America: A decade review. *Journal of Rural Health, 6*, 507–522.

Weigel, D. J., & Lloyd, A. P. (2002, March). *Mental health counseling practice in rural versus urban environments*. Poster session presented at the annual meeting of the American Counseling Association, New Orleans, LA.

York, R. O., Denton, T. T., & Moran, J. R. (1989). Rural and urban social work practice: Is there a difference? *Social Casework, 70*, 201–209.

17

Mental Health Services for Children with Chronic Illness

ANN M. McGRATH DAVIS and NGAN VUONG

The diagnosis of a chronic illness (CI) in a child can be a devastating blow to both a child and his or her family. Approximately 20% of children less than 18 years of age have a CI (Perrin & MacLean, 1988) for a total of 4–7 million children in the United States (Newacheck & Halfon, 1998). A CI has been defined as a "medically diagnosed ailment with a duration of 6 months or longer, which shows little change or slow progression" (Williams, 1997, p. 312). Ailments that fall into this category include juvenile rheumatoid arthritis, cancer, diabetes, and asthma, among others.

Clinical experience suggests that children and adolescents diagnosed with a CI may be likely to experience psychosocial difficulties. Research has repeatedly demonstrated, however, that children with CI experience only slightly elevated levels of psychosocial distress and that their scores on standardized instruments do not typically fall outside of the normal range on psychosocial measures and do not differ statistically from control groups (Bailey et al., 1993; Bennett, 1994; Hays et al., 1992; Meadows, McKee, & Kazak, 1989; Soliday, Kool, & Lande, 2000). These findings suggest that although children with a CI may experience slight increases in psychosocial distress, these increases are not statistically or clinically significant when compared to children without a CI. Whether these findings are the result of truly average levels of distress, or the result of low-end specificity problems with measurement remains a matter of debate (e.g., Phipps & Srivastava, 1997; Phipps & Steele, 2002).

ANN M. McGRATH DAVIS and NGAN VUONG • University of Kansas Medical Center, Kansas City, Kansas 66160.

The current chapter reviews the organization and delivery of mental health services for children and adolescents with a CI and their families. The chapter begins with the diagnostic process, then discusses the first 3–5 years following diagnosis, and finally the long-term issues associated with pediatric CI. Each of these three sections will begin by focusing on the mental health issues and services for the pediatric patient and move into discussion of issues and services available for parents. As there is little information available about siblings during the diagnostic process or regarding immediate adjustment, all sibling information will be discussed in the long-term issues section. The chapter ends with a discussion specific to hospitalization issues as many children with a chronic health condition are hospitalized repeatedly during the illness process.

THE MENTAL HEALTH ASPECTS OF THE DIAGNOSTIC PROCESS

The Process

The diagnostic process for children with a CI typically starts with a visit to the primary care physician followed by a referral to a pediatric subspecialist. During this process the child typically experiences medical symptoms varying in degree of severity, often including pain and accompanied by a decrease in functioning at school and at home. Once the child and family visit a pediatric subspecialist, the child typically undergoes a variety of tests that may or may not be painful in nature. When the tests are reviewed, the child and family receive news of their child's CI.

Effects on the Patient

Unfortunately, there are few data available to indicate the mental health needs of children during the diagnostic process. In fact, a recent meta-analysis indicates that most children who participated in studies on the psychosocial issues associated with CI were at least 5 years beyond the diagnosis of their medical condition (Kibby, Tyc, & Mulhern, 1998). However, the data that are available indicate that "open communication with children about life-threatening situations results in less emotional distress than protecting them from the difficult truth" (Stuber, 1996, p. 489). So, the family that is tempted to keep information from their child to protect them should be dissuaded from doing so. Also, results indicated that maternal distress significantly affects the ill child's appraisal of the situation (Stuber et al., 1994), suggesting that if a mother's distress could be decreased through intervention this may result directly in less distress for the ill child.

In a unique study of children diagnosed with juvenile rheumatoid arthritis and insulin-dependent diabetes mellitus, and healthy control children, Frank et al. (1998) assessed the adaptation of the children from diagnosis through the first 18 months of treatment. Child functioning indicated the highest scores immediately following diagnosis, although scores at all assessment points were still within normal limits. Parental distress also indicated the highest scores immediately following diagnosis that tended to regress to the mean by 6 months and remain there through the 18-month assessment point. These results support previous research that children with CI do have psychological functioning within normal limits, but highlight that distress may be most acute during the diagnostic process.

Despite the evidence indicating a likely increase in psychological distress during the diagnostic phase, no intervention studies could be found targeting this phase in the pediatric population. Looking to the adult literature, however, medical crisis counseling may present a treatment option. Medical crisis counseling (MCC; Pollin, 1994, 1995) was developed to decrease the psychological distress encountered by those recently diagnosed with a CI. The intervention uses cognitive coping strategies and increased social support in a brief focal treatment format that is reportedly easily integrated into medical care. In a randomized clinical trial with adults, Koocher, Curtiss, Pollin, and Patton (2001) compared the use of MCC to medical care alone. Results were difficult to interpret due to the low number of participants who agreed to participate in MCC (36%), but suggest that MCC may lead to increased perception of social support and increased satisfaction with treatment. Therefore, MCC may warrant further study with pediatric patients to determine whether it helps to ameliorate the increases in psychological difficulties experienced by children recently diagnosed with a CI (Schulz & Masek, 1996).

If children are admitted to the hospital for any part of the diagnostic process, they may encounter a mental health provider who is part of the inpatient medical care team (Williams & DeMaso, 2000). For example, at many institutions, a psychologist is routinely consulted for children who are newly diagnosed with cancer, diabetes, rheumatic disease, or any other CI. Although few data exist on the effectiveness of these services, or even their uniformity across sites, parents, referring pediatricians, and consultants indicate that inpatient mental health services do benefit the patient (Carter et al., 2003). Specifically, consultation services target improved management of health concerns, improved coping, and improved adjustment. The mental health consultant can also serve to coordinate care and facilitate communication between the patient, family, and team members (Williams & DeMaso, 2000).

Effects on Parents

As would be expected, the uncertainty that takes place during the diagnostic phase places a major stress on the family (Cohen, 1993), and if this process occurs in a technologically dense environment (such as a pediatric intensive care unit) parents are likely to report this as an additional stressor (Hughes & McCollum, 1994). In a review, Melnyk, Moldenhouer, Feinstein, and Small (2001) indicated that common parental reactions to child diagnosis with a chronic medical condition included shock, disbelief, denial, anger, despair, depression, frustration, confusion, guilt, decreased self-worth, and a lack of confidence. During this phase of CI, parents often have to miss work to take the child to the hospital or to medical appointments and may even find it necessary to quit their job. This causes a decrease in the financial stability of the family, which likely leads to increased stress. Also, parents often have to make child care arrangements for other children in the family and report feelings of guilt over not spending as much time with these siblings as they would like. However, research also suggests that families in this phase may experience some positive effects, including increased cohesion (Gonzalez, Steinglass, & Reiss, 1989). Stress may also decrease following the diagnosis as families have been experiencing increased worry since the patient's symptoms began, and getting a definitive diagnosis may bring them an explanation and therefore relief (Clubb, 1991).

Unfortunately, there have been few studies published that directly target improving parental mental health during the diagnostic process. Hakimi conducted a dissertation on the psychosocial adaptation of families and children following a diagnosis of insulin-dependent diabetes mellitus (IDDM; Hakimi, 1998). Children between the ages of 8 and 18 years who were newly diagnosed with IDDM were randomly assigned to an intervention group or a control group. Although not detailed in the abstract, the intervention was reportedly developmentally focused and family based. Unfortunately, the specific instrument used to measure adjustment was not mentioned but did suggest that differences in parent adjustment were not significant.

There are some clinical services currently available for parents of children undergoing diagnosis of a CI, despite the lack of research in this area. These services vary depending upon whether the diagnostic process takes place on an outpatient basis or in the hospital. For parents of children who are diagnosed on an outpatient basis, typically their physician will refer them for supportive services, but only if they request them. For parents of children who are diagnosed in the hospital, supportive services are typically provided by a social worker, chaplain, or pediatric psychologist who is part of the medical care team and visits the family on a regular basis during their hospital stay. The amount of contact that these parents have with supportive providers varies considerably across institutions and even across subspecialties within the same institution.

THE MENTAL HEALTH ASPECTS OF THE FIRST THREE TO FIVE YEARS POST-DIAGNOSIS

Effects on the Patient

Once a child has completed the diagnostic process and begun their treatment regimen, a number of changes take place. First, they must become accustomed to often invasive and painful treatments that can take place several times a day. They also begin to reintegrate into the life they had prior to becoming ill. This means returning home, returning to school, and resuming other childhood activities. However, accompanying them at this time may be stigmatizing treatments, such as medications, medication side effects (puffiness and weight gain), feeding tubes, etc. Children often have to leave class for medications or treatments, which may draw unwanted attention. And, they often are required to miss school regularly to attend doctor's appointments or return to the hospital for scheduled treatments and occasional exacerbations.

Initial research suggested that the most consistently significant predictor of psychological distress in chronically ill children is the number of physical stressors (Saylor et al., 1987). However, more recent research indicates that when other factors are considered, they often account for more of the variability in psychosocial distress than physical stressors. For example, Lavigne and Faier-Routman (1993) conducted a large meta-analysis assessing the factors related to adjustment to pediatric CI and found that disease factors were fairly poor predictors of adjustment. Reviewing 38 articles covering adjustment to pediatric CI, the authors found that disease severity, poor prognosis, and diminished functional status were the three disease factors most related to patient adjustment. However, both parent or family and child variables were much more highly related to adjustment than these disease factors. Parent or family and child variables included maternal maladjustment, increased family stress, child self-concept, low-IQ, and poor child coping. Interestingly, the authors also found that gender was significantly related to adjustment, with boys demonstrating lower levels of adjustment than girls across studies.

To decrease the difficulties experienced by the chronically ill child, Chernoff, Ireys, DeVet, and Kim (2002) designed a 15-month, community-based, family support intervention. This intervention was designed to reduce the risk for poor adjustment and mental health problems in children with a CI and their mothers. Specifically, the Family-to-Family Network, the intervention's title, was composed of both child and mother components. Children participated in group activities with child life specialists over the 15-month intervention period whereas mothers of newly diagnosed children met with mothers whose children had the same diagnosis, but had been diagnosed for a longer period of time ("veteran mothers"). Contacts included phone calls, home visits, community visits, group sessions, a regular newsletter, and occasional parties. Results indicate that this novel method of service delivery led to significant improvements in adjustment, especially for children who had low self-esteem regarding their physical appearance.

Effects on Parents

Once children begin treatment for their CI, parents often have to learn how to provide medical care for their child that is often painful, expensive, and time consuming. It is also possible that parents may have to become medically involved in the care of their child, likely decreasing their ability to care for their chronically ill child or other children. For example, in the case of pediatric liver transplant, parents are often considered optimal organ donors, who then may choose to undergo major surgery so as to donate an organ to their chronically ill child. In a study of parents who served as a donor for their child's liver transplant, Goldman (1993) found that marital dissolution was reported in two cases, adjustment disorder in one case, and other minor problems noted in several other patients, including in-law tensions, regression (immature coping), and suspected spousal abuse. These results suggest that parents may be in need of assessment at this point in their child's medical illness progression.

The example of parents serving as organ donor, however, is rare. It is more common for parents to have new responsibilities such as administering medications and therapies, scheduling appointments and coordinating medical care, as well as becoming an active member of the team making treatment decisions regarding their child. Research indicates that approximately 37% of mothers in this phase of their child's CI experience poor adjustment (Davis, Brown, Bakeman, & Campbell, 1998). Also, when parents are not equally dividing household tasks and child care tasks or when there is an imbalance in the amount of time spent in child care tasks compared to recreational activities couples are more likely to experience distress (Quittner, DiGirolamo, Michel, & Eigen, 1992; Quittner et al., 1998; Quittner, Opipari, Regoli, Jacobsen, & Eigen, 1992).

At least one promising intervention for parents during this phase of CI has been investigated: Sahler et al. (2004) reported on the results of a multisite investigation of a problem-solving skills therapy (PSST) for mothers of children undergoing treatment for cancer. The intervention involved 8 weekly 1-hour sessions that focused on teaching steps for solving mother-identified problems. Results indicated improved problem-solving skills and reduced distress (i.e., decreased depressive symptoms, mood disturbance, and posttraumatic stress symptoms) at the completion of therapy. Most of these gains were maintained 3 months after the completion of PSST.

Despite the apparent success of programs such as the PSST intervention, parents are rarely referred to a psychological provider at this time unless they directly make a request to their child's physician. The primary exception to this is when medical providers observe an indicator of problems within the family. At this time, they may choose to discuss referral to a psychological provider with the family. Because most of the stress experienced by parents during this phase of their child's CI have to do with financial issues, increased medical care demands and decreased recreational time and time with their spouse, it would be helpful if the services provided targeted these specific concerns.

THE LONG-TERM MENTAL HEALTH ASPECTS OF CI

Effects on the Patient

There are many factors that predict a child's long-term adjustment to CI. Previous research has indicated that both physical stressors

(Saylor et al., 1987) and functional impairment (Mulhern, Wasserman, Friedman, & Fairclough, 1989) are related to a long-term outcome in the chronically ill child, but that visible impairments are no more psychosocially damaging than psychosocial or psychological effects (O'Malley, Foster, Koocher, & Slavin, 1980).

In addition to the physical factors, studies indicate that it is the perception of stressors, rather than the actual nature of the stressors, that predicts long-term adjustment (Stuber, 1996). Despite these factors, however, survivors of pediatric CI apparently experience normal long-term mental health when compared to statistical norms and control groups (Kazak & Meadows, 1989). Some findings do indicate that children with a CI also report lesser social support and fewer peers in their social support networks than healthy children (Ellerton, Stewart, Ritchie, & Hirth, 1996).

Kazak et al. (1997) conducted a study on the mental health functioning of former leukemia patients and control participants. Using measures of posttraumatic stress, anxiety, family functioning, and social support, the authors found several differences between the two groups. For example, children who survived leukemia were significantly more likely to report symptoms of anxiety than control group children, and mothers and fathers were significantly more likely to report symptoms of posttraumatic stress than control group parents. However, children who survived leukemia were no more likely to report symptoms of posttraumatic stress than children in the control group, and family functioning and social support were not significantly different between groups. The authors reported that although parents and children indicate that they experience difficulties with anxieties and symptoms of posttraumatic stress, these symptoms did not interfere with their daily functioning, and thus may not indicate any sort of need for treatment.

Effects on Parents

Data on the long-term effects on parents of having a child with a CI indicate that these parents tend to experience no more stress overall than parents of nonchronically ill children (Leventhal-Belfer, Bakker, & Russo, 1993; Soliday et al., 2000). As mentioned in the previous section, certain long-term issues, such as symptoms of posttraumatic stress, have been reported in parents of chronically ill children (Kazak et al., 1997). Also, parents may experience stress due to disease-specific factors, such as fear of relapse among parents of cancer survivors (Leventhal-Belfer et al., 1993). Comparing 41 families of children with a chronic kidney disease to 34 healthy control children, Soliday et al. found that parents who reported higher levels of child behavior problems also tended to report higher parenting stress, which was also true for the control group. These authors also found that increased time since diagnosis correlated with decreased behavior problems, and that single parents tended to report increased child-externalizing behavior and increased parent stress. In qualitative analyses these authors found that parents of chronically ill children who were several years postdiagnosis were most concerned about child nonadherence to the medical regimen. When examined by age of the chronically ill child, qualitative analyses indicated that parents of younger children were concerned about acting-out behaviors and attention span, whereas parents of older children were concerned about academic issues.

Having a child with a chronic health condition may also negatively impact the marital relationship between parents. To combat such effects, Walker, Johnson, Manion, and Cloutier (1996) conducted an intervention with parents using emotionally focused therapy. This manualized treatment of ten 90-minute sessions was modified to focus on parents of children with a CI and was conducted with individual couples targeting nine specific steps throughout treatment. The steps included: (1) delineating conflict issues, (2) identifying the negative interaction cycle, (3) accessing unacknowledged feelings underlying interactional positions, (4) redefining problems in terms of underlying feelings and attachment needs, (5) promoting identification with disowned needs and aspects of experience in the redefined cycle, (6) promoting acceptance of the partner's experience and new interaction patterns, (7) facilitating expression of needs and wants to restructure interactions, (8) establishing the emergence of new solutions, and (9) consolidating new positions (Johnson & Greenberg, 1996). Comparing couples assigned to the intervention group to those assigned to a wait-listed control condition, the authors found that the intervention couples demonstrated significant decreases in marital distress at both post-treatment and 5-month follow-up.

Effects on Siblings

In recent years there has been increased attention to the effects of having a sibling diagnosed with a chronic health condition. A recent meta-analysis conducted by Sharpe and Rossiter (2002) indicates that the frequency of research on siblings of children with a CI is on the rise, but that sample size in these studies tends to be decreasing. Clinical knowledge would suggest that sources of stress include separation from parents, change in family routines, disruption in family relationships, lack of knowledge about the disease, and possibly exposure to the potentially painful treatments of the chronically ill sibling (such as insulin injections in the case of IDDM). As is the case with research on patients themselves, however, most research on siblings focuses on those who are several years postdiagnosis rather than studying siblings during the possibly traumatic diagnostic process.

Sharpe and Rossiter (2002) further reported that among those who have a sibling diagnosed with a chronic health condition, parent report is significantly more negative than sibling self-report. Siblings tended to display internalizing difficulties such as depression and anxiety rather than externalizing problems, possibly due to increased pressure to assist their parents in the caretaker role. Interestingly, the results indicated that siblings of children with a more severe illness were no more at risk for psychosocial difficulties when compared to those with a sibling with a less severe illness. However, the more the medical routine affects the day-to-day functioning of the chronically ill child, the more it is likely to impact the psychosocial functioning of the sibling.

Assessing siblings of cancer patients, Sargent et al. (1995) divided the 238 participating siblings into four groups; dysfunctional (22%), resilient (32%), intermediate-1 (those who had problems prior to the diagnosis that continued; 13%), or intermediate-2 (those who had no problems prior to diagnosis but developed minor problems postdiagnosis; 34%). These findings indicated that older siblings were more likely to indicate feeling more compassionate, caring, and mature since the diagnosis, whereas younger siblings were more likely to indicate feeling negatively.

To improve the difficulties associated with having a sibling diagnosed with a CI, Lobato and Kao (2002) conducted an intervention designed to improve sibling knowledge of and adjustment to CI. With a sample of siblings of children with a CI or developmental disability, the authors conducted six 90-minute group sessions for the siblings and their parents. The intervention was designed to improve sibling knowledge, family information exchange, identifying and managing emotions, meeting individual needs, and problem solving. Results indicated that this intervention improved both sibling knowledge and adjustment.

Outside of research studies, there are very few services regularly available for siblings. They are sometimes included during the diagnostic process, and given the factual information about their sibling's diagnosis by the medical team. However, beyond this, it is not typical for siblings to be included in mental health services. Just like parents, these siblings typically only receive such services if they express difficulty to such a significant degree that the parents or medical team become aware and request a referral, or if the child is sufficiently debilitated to request a referral on their own. These cases are rare, typically leaving siblings out of the mental health equation for children with CI.

MENTAL HEALTH ASPECTS OF HOSPITALIZATION

Effects on the Patient

The current literature supports that children, from preschoolers to school-age and adolescent children, experience psychological distress as a result of hospitalization (Bossert, 1994; Rossen & McKeever, 1996; Spirito, Stark, & Tyc, 1994). Distress is experienced both during and after the hospital stay. The majority of findings suggest that regardless of age or medical condition, the experience of negative stress is common during the 2-week period following hospital discharge (Thompson & Vernon, 1993), and can last up to 4 weeks for preschool-age children (Lynch, 1994; Zuckerberg, 1994). For preschoolers, signs of psychological distress may be manifested in behavioral symptoms including aggression, apathy, sleep disturbances, appetite changes, separation anxiety, and withdrawal from family members (Rossen & McKeever, 1996), whereas in older children, symptoms of distress may incorporate more internal manifestations including anger, sadness, and anxiety (Bossert, 1994; Spirito et al., 1994). The most significant risk factors for psychological distress include age, lack of information, separation from parents, perceived lack of control, and past negative experiences (Peterson, Mori, & Carter, 1985). Furthermore, psychological adjustment of a hospitalized child may be predicted by the number of physical stressors (e.g., illness-related symptoms, diagnostic procedures, and medical treatment procedures) that the child experiences during hospitalization (Saylor et al., 1987).

Coping with hospitalization from chronic childhood illness has been an aspect of concentrated research efforts within the field (Bossert, 1994; Savedra & Tesler, 1981; Spirito et al., 1994). Spirito and colleagues found that coping was dependent upon whether the child was in the school-age or adolescent developmental stage, and whether the child's illness was chronic or acute. Adolescents utilized more cognitive strategies such as problem solving whereas younger children engaged in more avoidant strategies such as wishful thinking and distraction. Chronically ill children were less likely to use maladaptive strategies, such as distraction and self-criticism, than children hospitalized for acute conditions. Anxious children engaged in more coping strategies than nonanxious children. Children experiencing sadness more frequently used active coping strategies, particularly social support and wishful thinking. Children experiencing anger also resorted to wishful thinking more frequently while utilizing self-blame and social withdrawal less often. The latter finding suggests that anger can be adaptive for children when dealing with the stressors of hospitalization. In a separate study of acutely and chronically ill children, Bossert (1994) found that in comparison to acutely ill children, chronically ill children perceived their coping as being less effective. However, consistent across the groups, two of the most common coping behaviors for these children were countermeasures (described as attempts to minimize distress by means of physical or cognitive escape, or by altering the situational effects) and support seeking.

Social support seeking as a common coping mechanism for hospitalized chronically ill children is not a surprising find, given the documented value of social support in relation to emotional functioning and self-worth in healthy children (Dubow, Tisak, Causey, Hyrshko, & Reid, 1991). In a review of 32 studies pertaining to childhood coping and illness, social support was the coping strategy most frequently reported by children with pediatric illnesses (Ryan-Wenger, 1996). Of the sources of social support that chronically ill children may rely upon, particularly the younger children, familial and parental supports are among the primary sources (Ellerton et al., 1996). Due to the bidirectional relation between stress and social support (Ellerton et al., 1996), and the family's close proximity to the stressful treatment demands of their chronically ill child, the child's illness-related stress can be a challenge for the family as well.

Effects on the Family

Stressors encountered by parents and families of chronically ill children are multifaceted and perpetual (Melnyk et al., 2001). A child's hospitalization is one stressor that introduces additional demands on an already taxing situation. Lifestyle changes are necessitated, normal routines are interrupted, and parents must divide their efforts between their hospitalized child and their daily responsibilities (Melnyk et al., 2001).

In a study of repeated hospitalizations of children with asthma, for example, a higher number of lifetime hospitalizations was related to an increased level of familial stress, increased family conflict, a negative impact upon the family's social network, and a negative impact on family finances (Chen, Bloomberg, Fisher, & Strunk, 2003). Parental perceptions of ability were also negatively affected by higher rates of hospitalization. With increased frequency of hospitalization, parents felt less able to stop their child's asthma once the attacks had begun, and less able to prevent the worsening of their child's asthma (Chen et al., 2003). This perceived helplessness from parents, in turn, was associated with a greater possibility of child hospitalization. Parents who perceived less confidence and less mastery of their own abilities to care for their child's asthma, who were also less "emotionally bothered" by their child's asthma, were more likely to rehospitalize their child during the year-long follow up (Chen et al., 2003).

Less researched are the positive aspects of a child's hospitalization upon the family. Kirkby and Whelan (1996) suggested that a child's hospitalization is not always necessarily viewed as negative. Rather, it can be viewed as a "socializing event"—one from which new coping strategies may formulate, and preexisting coping mechanisms employed by the family are further strengthened (Ogilvie, 1990; Parmalee, 1986). During times of a child's illness and hospitalization, parents are offered opportunities to better understand the effects of their child's illness, to nurture their children, and to feel more competent in the care of their children (Perrin, 1993). Although a family may be greatly affected by a child's illness and hospitalization, the family can be one source of support for the child, diminishing the illness-related stressors that the child may feel as a result of hospitalization.

Inpatient Treatments Available

Treatments for the psychological effects of hospitalization on children often include preadmission programs that prepare children for the hospitalization by familiarizing them to the experience. There are five major approaches identified for preparing children for pediatric hospitalization: (1) information giving, (2) encouraging emotional expression, (3) establishing a trusting relationship with hospital staff, (4) working to prepare parents, and (5) teaching coping strategies (Elkins & Roberts, 1983). This process of familiarization aims to diminish the potential psychological distress that children may feel due to their lack of information and the novelty of the hospital setting.

Some recent attempts to reduce children's hospital-related fears via preadmission preparations have been quite innovative, incorporating computer technology. Nelson and Allen (1999) examined the effectiveness of computer instruction, against more conventional means of instruction, in reducing children's fears surrounding the experience of going to the hospital. It was found that in this group of healthy children (in the 3rd grade), showing the educational slides on the computer was equally effective as conventional methods (i.e., viewing the same slide show on a projected screen) in reducing hospital-related fears. However, the children preferred the computer instruction, reporting significantly greater levels of satisfaction with the interactive format. Other approaches to familiarizing children with the hospitalization experience may also include more traditional methods such as educational books, modeling of appropriate coping behaviors, and role playing. More interactive approaches such as guided hospital tours and friendly visits with doctors may also be effective methods of familiarizing children to future hospitalization and diminishing their fears surrounding this potentially distressing experience.

In addition to the innovative methods, traditional psychological treatments such as cognitive behavioral treatments are in continued use in helping to reduce the distressing thoughts children may have due to their illness and hospitalization. Cognitive-behavioral methods have been effective in ameliorating negative thoughts and experiences surrounding pediatric illnesses such as diabetes, asthma, and pediatric cancer (Redlich & Prior, 1998), and have reduced hospital and emergency room admissions postintervention (Park, Sawyer, & Glaun, 1996). These services are typically provided by a child life specialist or social worker who is charged with providing front line psychological care for a hospital unit. These providers are on the floor and available on a daily basis to provide such services. If, however, these services are not available or there is a particularly difficult case, referral to a psychologist may be necessary.

Incorporation of the family has also been a component of treatment for hospitalized children (Clay, 1995). Research indicates that across different medical situations, a child's level of anxiety will reflect the anxiety level of his or her mother (Fosson, Martin, & Haley, 1990; Mabe, Treiber, & Riley, 1991). Therefore, it is important that any treatment for the hospitalized child, with incorporation of the family, should include a component addressing familial (e.g., parental and sibling) stress and coping, adequately preparing the family for a child's hospitalization (Melnyk, 1995). Any decrease in familial distress and anxiety will be reflected in the child's distress level as well. Unfortunately, these services are not regularly provided at the current time, despite the fact that the floor social worker or child life specialist would be ideally suited to do so.

CONCLUSIONS AND FUTURE DIRECTIONS

The mental health services for children with CI, their parents, and their siblings have been of increased importance in recent years due to increased survival rates and increased complexity and invasiveness of medical regimens. The organization and delivery of mental health services for these children is complicated, but follows directly with their CI progression. For this reason, the current chapter reviewed the delivery of mental health services to children with a CI throughout the diagnostic process, moving into the first 3–5 years postdiagnosis and finally, covering the long-term aspects of CI in children.

Overall, the studies are promising indicating that children and their families tend to function well, and in most cases report that they are doing as well as control groups and standardized norms (Bailey et al., 1993; Bennett, 1994; Hays et al., 1992; Meadows et al., 1989; Soliday et al., 2000). However, studies do indicate that there may be some areas in need of further attention. First, more research is needed to investigate the initial increase in stress and mental health concerns reported during and immediately following the diagnosis of a CI (Frank et al., 1998). Because families are in close contact with their child's medical providers at this point in time, these services would likely be best provided in this context. To best address these needs, a mental health provider, such as a nurse, social worker, or pediatric psychologist, should be part of the initial diagnostic team. This individual could meet with families on a regular basis at visits coinciding with their medical care, easing patient burden.

As families move through the adjustment process, data indicate that most families adjust well to their new routines and limitations and that most children do as well. However, there are some families who tend to have problems with increased child behavior problems (Soliday et al., 2000), decreased social support (Ellerton et al., 1996), and marital functioning (Walker et al., 1996), and possibly symptoms of anxiety and posttraumatic stress (Kazak et al., 1997). Ideally, the same mental health provider who was part of the diagnostic team would also be on the treatment team to regularly assess both patient and family for these difficulties throughout the treatment process. As a mental health prevention effort, this individual could facilitate a community-based, family support intervention effort similar to that of Chernoff et al. (2002) to be used for all families.

When difficulties are noted, it would be ideal for the mental health professional who is part of the medical team to conduct the psychological treatment. Treatment could be conducted in the form of individual meetings with the target child or in the form of patient groups. The mental health professional could also provide emotionally focused marital therapy to parents whose relationships are suffering, as Walker et al. (1996) found this service to be helpful. Finally, the provider could offer group services for siblings of children with CI, as these groups improve sibling knowledge, problem solving, and emotional functioning (Lobato & Kao, 2002).

Coordination of services between the medical team and the psychological treatment is especially important for children with CI as the medical issues and psychological issues are so closely related. For example, it is often important for mental health providers who treat children with CI to be intimately familiar with disease progression, treatment details, and potential side effects of each child's condition. If a child's hair is going to fall out, as it does during cancer treatment for many children, this may be an important issue to address in psychological treatment. Coordinating services between the medical and psychological providers would also decrease patient burden as visits to the two professionals could be coordinated. For these reasons, providing psychological treatment within the medical office is ideal for children and families during the treatment process. If this mental health service is not available on the medical team, it is necessary for families to seek a referral to an outside pediatric psychologist.

Finally, when children are feeling better and making the transition back to school and other activities, it would be helpful for the mental health provider to facilitate this transition. This individual could prepare children for the variety of reactions and questions they may receive from peers and other individuals they may not have seen in quite some time. If requested, this individual could even meet with peers prior to the child's return to the classroom, to prepare them for changes in the child's appearance, abilities, or needs. Finally, it is anecdotally reported that parents and teachers of children with CI may have trouble disciplining a chronically ill child. The mental health provider could train parents and teachers on appropriate expectations, as well as assist them in developing proper discipline strategies given the child's current functioning.

REFERENCES

Bailey, L. L., Gundry, S. R., Razzouk, A. J., Wang, N., Sciolaro, C. M., & Chiavarelli, M. (1993). Bless the babies: One hundred fifteen late survivors of heart transplantation during the first year of life. *Journal of Thoracic and Cardiovascular Surgery, 105,* 805–814.

Bennett, D. S. (1994). Depression among children with chronic medical problems: A meta-analysis. *Journal of Pediatric Psychology, 19,* 149–169.

Bossert, E. (1994). Factors influencing the coping of hospitalized school-age children. *Journal of Pediatric Nursing, 9,* 299–306.

Carter, B. D., Kronenberger, W. G., Baker, J., Grimes, L. M., Crabtree, V. M., Smith, C. et al. (2003). Inpatient pediatric consultation-liaison: A case-controlled study. *Journal of Pediatric Psychology, 28,* 423–432.

Chen, E., Bloomberg, G. R., Fisher, E. B., Strunk, R. C. (2003). Predictors of repeat hospitalizations in children with asthma: The role of psychosocial and socioenvironmental factors. *Health Psychology, 22,* 12–18.

Chernoff, R. G., Ireys, H. T., DeVet, K. A., & Kim, Y. J. (2002). A randomized, controlled trial of a community-based support program for families of children with chronic illness: Pediatric outcomes. *Archives of Pediatrics and Adolescent Medicine, 156,* 533–539.

Clay, R. A. (1995). Psychologists augment pediatric care. *APA Monitor, 26,* 23.

Clubb, R. L. (1991). Chronic sorrow: Adaptation patterns of parents with chronically ill children. *Pediatric Nursing, 17,* 461–466.

Cohen, M. H. (1993). The unknown and the unknowable: Managing sustained uncertainty. *Western Journal of Nursing Research, 15,* 77–96.

Davis, C. C., Brown, R. T., Bakeman, R., & Campbell, R. (1998). Psychological adaptation and adjustment of mothers of children with congenital heart disease: Stress, coping, and family functioning. *Journal of Pediatric Psychology, 23,* 219–228.

Dubow, E. F., Tisak, J., Causey, D., Hyrshko, A., & Reid. G. (1991). A two-year longitudinal study of stressful life events, social support, and social problem solving skills: Contributions to children's behavioural and academic adjustment. *Child Development, 62,* 583–599.

Elkins, P. E., & Roberts, M. C. (1983). Psychological preparation for pediatric hospitalization. *Clinical Psychology Review, 3*, 275–295.

Ellerton, M. L., Stewart, M. J., Ritchie, J. A., & Hirth, A. M. (1996). Social support in children with a chronic condition. *Canadian Journal of Nursing Research, 28*, 15–36.

Fosson, A., Martin, J., & Haley, J. (1990). Anxiety among hospitalized latency-age children. *Developmental and Behavioral Pediatrics, 11*, 324–327.

Frank, R. G., Thayer, J. F., Hagglund, K. J., Vieth, A. Z., Schopp, L. H., Beck, N. C. et al. (1998). Trajectories of adaptation in pediatric chronic illness: The importance of the individual. *Journal of Consulting and Clinical Psychology, 66*, 521–532.

Goldman, L. S. (1993). Liver transplantation using living donors: Preliminary donor psychiatric outcomes. *Psychosomatics, 34*, 235–240.

Gonzalez, S., Steinglass, P., & Reiss, D. (1989). Putting the illness in its place: Discussion groups for families with chronic medical illnesses. *Family Process, 28*, 69–87.

Hakimi, M. (1998). Psychosocial adaptation following the diagnosis of insulin-dependent diabetes mellitus: An intervention. *Dissertation Abstracts International: Section B: The Sciences and Engineering, 59*, 1852.

Hays, D. M., Landsverk, J., Sallan, S. E., Hewett, K. D., Patenaude, A. F., Schoonover, D. et al. (1992). Educational, occupational, and insurance status of childhood cancer survivors in their fourth and fifth decades of life. *Journal of Clinical Oncology, 10*, 1397–1406.

Hughes, M., & McCollum, J. (1994). Neonatal intensive care: Mothers' and fathers' perceptions of what is stressful. *Journal of Early Intervention, 18*, 258–268.

Johnson, S. M., & Greenberg, L. S. (1996). The effects of emotionally focused marital therapy: A response to a recent meta-analysis. Unpublished manuscript.

Kazak, A. E., Barakat, L. P., Meeske, K., Christakis, D., Meadows, A. T., Casey, R. et al. (1997). Posttraumatic stress, family functioning, and social support in survivors of childhood leukemia and their mothers and fathers. *Journal of Consulting and Clinical Psychology, 65*, 120–129.

Kazak, A. E., & Meadows, A. T. (1989). Families of young adolescents who have survived cancer: Social-emotional adjustment, adaptability, and social support. *Journal of Pediatric Psychology, 14*, 175–191.

Kibby, M., Tyc, V. L., & Mulhern, R. K. (1998). Effectiveness of psychological intervention for children and adolescents with chronic medical illness: A meta-analysis. *Clinical Psychology Review, 18*, 103–117.

Kirkby, R. J., & Whelan, R. J. (1996). The effects of hospitalisation and medical procedures on children and their families. *Journal of Family Studies, 2*, 65–77.

Koocher, G. P., Curtiss, E. K., Pollin, I. S., & Patton, K. E. (2001). Medical crisis counseling in a health maintenance organization: Preventive intervention. *Professional Psychology: Research and Practice, 32*, 52–58.

Lavigne, J. V., & Faier-Routman, J. (1993). Correlates of psychological adjustment to pediatric physical disorders: A meta-analytic review and comparison with existing models. *Developmental and Behavioral Pediatrics, 14*, 117–123.

Leventhal-Belfer, L., Bakker, A. M., & Russo, C. L. (1993). Parents of childhood cancer survivors: A descriptive look at their concerns and needs. *Journal of Psychosocial Oncology, 11*, 19–41.

Lobato, D. J., & Kao, B. T. (2002). Integrated sibling-parent group intervention to improve sibling knowledge and adjustment to chronic illness and disability. *Journal of Pediatric Psychology, 27*, 711–716.

Lynch, M. (1994). Preparing children for day surgery. *Children's Health Care, 23*, 75–85.

Mabe, A., Treiber, F. A., & Riley, W. T. (1991). Examining emotional distress during pediatric hospitalization for school-aged children. *Children's Health Care, 20*, 162–169.

Meadows, A. T., McKee, L., & Kazak, A. E. (1989). Psychosocial status of young adult survivors of childhood cancer: A survey. *Medical and Pediatric Oncology, 17*, 466–470.

Melnyk, B. M. (1995). Coping with unplanned childhood hospitalization: The mediating functions of parental beliefs. *Journal of Pediatric Psychology, 20*, 299–312.

Melnyk, B. M., Moldenhouer, Z., Feinstein, N. F., & Small, L. (2001). Coping in parents of children who are chronically ill: Strategies for assessment and intervention. *Pediatric Nursing, 27*, 548–558.

Mulhern, R. K., Wasserman, A. L., Friedman, A. G., & Fairclough, D. (1989). Social competence and behavioral adjustment of children who are long-term survivors of cancer. *Pediatrics, 83,* 18–25.

Nelson, C. C., & Allen, J. (1999). Reduction of healthy children's fears related to hospitalization and medical procedures: The effectiveness of multimedia computer instruction in pediatric psychology. *Children's Health Care, 28,* 1–13.

Newacheck, P. W., & Halfon, N. (1998). Prevalence and impact of disabling chronic conditions in childhood. *American Journal of Public Health, 88,* 610–617.

Ogilvie, L. (1990). Hospitalization of children for surgery: The parents' view. *Children's Health Care, 19,* 49–56.

O'Malley, J. E., Foster, D., Koocher, G., & Slavin, L. (1980). Visible physical impairment and psychological adjustment among pediatric cancer survivors. *American Journal of Psychiatry, 137,* 94–96.

Park, S. J., Sawyer, S. M., & Glaun, D. E. (1996). Childhood asthma complicated by anxiety: An application of cognitive behavioural therapy. *Journal of Paediatric and Child Health, 32,* 183–187.

Parmalee, A. H. (1986). Children's illnesses: Their beneficial effects on behavioral development. *Child Development, 57,* 1–10.

Perrin, E. C. (1993). Children in hospitals. *Journal of Developmental and Behavioral Pediatrics, 14,* 50–52.

Perrin, J. M., & MacLean, W. E. (1988). Children with chronic illness: The prevention of dysfunction. *Pediatric Clinics of North America, 35,* 1325–1337.

Peterson, L., Mori, L., & Carter, P. (1985). The role of the family in children's responses to stressful medical procedures. *Journal of Clinical Child Psychology, 14,* 98–104.

Phipps, S., & Srivastava D. K. (1997). Repressive adaptation in children with cancer. *Health Psychology, 16,* 521–528.

Phipps S., & Steele R. G. (2002). Repressive adaptive style in children with chronic illness. *Psychosomatic Medicine, 64,* 34–42.

Pollin, I. (1994). *Taking charge: Overcoming the challenges of long-term illness.* New York: Times Books.

Pollin, I. (1995). *Medical crisis counseling: Short-term treatment for long term illness.* Evanston, IL: Norton.

Quittner, A. L., DiGirolamo, A. M., Michel, M., & Eigen, H. (1992). Parental response to cystic fibrosis: A contextual analysis of the diagnosis phase. *Journal of Pediatric Psychology, 17,* 683–704.

Quittner, A. L., Espelage, D. L., Opipari, L. C., Carter, B., Eid, N., & Eigen, H. (1998). Role strain in couples with and without a child with chronic illness: Associations with marital satisfaction, intimacy, and daily mood. *Health Psychology, 17,* 112–124.

Quittner, A. L., Opipari, L. C., Regoli, M. J., Jacobsen, J., & Eigen, H. (1992). The impact of caregiving and role strain on family life: Comparisons between mothers of children with cystic fibrosis and matched controls. *Rehabilitation Psychology, 37,* 275–290.

Redlich, N., & Prior, M. (1998). Cognitive-behavioural interventions in pediatric chronic illness. *Behaviour Change, 15,* 151–159.

Rossen, B. E., & McKeever, P. D. (1996). The behavior of preschoolers during and after brief surgical hospitalizations. *Issues in Comprehensive Pediatric Nursing, 19,* 121–133.

Ryan-Wenger, N. A. (1996). Children, coping, and the stress of illness: A synthesis of the research. *Journal of the Society of Pediatric Nurses, 1,* 126–138.

Sahler, O. J., Fairclough, D. L., Katz, E., Varni, J., Phipps, S. et al. (under review). Problem solving skills training for mothers of children with newly diagnosed cancer: Report of a multisite randomized trial.

Sargent, J. R., Sahler, O. J. Z., Roghmann, K. J., Mulhern, R. K., Barbarian, O. A., Carpenter, P. J. et al. (1995). Sibling adaptation to childhood cancer collaborative study: Siblings' perceptions of the cancer experience. *Journal of Pediatric Psychology, 20,* 151–164.

Savedra, M., & Tesler, M. (1981). Coping strategies of hospitalized school-age children. *Western Journal of Nursing Research, 3,* 371–384.

Saylor, C. F., Pallmeyer, T. P., Finch, A. J., Eason, L., Trieber, F., & Folger, C. (1987). Predictors of psychological distress in hospitalized pediatric patients. *Journal of the American Academy of Child and Adolescent Psychiatry, 26,* 232–236.

Schulz, M. S., & Masek, B. J. (1996). Medical crisis intervention with children and adolescents with chronic pain. *Professional Psychology: Research and Practice, 27,* 121–129.

Sharpe, D., & Rossiter, L. (2002). Siblings of children with a chronic illness: A meta-analysis. *Journal of Pediatric Psychology, 27,* 699–710.

Soliday, E., Kool, E., & Lande, M. B. (2000). Psychosocial adjustment in children with kidney disease. *Journal of Pediatric Psychology, 25,* 93–103.

Spirito, A., Stark, L. J., & Tyc, V. L. (1994). Stressors and coping strategies described during hospitalization by chronically ill children. *Journal of Clinical Child Psychology, 23,* 314–322.

Stuber, M. L. (1996). Psychiatric sequelae in seriously ill children and their families. *The Psychiatric Clinics of North America, 19,* 481–493.

Stuber, M. L., Gonzalez, S., Meeske, K., Guthrie, D., Houskamp, B., Pynoos, R. et al. (1994). Post traumatic stress after childhood cancer II: A family model. *Psychooncology, 3,* 313–319.

Thompson, R. H., & Vernon, D. T. (1993). Research on children's behavior after hospitalization: A review and synthesis. *Journal of Developmental and Behavioral Pediatrics, 14,* 28–35.

Walker, J. G., Johnson, S., Manion, I., & Cloutier, P. (1996). Emotionally focused marital intervention for couples with chronically ill children. *Journal of Consulting and Clinical Psychology, 64,* 1029–1036.

Williams, J., & DeMaso, D. R. (2000). Pediatric team meetings: The mental health consultant's role. *Clinical Child Psychology and Psychiatry, 5,* 105–113.

Williams, P. D. (1997). Siblings and pediatric chronic illness: A review of the literature. *International Journal of Nursing Studies, 34,* 312–323.

Zuckerberg, A. L. (1994). Perioperative approach to children. *Pediatric Clinics of North America, 41,* 15–29.

18

Psychological Services for Children and Families Who Are Homeless

MARY E. WALSH and JULIE HEIM JACKSON

Persons who are homeless are not new to the streets of America. However, the documented existence of homeless children and families is a relatively recent phenomenon. With the exception of the Great Depression, families had not been a substantial part of the homeless population until approximately 1982 (Bassuk et al., 1996). Since the late 1980s homeless women with children have been identified as the most rapidly expanding segment of the homeless population (Bassuk et al., 1996). By 1995, it was estimated that about 744,000 school-age children in the United States were homeless over the course of a year (U.S. Department of Education, 1995). Although single males had traditionally dominated the homeless population, by 2002, families with children represented 41% of the homeless population—the same percentage as homeless single men (U.S. Conference of Mayors, 2002). This growing population of homeless children and families requires psychological services and resources that will assist them while they are homeless, help them to move to permanent housing, and ultimately, prevent future homelessness.

The goal of this chapter is to describe the current state of psychological services for children and families who are homeless. It is important to note that some of these services are directed primarily toward parents, others toward children, and some toward family intervention. For our purposes, "psychological services" are broadly conceptualized to include counseling interventions (e.g., family, group, and individual counseling), psychoeducational activities (e.g., parenting skills and life skills training),

MARY E. WALSH and JULIE HEIM JACKSON • Department of Counseling, Developmental, and Educational Psychology, Boston College, Chestnut Hill, Massachusetts 02467.

substance abuse treatments, cognitive developmental assessments and interventions, and other services that focus on prevention (e.g., early intervention programs). Psychological service providers include psychologists, psychiatrists, clinical social workers, mental health counselors, psychiatric nurses, pastoral counselors, school counselors, and school psychologists. The chapter will briefly review issues addressed in psychological services for homeless families, describe common models for delivery of these services and offer suggestions for service improvement.

ISSUES ADDRESSED BY PSYCHOLOGICAL SERVICES

Effective psychological services are largely shaped by the characteristics of the target population. The "typical homeless family" comprises a single mother in her mid-to-late 20s and 1–3 children who are generally under 6 years of age (Bassuk et al., 1996; Homes for the Homeless, 1998). Persons of color are heavily overrepresented among homeless families (U.S. Conference of Mayors, 2002). Most often, homeless mothers grew up in poverty, have experienced or witnessed domestic violence, and never completed high school (Homes for the Homeless, 1998). Most of the families have been homeless at least 9 months, and lived with a partner, their parents, or doubled up with friends before entering a shelter.

Largely left out of literature on homeless families, the typical father is 35 years old, a high school graduate, and not married (Homes for the Homeless, 2000). Data gathered in New York City indicated that fathers spent little or no time with their homeless children and provided little or no financial support, even if they were employed (Homes for the Homeless, 2000). The typical father often had children with multiple women. Over one third of homeless children's fathers had been violent toward their children or partners, nearly half had spent time in jail, and one third had a history of substance abuse. Overall, younger fathers were more likely to have contact and provide support for their children (Homes for the Homeless, 2000).

For homeless families, psychological services are ultimately designed to improve their quality of life and to assist them to gain and remain in permanent housing. The issues addressed by these services include the causes of the family's homelessness, the challenges of being homeless, and the stresses of transitioning to permanent housing.

Causes of Homelessness

Psychological services to homeless families assist families to understand, and, where possible, to prevent the recurrence of the conditions that led to their homelessness. Service providers recognize that poverty and the lack of affordable housing are the principal and ultimate causes of family homelessness. However, many families also commonly cite domestic violence and substance abuse as the more immediate reasons (Bassuk et al., 1996; Goodman, 1991). Research clearly demonstrates that poverty, domestic violence, and substance abuse are linked and can independently, or in combination, contribute to family homelessness (Salomon, Bassuk, & Huntington, 2002). Therefore, services need to be comprehensive to aid families who struggle with poverty, domestic violence, and substance abuse; they also need to be sufficiently flexible to assist families who present with only one of these issues.

Psychological Challenges of Being Homeless

Challenges Faced by Homeless Mothers

Caring for a family while living in temporary shelter (e.g., hotel, group shelter, automobile) presents substantial difficulties for mothers. A large portion of services for homeless families address the impact of homeless living conditions on children and families. An appreciation of these challenges and their impact on homeless families will lead to more targeted and comprehensive psychological services (McLoyd, 1998; Schmitz, Wagner, & Menke, 2001).

Psychological service providers focus particularly on parenting skills and the alleviation of mood disorders. Parenting skills are often severely challenged in shelter settings that crowd multiple families into a small space. These conditions can destabilize parenting skills and often result in less supportive parenting, more inconsistent discipline, and greater child maltreatment (Pianta, Egeland, & Erickson, 1989). Shelters are not typically designed to be developmentally appropriate environments in which children are encouraged to explore and become actively engaged in meaningful activities. As a result, managing children's behavior in an unstructured situation becomes many mothers' primary activity (Hausman & Hammen, 1993). They often report being criticized by other mothers and shelter staff for their children's behavior. In response, mothers may engage in "public mothering," which often includes angry punishment to demonstrate that they can control their child (Torquati, 2002). Children are overwhelmed by differing expectations, and they inevitably become demoralized after repeated failure in meeting these inconsistent demands (Walsh, 1992). Psychological service providers can support mothers as they learn to provide warmth, support, and effective behavior regulation under these exceedingly difficult conditions. Providers may also be in a unique position to collaborate with shelter staff to create more developmentally appropriate spaces and activities for children, improve parenting support, integrate community services, and institute rules that are flexible yet maintain safety.

It is important to note that some mothers indicate that their experience of parenting in a shelter is positive, indicating that they feel safe and supported, and that they appreciate the decent and comfortable living accommodations (Styron, Janoff-Bulman, & Davidson, 2000). Psychological service providers should be prepared for this diversity of responses to the shelter system and assist clients in reconciling conflicting feelings.

Through its daily trauma, uncertainty, and painful deprivations, homelessness not only challenges parenting skills but also produces or exacerbates profound feelings of sadness, hopelessness, and anxiety in mothers (Menke & Wagner, 1997b). Homeless mothers are more likely than women in general to be diagnosed with a major depressive disorder and have a greater prevalence of suicide attempts (Bassuk et al., 1996). Feelings of uncertainty, hopelessness, isolation, and urgency to find a home are common among homeless mothers and are likely to create or intensify depression and anxiety (Menke & Wagner, 1997b).

Also contributing to many homeless mothers' depression and anxiety is the potential for mother–child separation. Estimates of the percentage of homeless mothers and children who have been separated are as high as 60% (New York City Commission on Homeless, 1992). Children are either removed from their mothers' care by state officials or are separated from their mothers because of shelter policy. Often boys older than age 13, but sometimes as young as 10, are not allowed to stay at family shelters—forcing many homeless families to separate in order to obtain accommodation in emergency shelters (U.S. Conference of Mayors, 2002). Psychological service providers are increasingly addressing the separation that occurs in homeless families, and they could further work with shelters to develop ways to ensure the safety of all residents while allowing adolescent boys to remain with their family.

Psychological Challenges Faced by Homeless Children

Homeless children face their own set of psychological challenges that contribute to emotional, behavioral, cognitive, or academic problems (Menke & Wagner, 1997a). Becoming homeless appears to undermine two fundamental needs of children: a sense of predictability or continuity in their environment, and a belief that parents will provide the physical, social, and emotional resources that they require (Wall, 1996; Walsh, 1992). Witnessing a parent's inability to meet basic parenting roles leads children to have decreased confidence in their parent's ability to help them (Schmidtz et al., 2001; Walsh, 1992). Perhaps because of these experiences, homeless children are at an increased risk for internalizing problems (e.g., depression, anxiety, social withdrawal), out-of-home placement, and physical or sexual abuse, which are known to lead to posttraumatic stress disorder (Menke & Wagner, 1997a).

Although many homeless children react to the stressors of homelessness with anxiety or depression, some externalize their feelings. Externalization of feelings often results in behavioral outbursts, verbal and physical fights, and temper tantrums. Homeless children display more of these behavioral problems as compared to the general population (Masten, Miliotis, Graham-Bermann, Ramirez, & Neemann, 1993) and often lack the stable environment that usually helps children control their impulsive behavior (Walsh, 1990).

Psychological services include developmentally appropriate assessment, counseling, psychoeducation, and consultation for children. Mental health providers can closely monitor children's concerns, which could easily interfere with the child's ability to perform academically, form supportive relationships, and develop emotionally and behaviorally. They can also educate other professionals regarding mental health issues, and they can collaborate with schools and shelters to design and implement treatment plans for children.

A number of homeless children have been found to have significant cognitive delays. Bassuk, Rubin, and Lauriat (1986) found that half of preschool children in homeless shelters had one or more developmental delay. Compared to other children of the same age, homeless children are slower to develop in various areas such as gross motor skills, fine motor coordination, personal and social behaviors, and language (Walsh, 1990). Some children also manifest slowed physical growth as indicated by low-for-age weight and height (Walsh, 1990). These delays challenge psychological service providers to assess and recommend early intervention in treatment plans to lessen the long-term impact of the delay.

Further limiting academic achievement are obstacles such as residency requirements, lack of transportation, and lack of special education referrals, which often impede successful relationships between school systems and homeless families (Wall, 1996; Walsh & Buckley, 1994). Psychological service providers can attempt to provide continuity of services through communicating with teachers, administrators, and parents, coordinating paperwork and special education evaluations, and generally advocating for the student. They often are in a position to complete cognitive and socioemotional assessments of the children, increase communication between parents and teachers, and collaborate with school counselors in developing behavior plans and problem-solving strategies (Jackson & Walsh, 2004). Increasing these services will help to ensure that children who are homeless are provided with the educational opportunities that they will need to escape not only from homelessness but ultimately from poverty.

Issues in Transitioning to Permanent Housing

The final issue that effective psychological services must consider is the difficulty homeless families experience when transitioning to permanent housing. However, there is little research in this area (Dunlap & Fogel, 1998). Some of the more progressive shelter models (e.g., transitional housing and services-enriched housing) work to prepare families for living in permanent housing. Many of these shelters provide education, job training and placement, psychological services, and psychoeducational services such as parenting and independent living skills. Even with this preparation and support, reintegration into a permanent home is long and stressful and involves challenges and adjustments (Rog, Holupka, McCombs-Thornton, Brito, & Hambrick, 1997).

MODELS OF DELIVERY OF PSYCHOLOGICAL SERVICES FOR HOMELESS FAMILIES

Historically, service providers were solely focused on offering shelter to homeless families. Providers soon realized that permanent housing was not enough to combat homelessness because it only addressed a family's need for shelter and it did not address any of the underlying issues that contributed to the family's homelessness. This realization led providers to offer psychological and educational services. Although these services were generally separate from the housing services, interagency and cross-disciplinary collaboration has recently begun to address this fragmentation of services. Many programs have attempted to provide homeless families with "one stop shopping" for all of their educational, psychological, and housing needs. However, relative to the large number of homeless families, there are few programs that link comprehensive services to housing.

There is great variety in both the housing and the psychological services that homeless families are receiving today. Most cities have two levels of shelters for homeless families. Tier I shelters are generally short-term emergency housing and traditionally provide few services. Tier II shelters are more commonly called transitional housing and provide considerably more services. Most recently, "services-enriched housing" has been developed to meet the long-term needs of families, integrating comprehensive psychological services with long-term housing. Not all services for homeless families are linked to their housing. School systems that serve homeless children are beginning to provide school-based services for homeless families.

We will now review examples of psychological service programs that are linked to housing or located in schools. It is important to note that of the large number of such programs, only a few have been evaluated empirically (Fischer, 2000). There are even fewer programs in which the evaluation was rigorously conducted by an independent evaluator with a comparison control group and follow-up. Following are descriptions of programs that appear to have at least some data that support their effectiveness.

Services in Shelters

Many programs designed to meet the needs of homeless families provide brief interventions, typically focused on emergency services (Nabors, Proescher, & DeSilva, 2001). The shelter system is a good example. In general, traditional shelters are large emergency facilities where numerous families or single adults are housed overnight. In many cities, these shelters are identified as "Tier I," and they provide minimal services. Little mental health counseling is available because caseworkers assist as many as 60 families each. A few programs have been developed to address this gap in services. Two examples of services that can be implemented in shelters are the "respite camp" and the "therapeutic community program." The latter of which often specializes in drug rehabilitation.

Respite camp is designed as a temporary relief from the stress associated with homelessness and shelter living. The program provides outdoor camping experiences for homeless children and families. It is directed toward strengthening parenting skills and family communication (Kissman, 1999). The program is based on the assumption that a break from stress is beneficial to the parent–child relationship. Even a short respite can help mothers better apply parenting skills, such as positive reinforcement for desirable behavior and empathy toward their children's needs (Hausman & Hammen, 1993). Families attend a weekend or a 5-day session where parents participate in daily group discussions that are focused on parenting issues and facilitated by therapists. Kissman (1999) interviewed participating homeless mothers to qualitatively evaluate family satisfaction with the program. Overall, mothers reported that the program provides few new skills, but rather a respite from stress with the opportunity to engage in activities together as a family.

A modified therapeutic community is sometimes an option available to mothers who are in the shelter system and in need of drug rehabilitation. Therapeutic communities (TCS) have traditionally been employed in drug treatment centers. They have resulted in significant decreases in alcohol and drug use, reduced criminality, improved psychological functioning, and increased employment (Sacks, Sacks, Harle, & De Leon, 1999). The success of TCS has led to the implementation of modified TCS for homeless addicted mothers within the shelter system. The stay in these shelters is generally short in duration and focuses on engaging clients in the peer community and initiating treatment. Because addicted mothers have multiple needs, modified TC treatment programs incorporate educational, vocational, legal, and housing placement services. Modified TCS for women and children provide family-style housing, day care and after-school programs, parenting curriculum, and modifications of the daily program to accommodate the mother's parenting responsibilities (Sacks et al., 1999). Women in these programs have demonstrated decreases in alcohol and drug use, decreased depression, increases in employment, and improvement in other measures of mental health (Wexler, Cuadrado, & Stevens, 1998).

Transitional Housing

Unlike Tier I shelters, transitional housing (Tier II shelters) provide more services for a longer period of time. The Los Angeles Family Housing Corporation (LFHC), a private nonprofit organization, developed the first modern transitional housing programs for low-income families in 1983 (Lederman, 1993). Transitional housing was developed largely in response to the criticisms of emergency (Tier I) shelters. They are generally apartment-style facilities that offer services such as counseling, housing assistance, and recreation. The LFHC facilities originally provided 24-hour supervision, and cooperating social service agencies offered extensive counseling and case management services. From 1987 to 1990 the U.S. Department of Housing and Urban Development (HUD) awarded 534 Transitional Housing Program grants to nonprofit organizations, state, and local governments (Washington, 2002). Transitional housing programs go a step beyond emergency shelters by providing up to 12 months of structured housing together with a large range of supportive services to prepare homeless people to move into permanent housing (Washington, 2002). Although transitional housing programs are the most commonly used family shelter in the country, only a few have been evaluated.

Estival Place Transitional Housing Program

Estival Place was established in 1991, in Memphis, Tennessee. It provides homeless families with 38 temporary housing units for up to 12 months, plus life skills classes, financial counseling, school enrollment, job training, day care, after-school programs, mental health counseling, and case management services (Washington, 2002). The Metropolitan Inter-Faith Association (MIFA), a nonprofit faith-based agency, operates the program. The program's funding sources are the city of Memphis, MIFA, HUD, U.S. Department of Agriculture, and the Department of Health and Human Services (state and local). Estival Place screens its applicants; a positive drug screen or a felony conviction in the past 2 years prevents acceptance (Estival Place, 1994). All families are required to work or attend school and to attend weekly life skill meetings. Families are not charged rent, but are instead required to deposit 30% of their monthly income into savings accounts. Washington conducted qualitative interviews with individuals who were self-sufficient for 6–12 months after graduation from Estival Place. Family counseling, life skills classes, budgeting, job training, and leadership skills were the services that graduates found most helpful (Washington, 2002).

Hawkeye Area Transitional Housing Program

Using HUD grants, the Hawkeye Area Transitional Housing Program was established to provide transitional housing and family-centered supportive services to homeless families. It began in 1988 with 3 units, and by 1992 had 100 units and served 245 individual family members—37% of whom were children from 0 to 5 years of age (Richardson & Landsman, 1996). In 1993, a Homeless Head Start Project was added to the program. The Hawkeye Area Transitional Housing Program includes transportation services, substance abuse counseling, recreational services, family planning, and support groups. Richardson and Landsman found that those who successfully completed the program (as opposed who those who had not) experienced greater gains in income and were more likely to maintain stable housing 6 months to 1 year following completion of the program.

American Family Inns

The American Family Inns are Residential Educational Training (RET) Centers for the entire family. The Inns were developed by Homes for the Homeless in 1986, with the idea that all necessary services can be cost-effectively and efficiently provided for families, under one roof. Homes for the Homeless believes that to effectively break the cycle of homelessness and poverty, the underlying issues that lead to homelessness *all* must be addressed (Nunez, 1994). The American Family Inn is built on the assumption that providing educational and social services will address the underlying causes of homelessness. The American Family Inn offers comprehensive educational and training programs, which are supported by on-site services such as child care, family counseling, medical clinics, and substance abuse counseling. Parents are given the opportunity to complete their education, to acquire independent living skills, and to obtain job training before moving into permanent housing. At the same time, their children's education, recreation, and health care are assured and any family problems are addressed. American Family Inns tap the potential of the transitional shelters; they turn a long shelter stay into a productive, concentrated period of learning, recovery, and preparation, with all of the needed tools and support available on-site (Nunez, 1994).

The success of the American Family Inn demonstrates that shelters need not serve merely as waiting rooms between temporary bouts of housing. As a result of this education-based program (provided at the same cost as operating a traditional shelter in today's emergency shelter system), 94% of all families who graduate from the American Family Inns remain in permanent housing (Nunez, 1995).

Services-Enriched Housing

Services-enriched housing goes beyond transitional housing by providing long-term service-linked housing for homeless families. Services-enriched housing was developed in 1990 to address the long-term needs of families and individuals caught in the cycle of poverty. Although there are many similarities to transitional housing, the use of the term "services-enriched housing" refers primarily to permanent, basic rental housing for the general low-income population in which social services are available either by referral or on-site. In addition, residents are significantly involved in the decision-making process. Housing can be nonprofit, private, HUD-assisted, unsubsidized, mixed income, or any combination of the above (Beyond Shelter, 2003). Services-enriched housing allows residents to identify their own needs and concerns within a community-oriented housing structure. Residents themselves develop programs, services, and recreational and social activities often assisted by, but not necessarily originating from, an outside source. Yet, residents who maintain their rent and abide by basic landlord–tenant agreements do not risk losing their housing if they choose to bypass involvement in social services or other activities.

The services-enriched housing model can vary dramatically. It may be owned by a nonprofit organization or by a private landlord. Increasingly, nonprofit developers are contracting with social service agencies to provide services to residents in their buildings. Depending on size, services-enriched developments may have both on-site management and a part- or full-time services coordinator. Although not always possible, space may be provided for programs and activities on-site, including office space or classroom space, for both the services coordinator and resident groups to use. Services and community space may also be available to other residents in the neighborhood. The following is a description of two services-enriched housing projects—the Homeless Families Program and the Emerson-Davis Family Development Center.

The Homeless Families Program (HFP)

The first services-enriched housing project, the Homeless Families Program (HFP), was initiated in 1990 in nine sites across the country. It was a joint initiative of The Robert Wood Johnson Foundation and the U.S. Department of Housing and Urban Development. Each site received a $600,000 grant and 150 Section 8 certificates over 5 years. A major aspect of HFP is the combination of case management and subsidized housing for multiproblem families living in shelters or in other homeless situations (Rog et al., 1997). The program began with two goals: (1) to demonstrate a model of services-enriched housing for families and (2) to develop and restructure comprehensive systems of health services, support services, and housing for homeless families.

The HFP has received one of the few thorough evaluations of services for homeless families in the literature. The evaluation sought to determine the needs of the families served, how services and systems could be better organized and delivered, and how housing could be delivered to increase residential stability, increase service use, and move families toward self-sufficiency (Rog, 1999). The evaluation identified multiple service needs of families. Most pronounced were mental health and domestic violence services. Other service needs identified were physical health, substance abuse treatment, education, and training. Eighty-five percent of those in the HFP remained in stable housing for at least 18 months, with the percentage dropping slightly at 30 months. The evaluation determined that families demonstrated increased usage of services while in the program. The largest increase was in the use of mental health services and drug and alcohol treatment. Rog found some progress toward self-sufficiency, but the vast majority of families remained dependent on federal or state support. After leaving the program and receiving 1 year of case management services, 20% of the mothers were working as compared to 13% in a control group.

Rog (1999) also evaluated HFP's attempts at changing the systems. By developing and implementing many of the services that were found to be lacking within the community, the HFP successfully filled many of the gaps in the homeless system through services-enriched housing. Less often, HFP was able to make "system fixes," where services were increased or improved for homeless families who were both within and outside of the program. Major systems changes, however, were rare. The HFP officially ended after 5 years, in 1995, although some of the original sites continued beyond this point. Due to some of the success that the HFP enjoyed, other programs have begun to use the services-enriched model in conjunction with providing housing for homeless families.

Emerson-Davis Family Development Center

The Institute for Community Living opened the Emerson-Davis Family Development Center, known as "Emerson," in New York City in 1994. Emerson's goal is to reunite single parents separated from their children because of their mental illness or homelessness and to provide them with a healthy, safe home of their own. Emerson has a continuum of housing ranging from congregate residences with one- and two-bedroom apartments to stand-alone family apartments. Emerson serves the mental health needs of their clients in conjunction with other individual and family services needs. Residents are provided with housing services as well as case management, family, clinical, educational, and preventive services (Lieberman et al., 1999). Clinical interventions and support have allowed many of the parents with mental illness to attain competency in their parenting roles and thereby regain custody of their children.

Emerson is funded through the New York State Office of Mental Health, the New York City Department of Mental Health, the Stewart B McKinney Homeless Assistance Act funds from the Department of Housing and Urban Development, fees from client income and Medicaid, and private donations and foundations (Emerson-Davis Family Development Center, 2000). Between 1994 and 2000, Emerson has reunited 45 families with 63 children. Twenty-three out of 30 families who have moved out of the residence have departed with their family intact. Parents discharged from the program exhibit significantly improved parenting skills as well as improved daily living skills (Emerson-Davis Family Development Center, 2000).

School-Based Services

The Empowerment Zone Project

Although most services for homeless families are linked to their housing, schools are increasingly providing services for homeless children. School systems can be an important point of entry into an array of necessary services for homeless children. Schools that engage in a collaborative model, in which the school and community services are linked, are especially helpful in providing assessment and intervention for homeless children and families. The challenge for schools is, of course, that they must address these complex issues in conjunction with their primary mission of educating children. Coordinating interagency efforts primarily through the school can maximize the services by providing them in an environment that is familiar and accessible to children and parents (Wall, 1996).

The Empowerment Zone Project (EZ) is one example of a school-based program that addresses the needs of low-income and homeless families. Designed and implemented by Nabors, Proescher, and DeSilva (2001), the EZ project provides mental health prevention services to children during their school day. Teachers and mental health clinicians were involved in the development and implementation of the program. Prevention activities focus on conflict resolution, problem solving, coping with stress, anger management, violence and drug use prevention, and improving self-esteem and assertiveness skills. Clinicians also provide individual therapy services for homeless youth experiencing psychosocial or adjustment difficulties. Parents have a chance to participate in classes focused on teaching discipline techniques, dealing with defiant behavior, coping with psychological problems, and improving their children's coping (Nabors et al., 2001). Parents were paid a stipend based on the number of classes they attended ($10 per class).

The EZ project was evaluated during a summer program for low-income and homeless children where the EZ curriculum was incorporated into the school day as part of the children's "character education training" (Nabors et al., 2001). Parents reported a decrease in behavioral issues after the summer program; however, because the program was part of a larger effort, it is difficult to discern the impact of the EZ project itself.

SERVICE UTILIZATION

Although all of the programs described provide needed services to homeless families, they serve a relatively small number of all homeless families. Most homeless families do not demonstrate a high level of service use in general, and many who attempt to utilize services experience many barriers (Buckner & Bassuk, 1997; Shirley, 1995). Buckner and Bassuk found only modest rates of mental health-related service use within homeless families. Families with seriously emotionally disturbed youths were the least likely to utilize services. Yet, most of the mothers with seriously disturbed children did acknowledge their child's need for help.

There are many reasons why mothers, who may recognize the need for psychological services for their children, do not utilize the services. First, the services may not be available (Shirley, 1995). The previous review of services demonstrates that although many quality programs exist to assist homeless families, these programs are not widespread. The lack of comprehensive services is a major factor contributing to the poor psychological health of homeless children. Even when treatment is available, some homeless children do not access them. Single mothers, faced with the task of sustaining and raising children with few social supports and diminishing economic aid, have many pressing and competing demands (Buckner & Bassuk, 1997). For some families, a child's need for mental health treatment may be a low priority when compared to the need for shelter, food, and clothing.

When a family recognizes the need for psychological services and decides to seek treatment, there are often numerous barriers that they must be overcome, including transportation and child care (Buckner & Bassuk, 1997). Homeless mothers who have difficulty speaking English face yet another barrier to accessing services. Further, some immigrants fear engaging themselves and their children in services because of the possibility of deportation. Developing ways to eliminate these barriers should be a priority for mental health service providers.

Finally, the fragmentation of the system constitutes a significant obstacle to treatment. In many cities, service agencies fail to connect with one another. Families themselves are responsible for coordinating their multiple providers—for job placement, social security benefits, Medicaid, transitional assistance, housing, education assistance, childcare, and therapy.

Many times a week a homeless mother and all of her children (who are generally under 6 years of age) need to take buses all over the city to receive services. Between waiting for the buses, waiting within each of the agencies, and attempting to keep her children content and well behaved, the mother's resources are stretched very thin (Hatton, Kleffel, Bennett, & Gaffrey, 2001).

Even though integrated and comprehensive, quality services for homeless families are not the norm; there is much to be learned from the successful programs that do exist. As the trend in services for homeless families moves toward longer-term housing with increased integration of psychological services for all members of the family, it is vital to incorporate and improve upon the current successes.

CHARACTERISTICS OF SUCCESSFUL PROGRAMS

Successful psychological services appear to share a number of characteristics that can be incorporated into future service ventures. Some of these service characteristics are particular to the homeless population—others characterize effective psychological services to almost any population. Successful service programs are grounded in a comprehensive theoretical framework that informs their policies, services, and interactions with families (Lerner, 1995). Effective psychological services also include a focus on strengths and resilience and are not limited to "fixing" psychopathology (Lerner, 1995; Masten & Coatsworth, 1998). Despite the harmful consequences of homelessness for families, research on homeless children indicates that some children fare well despite these stressors (Masten & Coatsworth, 1998). Masten and Coatsworth found that social resources, including a supportive family and the availability of supportive persons outside the family are critical in contributing to the development of resilience in homeless children.

Successful psychological services integrate fragmented services through program implementation, collaboration among professionals and agencies, and coordination across services. Interprofessional collaboration and wraparound services are now becoming a standard of care, particularly among families living in poverty (Walsh, Brabeck, & Howard, 1999). Many programs for homeless families have linked a range of coordinated services to temporary housing in an attempt to increase the ease of service use for families as well as increase the ease of communication and collaboration among service providers (Nunez, 1994).

Provision of transportation and child care is also critical to the delivery of effective psychological services to homeless families. Consistent utilization of psychological services by this population will also require providers to address issues of insurance and free care since homeless families are unlikely to be able to afford to pay for such services (Buckner & Bassuk, 1997). Providers need to collaborate with other community service agencies to develop innovative ways to offer services to those with and without health coverage so that families may be empowered to break the cycle of poverty.

Successful psychological services also provide treatment and interventions that address the needs of each member of the family, including the children. Parenting skills for mothers, and to a lesser degree early intervention and preventative services for toddlers, are the type of psychological services most available to homeless families. The homeless family with school-aged and adolescent children, however, is in great need of psychological services. Although there is much focus on the runaway or "throwaway" homeless adolescent, there is virtually no literature on the homeless adolescent who is a part of a homeless family. The challenges and psychological issues facing these two groups of adolescents are different. Homeless adolescents living with their families would benefit from services that are targeted to their unique situation.

Effective psychological services also require ongoing program evaluations, ideally by an independent external evaluator. Although results of evaluations of programs that include psychological services are beginning to emerge, as yet there appear to be no evaluations of the outcomes of specific psychological services (e.g., cognitive-behavioral versus insight-oriented therapy, individual group or family treatment) for homeless families.

Finally, successful service programs develop ways to effectively sustain the programs and services that they offer. Most current programs are grant funded. Not only does grant writing require a considerable amount of time, energy, and knowledge on the part of the program staff, it is also very unpredictable. Often, as the economy turns downward and the greatest numbers of homeless families are in need of comprehensive services, grant funding is minimized or cut. Successful programs find ways to address sustainability and institutionalize services into traditional service delivery systems.

CONCLUSION

The rapidly increasing number of homeless families has demonstrated the need to assist these families to prevent future homelessness, to address the stress of being homeless, and to transition effectively to permanent housing. Effective psychological services are a critical component of the comprehensive and coordinated interventions that can offer homeless families a way out of homelessness and perhaps even out of poverty. The implementation and evaluation of a wide range of psychological services for homeless families have offered the beginnings of a knowledge base regarding the characteristics of effective psychological services for this population. Psychological service providers can build on this knowledge base as they continue to design and implement psychological services for this population.

REFERENCES

Bassuk, E. L., Rubin, L., & Lauriat, A. S. (1986). Characteristics of sheltered homeless families. *American Journal of Public Health, 76*, 1097–1101.

Bassuk, E. L., Weinreb, L. F., Buckner, J. C., Browne, A., Salomon, A., & Bassuk, S. S. (1996). The characteristics and needs of sheltered homeless and low-income housed mothers. *Journal of the American Medical Association, 276,* 640–646.

Beyond Shelter. (2003). *Beyond Shelter: Housing first, service enriched housing overview.* Retrieved April 26, 2003, from http://www.beyondshelter.org/aaa_housing_first/housing_first_SEH_overview.shtml

Buckner, J. C., & Bassuk, E. L. (1997). Mental disorders and service utilization among youths from homeless and low-income housed families. *Journal of the American Academy of Child & Adolescent Psychiatry, 36,* 890–900.

Dunlap, K. M., & Fogel, S. J. (1998). A preliminary analysis of research on recovery from homelessness. *Journal of Social Distress and the Homeless, 7,* 175–188.

Emerson-Davis Family Development Center. (2000). APA achievement awards, Gold Award: Supportive residential services to reunite homeless mentally ill single parents with their children. *Psychiatric Services, 51,* 1433–1435.

Estival Place. (1994). *Estival Place 1994 annual report.* Memphis, TN: Metropolitan Inter-Faith Association.

Fischer, R. (2000). Toward self-sufficiency: Evaluating a transitional housing program for homeless families. *Policy Studies Journal, 23,* 402–420.

Goodman, L. A. (1991). The prevalence of abuse in the lives of homeless and poor housed mother: A comparison study. *American Journal of Orthopsychiatry, 61,* 489–500.

Hatton, D. C., Kleffel, D., Bennett, S., & Gaffrey, E. N. (2001). Homeless women and children's access to health care: A paradox. *Journal of Community Health Nursing, 18,* 25–34.

Hausman, B., & Hammen, C. (1993). Parenting in homeless families: The double crisis. *American Journal of Orthopsychiatry, 63,* 358–369.

Homes for the Homeless. (1998). *Homeless families today: Our challenge tomorrow.* New York: Author.

Homes for the Homeless. (2000). *Multiple families: Multiplying problems. A first look at the fathers of homeless children.* New York: Author.

Jackson, J. H., & Walsh, M. E. (2004). School counseling. In C. B. Fisher & R. M. Lerner (Eds.), *Applied developmental science: An encyclopedia of research, policies, and programs.* Thousand Oaks: Sage.

Kissman, K. (1999). Respite from stress and other service needs of homeless families. *Community Mental Health Journal, 35,* 241–249.

Lederman, J. (1993). *Housing America.* Salem, MA: Probus Publishing.

Lerner, R. M. (1995). *America's youth in crisis: Challenges and options for programs and policies.* Thousand Oaks, CA: Sage.

Lieberman, H. J., Campanelli, P. C., Ades, Y., Cruz, T., Nagel, L., & Palmer, J. (1999). Reunifying single-parent families with special needs. *Psychiatric Rehabilitation Journal, 23,* 42–46.

Masten, A. S., & Coatsworth, J. D. (1998). The development of competence in favorable and unfavorable environments: Lessons learned from research on successful children. *American Psychologist, 53,* 205–220.

Masten, A. S., Miliotis, D., Graham-Bermann, S. A., Ramirez, M., & Neemann, J. (1993). Children in homeless families: Risks to mental health and development. *Journal of Consulting and Clinical Psychology, 61,* 335–343.

McLoyd, V. C. (1998). Socioeconomic disadvantage and child development. *American Psychologist, 53,* 185–204.

Menke, E. M., & Wagner, J. D. (1997a). A comparative study of homeless, previously homeless, and never homeless school-aged children's health. *Issues in Comprehensive Pediatric Nursing, 20,* 153–173.

Menke, E. M., & Wagner, J. D. (1997b). The experience of homeless female-headed families. *Issues in Mental Health Nursing, 18,* 315–330.

Nabors, L., Proescher, E., & DeSilva, M. (2001). School-based mental health prevention activities for homeless and at-risk youth. *Child and Youth Care Forum, 30,* 3–18.

New York City Commission on the Homeless. (1992). *The way home: A new direction in social policy.* New York: Author.

Nunez, R. (1994). *Hopes, dreams & promise: The future of homeless children in America.* New York: Homes for the Homeless.

Nunez, R. (1995). *An American family myth: Every child at risk.* Retrieved May 5, 2003, from http://www.homesforthehomeless.com/facts.html

Pianta, R., Egeland, B., & Erickson, M. F. (1989). The antecedents of maltreatment: Results of the Mother–Child Interaction Research Project. In D. Cicchetti & V. Carlson (Eds.), *Child maltreatment: Theory and research on the causes and consequences of child abuse and neglect* (pp. 203–253). New York: Cambridge University Press.

Richardson, B. B., & Landsman, M. J. (1996). *Community response to homelessness: Evaluation of the HACAP Transitional Housing Program. Final report.* Iowa City: The National Resource Center for Family Centered Practice.

Rog, D. J. (1999). The Evaluation of the Homeless Families Program. *American Journal of Evaluation, 20,* 558–561.

Rog, D. J., Holupka, C. S., McCombs-Thornton, K. L., Brito, M. C., & Hambrick, R. (1997). Case management in practice: Lessons from the evaluation of the RWJ/HUD Homeless Families Program. *Journal of Prevention & Intervention in the Community, 15,* 67–82.

Sacks, J. Y., Sacks, S. Harle, M., & De Leon, G. (1999). Homelessness prevention: Therapeutic community (TC) for addicted mothers. *Alcoholism Treatment Quarterly, 17,* 33–51.

Salomon, A. S., Bassuk, S. S., & Huntington, N. (2002). The relationship between intimate partner violence and the use of addictive substances in poor and homeless mothers. *Violence Against Women, 8,* 785–815.

Schmitz, C. L., Wagner, J. D., & Menke, E. M. (2001). The interconnection of childhood poverty and homelessness: Negative impact/points of access. *Families in Society, 82,* 69–77.

Shirley, A. (1995). Special needs of vulnerable and undeserved populations: Models, existing and proposed, to meet them. *Pediatrics, 96,* 858–863.

Styron, T. H., Janoff-Bulman, R., & Davidson, L. (2000). "Please ask me how I am": Experiences of family homelessness in the context of single mothers' lives. *Journal of Social Distress and the Homeless, 9,* 143–165.

Torquati, J. C. (2002). Personal and social resources as predictors of parenting in homeless families. *Journal of Family Issues, 23,* 463–485.

U.S. Conference of Mayors. (2002). *A status report on hunger and homelessness in America's cities: 2002.* Washington, DC: U.S. Conference of Mayors.

U.S. Department of Education. (1995). *Report to Congress on the education of homeless children and youth.* Washington, DC: Author.

Wall, J. C. (1996). Homeless children and their families: Delivery of educational and social services through school systems. *Social Work in Education, 18,* 135–144.

Walsh, M. E. (1990). Developmental and socio-emotional needs of homeless infants and preschoolers. In E. L. Bassuk, D. Mead-Fox, & M. Harvey (Eds.), *Designing programs for homeless families* (pp. 91–101). Newton, MA: Better Homes Foundation.

Walsh, M. E. (1992). *Moving to nowhere: Children's stories of homelessness.* Westport, CT: Auburn House.

Walsh, M. E., Brabeck, M. M., & Howard, K. A. (1999). Interprofessional collaboration in children's services: Toward a theoretical framework. *Children's services: Social Policy, Research, and Practice, 2,* 183–208.

Walsh, M. E., & Buckley, M. A. (1994). Children's experiences of homelessness: Implications for school counselors. *Elementary School Guidance & Counseling, 29,* 4–15.

Washington, T. A. (2002). The homeless need more than just a pillow, they need a pillar: An evaluation of a transitional housing program. *Families in Society, 83,* 183–189.

Wexler, H. K., Cuadrado, M., & Stevens, S. J. (1998). Residential treatment for women: Behavioral and psychological outcomes. *Drugs & Society, 13,* 213–233.

19

Telehealth/Internet Services for Children, Adolescents, and Families

HEIDI J. LISS

As technology advances, innovative methods of service delivery become available. Telehealth, or the use of technology to provide health-related services, is emerging as a potential avenue for the provision of health and mental health services. As the word suggests, the term "telehealth" was originally coined to describe the provision of health services at a distance. Today, however, the term has come to describe not just the provision of services at a distance, but also the use of various forms of technology to assist in the provision of medical, health, and mental health services.

The movement to develop telehealth programs likely was motivated by several factors. The first factor was the lack of local or easily available services for large segments of the population. Good examples of this phenomenon are military personnel, prisoners, and rural residents, citizens who would otherwise have difficulty receiving specialty services due to inaccessibility of providers. A second factor was the need to provide services in a more efficient, cost-effective way. One way that telehealth could help in this regard is that it can allow for a single provider to consult with patients in various locations without the need to travel, thereby saving both time and travel costs. Finally, a need to support isolated providers or consumers has led to a desire to use technology to enhance or supplement traditional services. For example, online support groups may provide a supplemental service to people who already receive psychotherapy, or can serve as a way to provide collegial support to isolated psychotherapists.

HEIDI J. LISS • National Rural Behavioral Health Center, University of Florida, Gainesville, Florida 32610.

Already various media have been utilized to provide telehealth services, such as teleconferencing, the Internet, telephones, computer programs, virtual reality, and handheld devices. The types of new technology that can be utilized for service delivery are constantly increasing as technology improves and evolves over time. One of the earliest known uses of telehealth occurred in Sweden in 1922, when a hospital communicated by wire with sailors to provide treatment advice (Hakansson & Gavelin, 2000). From the 1950s through the 1970s, telehealth programs using interactive video were tried and discontinued due to high cost (Grigsby & Sanders, 1998). Although technically telehealth has been in existence for some time, it is only in the past few decades that research and program development in this area have blossomed.

One of the challenges to telehealth research and programs is the rapid rate of technology development: by the time a research or service program has been created and studied, the technology used could be obsolete. Another, and related, challenge is determining the acceptability of usage by consumers. This is difficult because usage patterns change at a rapid rate. Therefore, data obtained on usage patterns and acceptability only a few years ago might now be irrelevant, as acceptability of technology likely increases along with its use in the population.

As with most areas of study (Hammen & Compass, 1994), the examination of services and treatment for children and their families in the realm of telehealth lags behind the adult literature (Alessi, 2000). Nevertheless, although the literature on telehealth with children is in its infancy, some research in this area has begun, and various programs have been devised. Some of the programs have been designed specifically for use with children and their families, whereas others are adaptations of techniques developed for adults. The purpose of this chapter is to describe and comment on the primary uses of telehealth with children and their families to date, with a special focus on its use for mental health purposes. The following uses of telehealth with children and families will be described: (1) psychological or psychiatric assessment and intervention, (2) prevention programs, and (3) use as an aid to providers. Finally, a summary of the current uses of technology will be provided, along with a commentary on the needs for future research in this area.

PSYCHOLOGICAL OR PSYCHIATRIC ASSESSMENT AND INTERVENTION

Psychological or psychiatric assessment and intervention often have limited availability in remote areas. The main type of technology used to assist in the provision of mental health services to children in remote areas is videoconferencing. The focus of this section is to describe the findings of a selection of seminal programs in which videoconferencing with children has been performed.

Several Australian researchers have reported on the use of videoconferencing for child psychiatric care. Gelber and Alexander (1999) reported on user satisfaction and utilization of teleconferencing services over a 2-year period. Survey respondents (remote health and mental health professionals) indicated that the equipment most frequently was used for consultation and clinical care, but it also was used for supervision of remote personnel, teaching, and administration. Approximately 52% of survey respondents reported feeling depersonalized due to the use of the teleconferencing, and 40% reported problems with the technology. However, 52% of respondents indicated that the system allowed for cost and time savings due to reductions in travel, and 50% reported improvement in consultation.

Another group of Australian researchers, Kopel, Nunn, and Dossetor (2001), evaluated satisfaction with a videocounseling psychiatry program. Psychiatrists at the hub site, and patients and mental health workers at the remote sites, were surveyed on their comfort with the technology, quality of the interaction, and overall satisfaction. A very high percentage (93–99%) of respondents reported high comfort levels with the technology. Most respondents (91–94%) also reported high levels of satisfaction with the videoconferencing program compared with face-to-face interaction. Consistent with other studies, the medical professionals providing consultation were more likely than patients or remote clinicians to feel that the technology interfered with the consultation.

Similarly, Elford et al. (2000) examined the reliability of psychiatric video-interview for assessment purposes, as well as user satisfaction with the video assessment. Twenty-three patients (ages 4–16) were assessed both by video and in-person assessments (order of assessment was randomized). There was a 96% agreement in diagnosis and treatment evaluation when assessment results were compared. This suggests that videoconferencing may provide an alternative, reliable means for conducting psychiatric evaluation. Although children and their parents reported comfort with the videoassessments, psychiatrists reported a preference for live patient interviews. Therefore, although use of video did not appear to affect the accuracy of diagnosis, the ability to see a patient in person appears to be valued by psychiatrists. This is consistent with other reports of physician satisfaction.

In one of the few studies to examine mental health treatment effectiveness with telehealth, Glueckauf et al. (2002) conducted a study of psychotherapy treatment effectiveness using telehealth with a sample of rural, American adolescents with epilepsy and their families. Teens and their families ($n = 39$) initially received an in-person intake assessment, and then were assigned to one of three conditions: videocounseling conducted at home, speakerphone counseling conducted at home, or in-person counseling conducted in a traditional office setting. All families received five sessions of postassessment family counseling, and level of participation, satisfaction, and perception of problem severity were assessed during treatment, at the end of counseling, and at 6-month follow-up. It was found that dropout was associated with being assigned to the in-person condition, which necessitated lengthy travel by families. This occurred despite offering compensation to participants for travel expenses.

Significant therapeutic gains (as reported by teens, their parents, and teachers) were found for all methods of therapy presentation, with no differences noted in effectiveness among the treatment methods. Treatment adherence did not improve when psychotherapy was conducted in-home (via telephone or video).

Preliminary results indicate that videoconferencing provides a reliable way of conducting mental health and psychiatric evaluation for children. It also appears to provide an effective means of providing mental health treatment. Patients and staff report comfort with the technology and general satisfaction with the approach to assessment and treatment. However, it is notable that consulting physicians are more likely to view the technology as interfering with their ability to perform their evaluations, although patients and support staff do not report concern about this issue. Furthermore, one study (Gelber & Alexander, 1999) reported that a sense of depersonalization was described by a large proportion of service consumers and providers. This is a finding that should be examined more closely in future research, as it could potentially have a negative impact on patient treatment. Additionally, it is unclear whether video counseling or video assessment services truly provide a savings in cost to either provider or consumer in practice. Finally, it is notable that one study reported problems with the technology itself. It is possible that the specific technology in use at the time (which might now be outdated) was not optimal, but this could also suggest that technology in general is not yet in place for optimum use in providing real-time mental health treatment and evaluation.

PREVENTION SERVICES

This section focuses on the use of telehealth as a means of providing prevention services to children and their families. The types of prevention programs examined in this section vary from primary prevention to tertiary prevention programs. Types of problems that have been targeted by telehealth prevention programs vary widely, and include academic performance, health-related behavior, emotional problems related to health problems, and child abuse.

Fels, Williams, Smith, Treviranus, and Eagleson (1999) developed a remote-controlled videoconferencing system called Providing Education By Bringing Learning Environments to Students (PEBBLES), which allows hospitalized students to participate in their regular classroom activities. The system involves two-way video and audio communication between the classroom and the student, as well as a control panel for students, which allows zoom and video manipulation, as well as responses to questions using a keypad. It was expected that this would assist students both academically and psychologically. Being able to attend academic classes remotely should facilitate academic achievement and keep students from falling behind in class work. Furthermore, maintaining a presence in the classroom should reduce the sense of isolation a child may feel while hospitalized for long periods of time, enhancing social involvement with others outside of the hospital. It also can be comforting to maintain routines, providing a sense of "normal" in an otherwise stressful and abnormal circumstance.

Multiple short-term studies were conducted using the PEBBLES system. Initially, the system was tested with a few nonhospitalized children who participated in learning experiences remotely. Later studies involved using the system with single students who were hospitalized for long periods of time. Students would use the system daily for two 1-hour sessions. Although there were occasional problems with the technology, such as poor audio and video quality, overall, the system appeared to effectively provide a means for students to remain involved in the classroom. It is notable that a large degree of coordination with and support from the classroom teacher would be necessary to institute this system effectively. Children who participated became bored when they could not perform the classroom activity, so efforts would need to be made to emphasize activities in which the child could participate remotely during their classroom observation periods. Furthermore, finding a way to remotely provide children with homework sheets would help facilitate participation. Teachers reported the equipment to be disruptive to the class at first, but that this subsided after usage became routine. Overall, the system appeared to provide a nice supplement to existing hospital tutoring, rather than providing a replacement for such services. Although this innovative use of technology is promising, further study of this system with larger samples and more diverse age groups should be done. More structured measures of effectiveness and psychological benefit would also be helpful in determining usefulness of PEBBLES technology.

Another group that has developed interventions specifically for children with serious illnesses is the STARBRIGHT Foundation. The types of STARBRIGHT interventions are varied, but the overarching goal of the interventions is to prevent the negative physical or psychological impacts associated with chronic illness and hospitalization (Bush & Simonian, 2002). One intervention, called STARBRIGHT World, is a private online computer network that connects hospitalized children with one another (Bush, Huchital, & Simonian, 2002). In addition to providing a means for connecting with other chronically ill children, it also provides opportunities for children to learn about their disease and coping skills for disease management, as well as distract themselves with pleasurable activities, such as games and art projects. Five areas targeted by the system are interpersonal communication, peer support, self-expression, knowledge and information, and distraction-affective elevation. The network is large, and includes most of the functions that are generally available on the Internet, but websites and functions available are restricted to those that are pre-screened. The system components are child and health focused, allowing children to explore in a safe environment in which their needs might more easily be met than the general Internet. The STARBRIGHT World system has been instituted at hospitals across the United States and Canada, and will be expanding internationally.

Research on STARBRIGHT World can be challenging due to the difficulties in maintaining control over the implementation (i.e., each child will have a unique experience with the system). Battles and Wiener (2002) examined the use of STARBRIGHT World with children who had life-threatening illnesses, and examined the variables of loneliness, problem behavior, and willingness to return to the hospital for treatment. Parental report suggested that the system was helpful in reducing loneliness and depressive symptoms for children with life-threatening illnesses, as well as reducing their resistance to returning to the hospital for treatment. Hazzard, Celano, Collins, and Markov (2002) used STARBRIGHT World to provide a more structured curriculum to children with sickle cell disease or asthma, and compared this form of intervention with traditional recreational and educational activities provided at the hospital. Although children who received STARBRIGHT showed gains, measures used in this study did not identify significant differences from gains shown by traditional hospital services. Authors hypothesized that this could be due to the less intensive nature of the curriculum as presented in this study, although they noted that conducting research on a hospitalized population is challenging in general due to difficulties in standardization and having less control over intervention presentation due to conflicts with hospital treatment protocols.

A second STARBRIGHT intervention is called STARBRIGHT Hospital Pals. This program was developed to target young children undergoing radiation treatment for cancer. The intervention includes a preprocedure video in which good coping and appropriate behavior are modeled with the child character Barney. A toy Barney is with them during the video presentation providing auditory messages to them via infrared communication from the video system. Then during radiation treatment a plush Barney toy is given, which provides supportive messages and distracting stories throughout the procedure. Only preliminary research has been conducted on this type of intervention, but it appears to provide reductions in child and parent distress related to radiation treatment (Tyc et al., 2000).

In addition to the use of Internet-based prevention services with hospitalized children, it also has been used as a prevention tool with other child populations. As the Internet has increased in availability, the number of Websites dedicated to health and health-related information has increased. The initial target audience for these Websites was the adult population, but Websites providing information and support to youngsters are growing in number. One good example of this is a Website developed by researchers who initially developed a health-based Internet site for adults (CHESS; Gustafson et al., 1999). "Stomp Out Smokes" (SOS) is an Internet-based smoking cessation program for children and adolescents ages 11–17 years (Meis et al., 2002). In their report of the development of this program, the authors noted that very little research had been done previously in the area of smoking cessation with preadolescents and adolescents. For the purposes of this project, efforts were made to take into account developmental issues when tailoring the smoking cessation program for this population and designing the Web site. To start, a panel of 17 adolescents provided feedback on potential Web site features and design. Second, the positive and negative aspects of smoking, as viewed by adolescents, were presented, along with alternative ways to obtain the positive aspects of smoking. Third, efforts were made to use language that was direct, simple, clear, nonjudgmental, colloquial, and specific. Fourth, the program allowed teens to have a sense of autonomy by allowing them to design their own cessation programs. Overall, the website provides a system of smoking cessation, general information, discussion groups, live chat, journaling, a gallery for posting artwork, and an ask-an-expert forum. At the time information about this program was published, formal evaluation of the sos program had not been conducted. However, pilot participants provided positive feedback about the program, and the authors planned to examine the effectiveness of the system by comparing it to office-based smoking cessation treatment in a formal research study.

Finally, teletechnology has been used as a tool for prevention efforts with children and their families in the realm of child abuse. Due to the success of home visitation programs instituted to prevent child abuse, attempts have been made to duplicate results by using telehealth technology. Pilot work in this area was conducted by Inouye, Cerny, Hollandsworth, and Ettipio (2001). A sample of 20 at-risk military families were nonrandomly chosen to participate in a 6-month trial of home-based videophone meetings, in addition to nurse-provided education and assistance with typical parental responsibilities (e.g., breastfeeding, infant care). Participants engaged in a video visit with their assigned nurse at least once weekly. Satisfaction ratings obtained from both nurses and parents did not change significantly between the beginning and end of the study. It is notable that parents' ratings of satisfaction with the equipment were lower than those of nurses. Both nurses and parents reported difficulty with using the technology, and in one case a family withdrew from the study due to safety concerns (the child was repeatedly tripping on the equipment cord). Difficulty setting up the equipment and problems with hearing accurately were reported by both nurses and parents. Nurses reported enjoying the greater flexibility allowed by video use. Additionally, they reported that less time was wasted when a family did not show for an appointment, and they felt more comfortable working through video with violent families, particularly after hours. Families reported feeling that video allowed better access to their nurse and less isolation. Overall, video home visits appear to be feasible and provide advantages to both families and nurses, although the technology used in this study was not optimal.

USE AS AN AID TO PROVIDERS

Teletechnology has also been used to support the provision of services to children and their families by providing assistance and support to professionals who work with children and their families. One example of this is the use of videoconferencing equipment to provide professional development opportunities to isolated child and adolescent mental health providers in Australia. In a study by Mitchell, Robinson, Seiboth, and Koszegi (2000), videoconferencing was used for professional case consultation (e.g., with a psychiatrist), staff development and training, remote interviews of patients by professionals (e.g., psychologist), and administrative meetings. Participants in the network were surveyed, and their responses indicated that they viewed this network as providing them with good opportunities for networking and peer support, more efficiency in providing health services, and reductions in travel cost and time. They also noted that the cost of providing the Integrated Services Digital Network (ISDN) used in teleconferencing was very high, that it was difficult to receive technical assistance at remote locations, and that the equipment necessitated additional training for staff members.

Another way in which telehealth has been used by health care professionals is to provide consultation and support services to rural health and mental health facilities in cases of suspected child abuse. Faculty at the University of Kentucky Chandler Medical Center developed the Child Advocacy Outreach Project in an effort to provide improved availability and quality of care for child victims of sexual abuse living in rural areas (Burton, Stanley, & Ireson, 2002). A brief report was given on the utilization of services and user satisfaction. Internet-based and telephone-based services were utilized to conduct case conferences and consultation with experts located at the hub site, and equipment was available for video colposcopy. Over the initial 2 years of the project, the number of sexual abuse physical examinations conducted by qualified physicians more than quadrupled (from 77 to 339), and the number of expert consultations conducted increased dramatically (from 0 to 74). Although details regarding procedures used in obtaining clinician ratings were unavailable, the authors reported that rural clinicians receiving consultation felt comfortable with the equipment and were very satisfied with the service. Physicians providing consultation to rural providers reported more concerns about the ease of the service, including problems with locating the rural providers, learning how to use the equipment, and difficulties with the software, but felt that they could provide accurate diagnoses based on information received. One significant advantage of this method of service support is that it prevented children, who likely were already traumatized by abuse, from having to make a long trip to an unfamiliar location in order to undergo abuse-related physical examinations.

Beyond treatment and consultation, the creation of a virtual reality environment for the purpose of assessment has been of use to providers (Rizzo et al., 2000). Rizzo and colleagues created the "virtual classroom" in an effort to actively assess symptoms of Attention Deficit Hyperactivity Disorder (ADHD). The classroom is presented through a head-mounted device that provides a three-dimensional classroom environment (desks, blackboard, windows, people, etc.). This allows for experimental control and presentation of distracters to determine task performance speed and accuracy under various conditions, as well as measure the number of incidents of physical distraction (head turning, motor movement, etc.).

Only initial findings of the virtual classroom trial were available at the time that this chapter was written. The trial consisted of an initial time period in which the participants familiarized themselves with the scenario and equipment, and then the presentation of three 10-minute conditions.

The first condition entailed a visual discrimination task with no distraction present. The second condition utilized the same task, but with different types of distracters, both auditory and visual. The third condition required recognition, with changing response requirements over the course of the task. Also, a combination of both auditory and visual distracters was utilized in this condition. Initial anecdotal results suggest that children were able to use the equipment without negative results (e.g., nausea or dizziness associated with virtual reality usage), and appeared comfortable with the equipment. The use of virtual reality might enhance the accuracy of diagnosis, and provide greater information about the conditions under which children have difficulty concentrating. Furthermore, the authors anticipate that the same equipment could be used to provide attention training to children with attention deficits. Although further research is necessary, initial program reports suggest that virtual reality is a promising way of conducting assessment of ADHD in children, and might even be usable as a means of treating attentional problems.

SUMMARY

Overall, preliminary research suggests that telehealth has the potential to adequately provide services to children and families, and even act as a replacement for traditional services. It also provides a vehicle for conducting preventive interventions and supporting those professionals who work with children and families. Due to the newness of this field, particularly its use with children, much of the research that has been done is more descriptive in nature, or provides demonstration of the use of the new technology. Many reports available on telehealth programs for children and families simply entail a description of the program, pilot research, or only a rudimentary study of cost-effectiveness or feasibility. Clearly, there is sufficient evidence to show that the use of telehealth is feasible; however, more rigorous research work is needed to determine which services work best with each population, and under what circumstances.

In addition to the question of effectiveness, it is important to find out whether this technology provides a financially sound alternative to traditional, office-based services. A key question to answer is, do the benefits that may be gleaned by providing services to remote locations outweigh the financial costs associated with such technology? Further studies using cost–benefit analysis are needed to answer this question. However, it is notable that with the rapid changes in technology, and the cost of technology, it may be challenging to answer this question in a meaningful way.

It is notable that the technology currently available has not been ideal for use in assessment, treatment, or consultation. Several studies reported significant difficulties with transmission, which could have an impact on service success and can cause general frustration among both service providers and recipients. Technology is improving at a rapid pace, so it is unclear whether this issue will continue to be problematic.

Another area that has not been fully examined is the social or emotional impact of the use of teletechnology versus face-to-face services. A related factor, user satisfaction, has been examined to some degree in most of the research studies presented, and overall, both providers and care recipients had positive reports about use of the new technology. This does not mean, however, that there is no difference between providing services face-to-face and providing them through telehealth. In one study (Kopel et al., 2001) a large percentage of participants reported feeling dehumanized by the use of teletechnology. Technology potentially causing a sense of dehumanization is an area of concern, and certainly this report suggests that it should be studied further.

Finally, it is notable that developmental issues in the use of telehealth have not been explored. Age-related differences in understanding and acceptance of the technology were not mentioned or examined in the existing literature, nor were any age-related difficulties reported. For example, one might expect that it could be confusing for younger children to be able to talk to the TV OR computer only some of the time. Another possibility is that it could be challenging for children to maintain attention without immediate stimulus cues that provide reinforcement when a person is physically present. It is unclear whether developmental differences in this area of telehealth do not exist, if the newness of the field has left this aspect as yet unexamined, or if this topic has been virtually ignored by researchers.

REFERENCES

Alessi, N. (2000). Child and adolescent telepsychiatry: Reliability studies needed. *CyberPsychology & Behavior, 3,* 1009–1015.

Battles, H. B., & Wiener, L. S. (2002). STARBRIGHT World: Effects of an electronic network on the social environment of children with life-threatening illnesses. *Children's Health Care, 31,* 47–68.

Burton, D. C., Stanley, D., & Ireson, C. L. (2002). Child advocacy outreach: Using telehealth to expand child sexual abuse services in rural Kentucky. *Journal of Telemedicine and Telecare, 8*(Suppl. 2), 10–12.

Bush, J. P., Huchital, J. R., & Simonian, S. J. (2002). An introduction to program and research initiatives of the STARBRIGHT Foundation. *Children's Health Care, 31,* 1–10.

Bush, J. P., & Simonian, S. J. (2002). New directions in research on STARBRIGHT interventions. *Children's Health Care, 31,* 87–91.

Elford, R., White, H., Bowering, R., Ghandi, A., Maddiggan, B., St. John, K. et al. (2000). A randomized, controlled trial of child psychiatric assessments conducted using videoconferencing. *Journal of Telemedicine and Telecare, 6,* 73–82.

Fels, D. I., Williams, L. A., Smith, G., Treviranus, J., & Eagleson, R. (1999). Developing a video-mediated communication system for hospitalized children. *Telemedicine Journal, 5,* 193–208.

Gelber, H., & Alexander, M. (1999). An evaluation of an Australian videoconferencing project for child and adolescent telepsychiatry. *Journal of Telemedicine and Telecare, 5*(Suppl. 1), 21–23.

Glueckauf, R. L., Fritz, S. P., Ecklund-Johnson, E. P., Liss, H. J., Dages, P., & Carney, P. (2002). Videoconferencing-based family counseling for rural teenagers with epilepsy: Phase I findings. *Rehabilitation Psychology, 47,* 49–72.

Grigsby, J., & Sanders, J. H. (1998). Telemedicine: Where it is and where it's going. *Annals of Internal Medicine, 129,* 123–127.

Gustafson, D. H., Hawkins, R., Boberg, E., Pingree, S., Serlin, R. E., Graziano, F. et al. (1999). Impact of a patient-centered, computer-based health information/support system. *American Journal of Preventive Medicine, 16*, 1–9.

Hakansson, S., & Gavelin, C. (2000). What do we really know about the cost-effectiveness of telemedicine? *Journal of Telemedicine and Telecare, 6*(Suppl. 1), 133–135.

Hammen, C., & Compass, B. E. (1994). Unmasking unmasked depression in children and adolescents: The problem of comorbidity. *Clinical Psychology Review, 14*, 585–603.

Hazzard, A., Celano, M., Collins, M., & Markov, Y. (2002). Effects of STARBRIGHT World on knowledge, social support, and coping in hospitalized children with sickle cell disease and asthma. *Children's Health Care, 31*, 69–86.

Inouye, J., Cerny, J. E., Hollandsworth, J., & Ettipio, A. (2001). Child abuse prevention program with POTS-based telehealth: A feasibility project. *Telemedicine Journal and e-Health, 7*, 325–332.

Kopel, H., Nunn, K., & Dossetor, D. (2001). Evaluating satisfaction with a child and adolescent psychological telemedicine outreach service. *Journal of Telemedicine and Telecare, 7*(Suppl. 2), 35–40.

Meis, T. M., Gaie, M. J., Pingree, S., Boberg, E. W., Patten, C. A., Offord, K. P. et al. (2002, April). Development of a tailored, Internet-based smoking cessation intervention for adolescents. *Journal of Computer-Mediated Communication, 7*. Retrieved March 20, 2003, from http://www.ascusc.org/jcmc/vol7/issue3/

Mitchell, J., Robinson, P., Seiboth, C., & Koszegi, B. (2000). An evaluation of a network for professional development in child and adolescent mental health in rural and remote communities. *Journal of Telemedicine and Telecare, 6*, 158–162.

Rizzo, A. A., Buckwalter, J. G., Bowerly, T., Van der Zaag, C., Humphrey, L., Neumann, U. et al. (2000). The virtual classroom: A virtual reality environment for the assessment and rehabilitation of attention deficits. *CyberPsychology & Behavior, 3*, 483–499.

Tyc, V. L., Merchant, T. E., Srivastava, D. K., deArmendi, A. J., Klosky, J. L., Kronenberg, M. E. et al. (2000, August). An intervention for reducing radiation therapy-related distress among pediatric patients. In R. Brown's (Chair), *Technology innovations in pediatric psychology: Research on STARBRIGHT initiatives.* Symposium conducted at the 108th Annual Convention of the American Psychological Association, Washington, DC.

20

Therapeutic Camping Programs

KERI J. BROWN

Camps are a childhood summer pastime and an estimated 10,000 camps are in existence. On the most basic level, camps are thought to provide increased supervision, and social opportunities for attendees. Specifically, for children and adolescents with mental health, behavioral, or pediatric health needs, summer camps can provide a unique venue in which to deliver concentrated therapeutic services in a nonclinical environment. Therapeutic camps differ along many dimensions including the population served, camp duration, counselor expertise, therapeutic components, and camp goals (Levitt, 1994). However, most camps include traditional camp experiences such as fishing, campfires, and sleeping in tents or cabins. This chapter will report on the organization, delivery, and evaluation efforts as they relate to four types of therapeutic camps: (1) wilderness-based camps, (2) camps for children with emotional and behavioral needs (Without Wilderness therapy component), (3) camps for children with chronic illness, and (4) camps for children who are bereaved. Although these are not mutually exclusive categories, they provide an organization to review the camp components and evaluation in these areas. This examination of the extant literature is not exhaustive, rather selected works are presented to serve as examples of the service and research efforts in therapeutic camping. In particular, a report on military-style boot camps is not included and interested readers are referred to Tyler, Darville, and Stalnaker (2001) for a review of these interventions.

KERI J. BROWN • Department of Psychology, Columbus Children's Hospital, Columbus, Ohio 43215.

WILDERNESS THERAPIES

Definition

Wilderness therapy lacks a coherent definition and can be found under multiple names including adventure-based counseling, outdoor experiential learning, wilderness adventure therapy, and derivations thereof. As the name suggests, wilderness therapies utilize the intensity of the outdoors to provide a naturalistic setting to explore the dynamics of group relationships, natural consequences for unproductive behaviors, and enhancement of problem-solving skills (Behar & Stephens, 1978). Most of the theory behind wilderness camps is grounded in the tradition of experiential education (Carver, 1996; Gass, 1993) and it is theorized that these participants "learn by doing." Thus the provision of multiple novel opportunities for campers to "do" is thought to provide the maximum potential for therapeutic growth. The incorporation of such elements as building trust, setting goals, giving consistent feedback, and designing challenging situations is also present in many programs (Bacon & Kimball, 1989). Though many of these children and adolescents have maladaptive externalizing behaviors (and hence the reason they were referred for camp), the focus is often on the positive and adaptive skills of the camper that will help him or her succeed in the difficult and potentially risky task at hand. Additionally, "nature" is thought to be a haven from the stressors of modern society and thus the ideal place for experiential learning.

Russell and Phillips-Miller (2002) defined four key components for therapeutic wilderness camps aimed at addressing psychological needs of attendees: (1) the intervention(s) provided should have clear and well-defined therapeutic components; (2) clinical assessment should be used to select appropriate camp participants and individual treatment plans should be devised; (3) qualified professionals should deliver treatments and assess therapeutic progress during camp; and (4) a post-camp psychological plan should be devised to help maintain any therapeutic gains.

The Camp Experience

Most wilderness programs are between 7 and 28 days long and require skills from each camper to achieve the *group* goals of the day. The adventure-based counselors choose activities that are "risky enough to provide an adventurous learning experience and engaging enough to challenge participants, but appropriate for reducing the actual risks encountered" (Priest & Gass, 1997, p. 110). Generally, tasks become more complex as the camp progresses. For example, in planning the camp adventure experiences, the maturity of campers, physical limitations, social and cognitive abilities, and skill levels are considered (Fletcher & Hinkle, 2002). Campers are expected to participate in challenges such as hiking, spelunking, orienteering, and bicycling. Some camps have reported additional (and arguably more risky) activities such as skydiving, hang gliding, and white-water rafting (Ewert, 1989). Because of the inevitable risks involved in the wilderness activities, guidelines for risk management from the Association for Experiential Education have been established (Leemon, Schimelpfening, Gray, Tarter, & Williamson (1998)). Most wilderness programs require that counselors have a background in counseling or clinical psychology ("soft skills") as well as an understanding and mastery of wilderness survival ("hard skills"). See Fletcher and Hinkle (2002) for a review of ethical considerations given the nontraditional elements of the therapeutic relationship.

Wilderness camps target adolescents with various behavioral, psychological, academic, or family problems (Moote & Wodarski, 1997) and have been used with adolescents with chemical dependency (Gillis & Simpson, 1991), delinquent behaviors (Wilson & Lipsey, 2000), sexual offenders (Kjol & Weber, 1993), and children who are victims of abuse and neglect (McNamara, 2002). Youth are referred by social service workers, mental health agencies, juvenile correctional facilities, schools, and psychiatric facilities (Levitt, 1994). Most campers have often received some form of mental health services at some point, although for some adolescents, these camps will be their primary mental health intervention as they offer an attractive alternative to those adolescents resistant to traditional therapeutic efforts (Russell & Phillips-Miller, 2002).

How does therapeutic change occur in wilderness camps? Recently, Russell and Phillips-Miller (2002) examined key change agents in a multisite study of four adventure programs that were intensive, lengthy (average of 38 days), and staffed with licensed clinicians. In an impressive study that utilized advanced means of capturing qualitative data, the researchers noted four key process findings from camper interviews. First, the nonconfrontive and nurturing approach of the counselors was noted as important in the creation of campers' desire to change. Second, campers felt that the peer and group dynamics of the program were important vehicles for change. Third, time alone during the wilderness experience facilitated reflection on life. Last, campers noted the challenging aspect of the wilderness therapy as being beneficial.

Evaluation Efforts

Improvements in self-confidence, self-esteem, and social interactions have been demonstrated by previous research (Davis-Berman & Berman, 1989; Durkin, 1988; Hattie, Marsh, Neil, & Richards, 1997; McNamara, 2002). Additionally, a recent meta-analysis of programs designed for delinquent youth found lower recidivism rates for participants than control adolescents (Wilson & Lipsey, 2000). In this study, lengthier programs (> 10 weeks) showed smaller effects than those that were shorter in duration. The intensity of the wilderness activities and the inclusion of a distinct therapeutic component in the camp (regardless of therapy type) were found to be the most facilitative for positive change.

A noteworthy study examined 1-year outcomes for 277 participants in a wilderness therapy program for inpatient adolescents in Utah (Hoag, Burlingame, Parsons, & Hallows, 2003). Camp participants were found to have clinically significant changes in behavioral functioning following the intervention, and at 3, 6, and 12-month reassessments. Although the authors noted high attrition rates, this study exemplifies the rigor of research needed in demonstrating the therapeutic benefits of wilderness camping.

CAMPS FOR CHILDREN WITH BEHAVIORAL AND EMOTIONAL NEEDS

Definition

Camps for children with emotional and behavioral needs are often provided as a therapeutic intervention in conjunction with ongoing community mental health services. Like wilderness camps, the curriculum is designed to optimally challenge campers, providing opportunities for campers to practice appropriate behaviors with like-peers in a controlled setting. There are several noted advantages to providing psychological services in a camp setting: daily interaction with children, assessment in a realistic living situation, monitoring of responses to challenges, removal of the child or adolescent from a potential disturbing environment, and the presence of adult role models (Morse, 1947).

Therapeutic camps offer specialized treatment for children and adolescents with a myriad of behavioral and emotional problems including attention deficit problems, anxiety, depression, learning disabilities, and behavioral disorders. Some camps target specific diagnostic groups whereas others include children with diverse psychological difficulties.

The Camp Experience

Most camps occur in outdoor settings in a camping facility, although some programs can take place in community recreation centers, schools, or other community spaces. Camps for emotional and behaviorally challenged youth can last for a week or more as either day or overnight camps. The provision of therapeutic services is most often by a licensed social worker or psychologist, with volunteers providing increased supervision and support. Camps with low camper-to-counselor ratios have been found to be more successful (Wetzel, McNaboe, & McNaboe, 1995).

Typically, the entire camp participates in more traditional camping activities (e.g., swimming, campfires); smaller groups are formed for therapeutic exercises and group-building activities. The mental health providers generally formulate individualized treatment goals with weekly goal tracking for youth with more severe pathology. Some programs communicate progress on these goals to the referring community mental health centers and families for increased continuity of care (McCammon, 1983).

Camp goals vary widely depending on the needs of the camp population. For example, a 3-week camp for adolescents with learning disabilities and social difficulties was designed to increase camper self-confidence, decrease feelings of isolation, and increase social competencies through traditional camp activities and group therapy (Michalski, Mishna, Worthington, & Cummings, 2003). In another camp, a behavioral management and skills program was used to increase sportsmanship behaviors in children with attention deficit hyperactivity disorder (ADHD) at a basketball camp (Hupp & Reitman, 1999). In a third example, a "Bracelet Behavior Program" was successfully utilized to increase prosocial behaviors in homeless children during a day camp designed to enrich reading skills (Nabors, Hines, & Monnier, 2002).

Therapeutic camps also can be designed to foster resiliency in at-risk children. In a 6-week camp for inner-city youth, the goals included the prevention of risk-taking behaviors (e.g., drug and alcohol use, truancy) and increasing self-competency and hope (Brown & Roberts, 2002). Camp components included intensive training in dance and other artistic mediums, minority role models, on-site mental health professionals, and performance opportunities. Campers also participated in group therapy sessions on a variety of psychosocial issues related to their life experiences.

Evaluation Efforts

More extensive and systematic research on the impact of therapeutic camps for children with behavioral and emotional difficulties is needed. Most of the outcome data have addressed changes in self-esteem, self-competency, and social skills. For example, Michalski and colleagues (2003) used standardized instruments, camp-specific satisfaction measures, and parent interviews to assess the impact of a 3-week overnight camping program for children and adolescents with learning and behavioral problems. They found that participants reported improved self-esteem, high camp satisfaction, and were less socially isolated during camp. Parents reported that upon return to the home, children showed improvement in cooperation, responsibility, and self-control; however, the majority of the positive outcomes faded over time. Another study reported significant increases in hope, postcamp peer contact, and arts-related competency, although academics and school attendance were not found to be effected by the 6-week intervention (Brown & Roberts, 2002). Little is known about the stability of psychosocial changes attributed to camp interventions.

CAMPS FOR CHILDREN WITH CHRONIC ILLNESS

Definition

Children with pediatric illnesses have intensive medical regimens that often prohibit inclusion in traditional summer camp experiences (Klee, Greenleaf, & Watkins 1997). To meet that need, a number of pediatric organizations have developed summer programs to provide children with pediatric illnesses a "normal" summer experience while providing disease-specific care. As such, fun is a high priority for many camp facilitators and campers alike. Illness groups most cited in the camping literature are cancer, diabetes, and asthma, although camps for children with end-stage renal disease (Klee et al., 1997), sickle cell (Powars & Brown, 1990), epilepsy (Sawin, Lannon, & Austin, 2001), and hemophilia (Thomas & Gaslin, 2001) have also been organized. Camp staff often includes physicians, nurses, hospital social workers, pediatric psychologists, and dieticians. In addition, camp volunteers can consist of college, graduate students, or past campers. Reference items such as camper and counselor manuals are available to the prospective camp coordinator (Thomas & Gaslin, 2001).

The Camp Experience

Activities such as talent shows, survival hikes, dinner and dance with tuxedoed waiters, and water balloon fights have been documented (Warady, Carr, Hellerstein, & Alon, 1992). Ironically, camp activities for children with a chronic illness are often enhanced by what is *not* there. For example, children with renal disease plan a camp-out with the scheduled absence of dialyses. Doctors, nurses, and other medical staff often participate in the fun of camp so that campers (i.e., patients) feel more connected with the health care team. Activities such as role playing, quizzes, and debates can be used as alternative ways to teach disease-related information (Travis & Schreiner, 1984).

In addition to the primary goal of "having fun" (Sawin et al., 2001), time at camp can be used to address additional medical and psychological needs such as adjustment to the chronic illness, adherence, education and disease knowledge. In a review of 23 articles describing camps for children with asthma or diabetes, researchers found that an increase in adaptation to their illness was a primary target of most of these programs (Plante, Lobato, & Engel, 2001). Other prominent goals included increasing disease knowledge, improving self-care skills and adherence, providing parent respite, and creating opportunities for peer socialization (Klee et al., 1997). Decreasing anxiety and depression (Swenson, 1988) has also been cited as a goal with secondary goals of staff education (Swenson, 1988; Warady et al., 1992). Although the literature provides much anecdotal evidence to suggest some strides toward meeting one or more of the above goals, few studies have systematically evaluated these efforts (Punnett & Thurber, 1993).

For some illness groups, physiological measurements have been used to examine the camp goal of increased adherence and better disease management. Singh, Kable, Guerrero, Sullivan, and Elsas (2000) examined the effect of a 1-week educational intervention on metabolic control in adolescent girls with phenylketonuria (PKU). Camp interventions included diet and disease education, sessions on reproductive development, and therapeutic recreation. A pediatric psychologist and nutritionist conducted group sessions targeting disease attitudes and perceptions of PKU. Significant short-term effects were found on plasma pheylalanine (Phe) levels, knowledge of PKU, and attitudes toward their disease.

Evaluation Efforts

The literature in the area of therapeutic camping for pediatric illnesses is replete with quotes from children and families proclaiming the benefits of camp and concurring anecdotal accounts from medical staff (Hvizdala, Miale, & Barnard, 1978). Other studies have used nonstandardized forms to assess parent and child perceptions of camp or opinions regarding outcome (Smith, Gotlieb, Gurwitch, & Blotcky, 1987). Few studies have utilized standardized assessment tools. In short, participation in camps has been found to increase positive attitudes toward illness (Briery & Rabian, 1999; Sawin et al., 2001), improve postcamp social activities (Smith et al., 1987), decrease reports of depression (Warady et al., 1992), and decrease anxiety (Briery & Rabian, 1999). However, results on improvements in disease-related knowledge and skill have been inconclusive (Koontz, 2002; Wolanski, Sigman, & Polychronakos, 1996).

BEREAVEMENT CAMPS

Definition

Bereavement camps have been introduced to help children and their families cope with the death of a family member. A second aim is to help decrease the incidence of secondary behavioral problems including enuresis, headaches, peer problems, academic problems, depression, fear, sleep problems, sense of isolation, and somatic complaints (Walker, 1993). These therapeutic camps are relatively short in duration, usually lasting from 1 to 5 days. Simultaneous parent groups are also common. Most of these camps are provided by oncology groups and pediatric hospitals for families after the death of child to a terminal illness and are free to participating families. Camp staff often includes psychosocial coordinators, social workers, bereavement specialists, and child life specialists. Additional staff may include music and art therapists (Creed, Ruffin, & Ward, 2001).

The Camp Experience

Activities for bereavement camp target feelings of isolation, coping with grief-related anger, and the expression of remembering the lost loved one in a healthy way (Creed et al., 2001). To reduce feelings of isolation, campers are encouraged to interact with other bereaved youth through participation in games, rope course challenges, and storytelling activities. To help the campers process their grief, activities include the creation of memory items, such as scrapbooks or memory boxes. Other activities focus on helping the camper cope with intense feelings associated with grief. Grief counselors attempt to help children identify ways to celebrate the loved one's life (e.g., plant a tree) and learn strategies to defuse anger. Because grief camps often include children of all ages, it is important for activities to be planned based on developmental considerations. For example, to help younger campers express feelings, they create masks of their "inner feelings," whereas older students compose lyrics to a song. Most bereavement camps feature a family time, usually near the closing of camp. During this session, the family remembers the loved one by lighting candles, making memory boards, or reading poetry (Creed et al., 2001; Stokes, Wyer, & Crossley, 1997).

Evaluation Efforts

There has been a shortage of research on bereavement camps. Most of the reports include only results of satisfaction surveys of parents and children. Generally, parents have reported positive feelings toward the camp experience and noted increased communication about the death in their family and additional social support from other camp attendees (Creed et al., 2001). One study examined behavioral outcomes and found no differences in children after the camp experience (Stokes et al., 1997). The lack of research has been explained, in part, by the ethical considerations of conducting bereavement research (Stokes et al., 1997).

FUTURE RESEARCH DIRECTIONS

In each of the four subtypes of therapeutic camping, the majority of published works focused on camp descriptions and satisfaction surveys. Of those that provided results, few of the studies reported research methodology with the rigor necessary to make any conclusive comments about either process or outcome variables associated with therapeutic camping designs.

How have camping programs that have existed for decades escaped empirical evaluation? Given the long-standing nature of therapeutic camps and pervasiveness of positive anecdotal accounts, the scientific community may have the misconception that the efficacy of these programs has already been documented. In a meta-analysis of adventure-based camps for delinquent youths, 64% of the studies identified were unpublished dissertations or technical reports (Wilson & Lipsey, 2000). Why are these studies not published in peer-reviewed journals? Is it that editors feel it is "old news" or do the authors not feel motivated to submit for publication?

Ironically, the multidisciplinary team members that are the think tanks behind some of the camp interventions may interfere with the integrity of the research conducted. Team members (and funders) may have different views of "successful interventions." For example, one core goal for a Colorado-based asthma camp was "to avoid the professional temptation to use the ChampCamp activity as a research opportunity in a way that might even remotely detract from a child's camp experience" (Silvers et al., 1992, p. 122). Similarly, a published description of a Texas diabetes camp that has been in existence for 25 years noted "Thus, as long as the rules are followed and the investigative studies do not interfere with the overall primary goals of the camp, observational investigations seem to be warranted. Interventional research must be considered differently" (Travis & Schreiner, 1984, p. 14). If these sentiments are pervasive among therapeutic camp planners, then it may be difficult to gain the consensus and team support necessary to conduct a comprehensive program evaluation.

A related barrier to empirical research is the notion that if "it ain't broke, don't fix it." Typically, programs are evaluated when they fail. If, however, a program is apparently running smoothly and anecdotal notes from counselors, parents, and campers are positive, is it necessary to document this intervention in a methodological fashion? This justification for limited research is paired with the old adage that "idleness" or "undirected activity" is destructive (McNeil, 1957, p. 3); then it seems only logical that something (i.e., camp) is better than nothing.

For providers of therapeutic camping programs to prove they aren't "beating around the bush" (Winterdyk & Griffiths, 1984), researchers must (1) identify the problems most treatable in a camp mileu and how to maintain those treatment gains; (2) examine which camp components are core in producing change; (3) identify what youth are most likely to respond to specific camping interventions, including gender differences; (4) recognize and evaluate potential effects of homesickness (Thurber, 1999) on intervention efforts; and (5) document cost-effectiveness.

The efforts to provide therapeutic camping experiences to children and adolescents with emotional, behavioral, or physical needs are laudable. The logistics of planning, funding, and recruiting potential campers alone is a heroic endeavor. This same energy must be funneled into empirically validating those efforts.

REFERENCES

Bacon, S., & Kimball, R. (1989). The wilderness challenge model. In R. Lyman, Prentice-Dunn & Gabel (Eds.), *Residential and inpatient treatment of children and adolescence* (pp. 115–144). San Diego: Academic.

Behar, L., & Stephens, D. (1978). Wilderness camping: An evaluation of a residential treatment program for emotionally disturbed children. *American Journal of Orthopsychiatry, 48,* 644–653.

Briery, B. G., & Rabian, B. (1999). Psychosocial changes associated with participation in a pediatric summer camp. *Journal of Pediatric Psychology, 24,* 183–190.

Brown, K. J., & Roberts, M. C. (2002). *An evaluation of the Alvin Ailey Dance Camp, Kansas City Missouri.* Unpublished manuscript, University of Kansas.

Carver, R. (1996). Theory for practice: A framework for thinking about experiential education. *The Journal of Experiential Education, 19,* 8–13.

Creed, J., Ruffin J. E., & Ward, M. (2001). A weekend camp for bereaved siblings. *Cancer Practice, 9,* 176–182.

Davis-Berman, J., & Berman, D. S. (1989). The Wilderness Therapy Program: An empirical study of its effects with adolescents in an outpatient setting. *Journal of Contemporary Psychotherapy, 19,* 271–281.

Durkin, R. (1988). A competency-oriented summer camp and year-round program for troubled teenagers and their families. *Residential Treatment for Children and Youth, 6,* 63–85.

Ewert, A. W. (1989). *Outdoor adventure pursuits: Foundations, models, and theories.* Columbus, OH: Publishing Horizons.

Fletcher, T. B., & Hinkle, J. S. (2002). Adventure based counseling: An innovation in counseling. *Journal of Counseling & Development, 80,* 277–285.

Gass, M. A. (1993). Foundations of adventure therapy. In M. A. Gass (Ed.), *Adventure therapy: Therapeutic applications of adventure programming* (pp. 3–10). Dubuque, IA: Kendall Hunt.

Gillis, H. L., & Simpson, C. (1991). Project Choices: Adventure-based residential drug treatments for court-referred youth. *Journal of Addictions and Offender Counseling, 12,* 12–27.

Hattie, J., Marsh, H. W., Neil, J. T., & Richards, G. E. (1997). Adventure education and Outward Bound: Out-of-class experiences that make a lasting difference. *Review of Educational Research, 67,* 43–87.

Hoag, M. J., Burlingame, G. M., Parsons, P., & Hallows, G. (2003). The efficacy of wilderness therapy: Analysis of change using the Y-OQ. Unpublished manuscript.

Hupp, S. D., & Reitman, D. (1999). Improving sports skills and sportsmanship in children diagnosed with attention-deficit/hyperactivity disorder. *Child and Family Behavior Therapy, 21,* 35–51.

Hvizdala, E. V., Miale, T. D, & Barnard, P. J. (1978). A summer camp for children with cancer. *Medical and Pediatric Oncology, 4,* 71–75.

Kjol, R., & Weber, J. (1993). The 4th fire: Adventure-based counseling with juvenile sex offenders. In M. A. Gass (Ed.), *Adventure therapy: Therapeutic applications of adventure programming* (pp. 103–110). Dubuque, IA: Kendall Hunt.

Klee, K., Greenleaf, K., & Watkins, S. (1997). Summer camps for children and adolescents with kidney disease. *ANNA Journal, 24,* 57–61.

Koontz, A. D. (2002). A mission-based program evaluation and outcome study of a diabetes summer camp. *Dissertation Abstracts International, 62,* 4792.

Leemon, D., Schimelpfening, T., Gray, S., Tarter, S., & Williamson, J. (Eds.). (1998). *Adventure Program Risk Management Report: 1998 Edition.* Boulder, CO: The Association of Experiental Education.

Levitt, L. (1994). What is the therapeutic value of camping for emotionally disturbed girls? *Women and Therapy, 15,* 129–137.

McCammon, S. (1983). *Summer camp as therapeutic context: The Camp Logan Program.* Atlanta, GA: Southeastern Psychological Association Annual Meeting. (ERIC Document Reproduction Service No. ED244201)

McNamara, D. N. (2002). Adventure-based programming: Analysis of a therapeutic benefits with children of abuse and neglect. *Dissertation Abstracts International Section A: Humanities & Social Sciences, 62,* 2353.

McNeil, E. B. (1957). The background of therapeutic camping. *Journal of Social Issues, 13,* 3–14.

Michalski, J. H., Mishna, F., Worthington, C., & Cummings, R. (2003). A multi-method impact evaluation of a therapeutic summer camp program. *Child and Adolescent Social Work Journal, 20,* 53–76.

Moote, G. T., & Wodarski, J. S. (1997). The acquisition of life skills through adventure-based activities and programs: A review of the literature. *Adolescence, 32,* 143–167.

Morse, W. (1947). From the University of Michigan Fresh Air Camp: Some problems with therapeutic camping. *Nervous Child, 6,* 211–224.

Nabors, L., Hines, A., & Monnier, L. (2002). Evaluation of an incentive system at a summer camp for youth experiencing homelessness. *Journal of Prevention and Intervention in the Community, 24,* 17–31.

Plante, W. A., Lobato, D., & Engel, R. (2001). Review of group interventions for pediatric chronic conditions. *Journal of Pediatric Psychology, 26,* 435–453.

Powars, D. R., & Brown, M. (1990). Sickle cell disease. Summer camp. Experience of a 22-year community-supported program. *Clinical Pediatrics, 29,* 81–85.

Priest, S., & Gass, M. A. (1997). *Effective leadership in adventure programming.* Champaign, IL: Human Kinetics.

Punnett, A. F., & Thurber, S. (1993). Evaluation of the asthma camp experience for children. *Journal of Asthma, 30,* 195–198.

Russell, K. C., & Phillips-Miller, D. (2002). Perspective on the wilderness therapy process and its relation to outcome. *Child and Youth Care Forum, 31*, 415–437.

Sawin, K. J., Lannon, S. L., & Austin, J. K. (2001). Camp experiences and attitudes toward epilepsy: A pilot study. *Journal of Neuroscience Nursing, 33*, 57–64.

Silvers, W. S., Holbreich, M., Go, S., Morrison, M. R., Dennis, W., Marostica, T. et al. (1992). Champ Camp: The Colorado children's asthma camp experience. *Journal of Asthma, 29*, 121–135.

Singh, R. H., Kable, J. A., Guerrero, N. V., Sullivan, K. M., & Elsas, L. J. (2000). Impact of a camp experience on phenylalanine levels, knowledge, attitudes, and health beliefs relevant to nutrition management of phenylketonuria in adolescent girls. *Journal of the American Dietetic Association, 100*, 797–802.

Smith, K. E., Gotlieb, S., Gurwitch, R. H., & Blotcky, A. D. (1987). Impact of a summer camp experience on daily activity and family interactions among children with cancer. *Journal of Pediatric Psychology, 12*, 533–542.

Stokes, J., Wyer, S., & Crossley, D. (1997). The challenge of evaluating a child bereavement programme. *Palliative Medicine, 11*, 179–190.

Swenson, T. G. (1988). A dose of Camp Dost: Meeting the psychosocial needs of children with cancer. *Issues in Comprehensive Pediatric Nursing, 11*, 29–32

Thomas, D., & Gaslin, T. (2001). "Camping up" self-esteem in children with hemophilia. *Issues in Comprehensive Pediatric Nursing, 24*, 253–263.

Thurber, C. A. (1999). The phenomenology of homesickness in boys. *Journal of Abnormal Child Psychology, 27*, 125–139.

Travis, L. B., & Schreiner, B. (1984). Camps for children with diabetes: A philosophy and its application. *The Diabetes Educator, 10*, 13–20.

Tyler, J., Darville, R., & Stalnaker, K. (2001). Juvenile boot camps: A descriptive analysis of program diversity and effectiveness. *Social Science Journal, 38*, 445–460.

Walker, C. L. (1993). Sibling bereavement and grief responses. *Journal of Pediatric Nursing, 8*, 325–334.

Warady, B. A., Carr, B., Hellerstein, S., & Alon, U. (1992). Residential summer camp for children with end-stage renal disease. *Child Nephrology and Urology, 12*, 212–215.

Wetzel, M. C., McNaboe, C., & McNaboe, K. A. (1995). A mission based ecological evaluation of a summer camp for youth with developmental disabilities. *Evaluation and Program Planning, 18*, 37–46.

Wilson, S. J., & Lipsey, M. W. (2000). Wilderness challenge programs for delinquent youth: A meta-analysis of outcome evaluations. *Evaluation and Program Planning, 23*, 1–12.

Winterdyk, J. & Griffiths, C. (1984, Fall). Wilderness experience programs: Reforming delinquents or beating around the bush? *Juvenile & Family Court Journal*, 35–44.

Wolanski, R., Sigman, T., & Polychronakos, C. (1996). Assessment of blood glucose self-monitoring skills in a camp for diabetic children: The effects of individualized feedback counseling. *Patient Education and Counseling, 29*, 5–11.

21

Implementation of the Felix Consent Decree in Hawaii[†]

The Impact of Policy and Practice Development Efforts on Service Delivery

BRUCE F. CHORPITA and CHRISTINA DONKERVOET

Hawaii's unique environment combines geographic isolation with a richness of cultural and economic diversity. The state is a veritable mosaic of interests, ethnicities, cultures, communities, and values. According to the Hawaii's Vital Statistics 2001 Report (Hawaii Department of Health, 2002), 19.8% of general population is Caucasian, 21.3% are Hawaiian, 21.6% are Japanese, 15.7% are Filipino. A large group of Hawaii's residents identify themselves as being of other ethnic groups or mixed ethnicity (21.5%). There is a wide variance in community structure as well. Honolulu is one of the largest cities in the United States, with more than 1 million people in the greater metropolitan area. The city faces many of the challenges that plague other urban areas in the United States, including poverty, homelessness, substance abuse, and unemployment. Outside of Honolulu, Hawaii is primarily composed of isolated small towns and rural communities. These communities struggle with common challenges facing rural areas, such as poverty, unemployment, substance abuse, and scarcity of resources.

Hawaii also has an informed and critical attitude toward change. The anthropology and social science literature is replete with examples of

BRUCE F. CHORPITA • Department of Psychology, University of Hawaii at Manoa, Honolulu, Hawaii 96822.   **CHRISTINA DONKERVOET** • Child and Adolescent Mental Health Division, Hawaii Department of Health, Honolulu, Hawaii 96813.

[†]The authors wish to thank Eric Daleiden and Jacquelyn Trumbull for their assistance and organization of some of the data used in this chapter.

"progress" leading to negative social and cultural consequences for communities (e.g., Pelto, 1973), and Hawaii is no exception. Given Hawaii's history with colonialism and commercial development, there is a healthy skepticism regarding externally imposed initiatives or innovations. Business is generally conducted in a manner that prioritizes relationships and local trust. It is in this context that significant innovations and changes were to be introduced into Hawaii's education and mental health systems. These changes have subsequently impacted service delivery in ways that we are just now beginning to identify and document, and they appear to be significant.

THE FELIX CONSENT DECREE

In 1993, Hawaii's children's mental health system faced a class action lawsuit concerning inadequacies in the state's education system and the related mental health services provided to disabled children. In 1994, this suit was settled with all parties in agreement. The settlement, known as the Felix Consent Decree, identified that children and youth with educational disabilities who need mental health services to benefit from their public education must receive assessment and treatment services within a system of care. As part of the Felix Consent Decree, the state agreed to provide all necessary services for youth certified as eligible under the Individuals with Disabilities Education Act (IDEA) or under Section 504–Subpart D of the Vocational Rehabilitation Act of 1973 (as amended in 1974) to benefit from their free and appropriate public education. The state was mandated to establish a statewide system of care in accordance with the Child and Adolescent Service System Program (CASSP) principles (Stroul & Friedman, 1986). The CASSP principles emphasize such values as family strengths, youth participation in care, straightforward access to services, the use of least restrictive environments, continuity of care, and cultural sensitivity.

HAWAII'S EFFORTS TO COMPLY: THE STAGING OF COMPLIANCE

Nationally, the impact of class action lawsuits on broad systems change has been mixed (e.g., Weisz et al., 1990). Typical of some larger settlements is a rapid increase in funding allowing for infusion of new services, programs and expertise. However, little is known about the sustainability of these systems following the closure of the suit (cf. Rogers, 1995). In the initial stages of Hawaii's effort to comply with the Felix Consent Decree, much of the leadership was provided externally by the federally appointed court monitor, who assembled a group of technical assistants to aid him in carrying out his role. At that time, the state's child mental health system was primarily in a position of responding to external guidance.

Although the Felix Consent Decree was based on the federal education law (i.e., IDEA and Section 504), the leadership of the state's education
system was not significantly involved at that time. In the initial years following this lawsuit, much of the leadership came from the Court Monitor
and the Director of the Department of Health. One of unique characteristics of managing change in a lawsuit environment is the clarity of the
mandate for change. The consent decree externally imposed changes that
would be rare if not impossible in self-governing systems. Although such
external stimulus for change may initially carry more influence, it can also
be met with resistance and concern, particularly in the context of Hawaii's
community values outlined above.

The task, then, was to capitalize on the stimulus for change to achieve
genuine progress and innovation, while planning for and managing the
known risks associated with mandated change in social systems. This required a staging of change that balanced federal mandates, science-based
initiatives, the establishment of community and state partnerships and
trust, and carefully managed social and community influence strategies.
The four stages in the implementation of the consent decree are outlined
below.

STAGE I (1994–1995): PREPARING THE ENVIRONMENT FOR CHANGE

Following the court mandate, there was an immediate need for the
state leadership to provide information and define responsibilities. System
change is an inherently social process (Rogers, 1995), and this initial period
required trust and relationship building among families, providers, and
state agencies.

Research has shown that a variety of factors are associated with a
greater rate of change in systems (Rogers, 1995). Such factors include
amount of effort on the part of the change agent, compatibility of the change
with the system to be impacted, engagement of opinion leaders within the
system, integration with indigenous knowledge, and the observable relative advantage of the proposed change. In the first stage of change, most
of these strategies were deployed.

The court monitor took the lead in identifying community leaders and
critical stakeholders. A technical assistance council was appointed to establish community meetings and focus groups. Seventeen formal meetings
were held, which involved the introduction and review of the system-of-care
principles as a guiding framework for building a new education or mental
health infrastructure.

One of the best examples was the "reinvention" of the CASSP principles
outlined by Stroul and Friedman (1986) to be compatible with local needs
and values. The original CASSP principles, as outlined in *A System of Care
for Severely Emotionally Disturbed Children and Youth*, were modified to
reflect the language preferences of Hawaii's communities, but remained
true to the original principles. This important exercise not only yielded a

definitive framework for change, but the process drew in key figures from the communities to participate in the agenda for change. These local opinion leaders, whether families, educators, or community leaders, carry significant power to influence other members of systems to adopt new programs and strategies, far more than that carried by state administrators or even the federal court. Equally importantly, the development of the Hawaii CASSP principles ensured a respect for local knowledge and a compatibility with local values that would prove to be critical to the sustainability of the new mental health service infrastructure. It was these early stakeholder meetings that laid the foundation for the successful changes that were to follow.

STAGE II (1996–1998): BUILDING A SYSTEM OF CARE

Structure of the System

Given the priorities identified in Stage I, a system was organized to facilitate access to services, continuity of care, and support to families. This model involved the establishment of seven regional Family Guidance Centers (FGCs), staffed by care coordinators (cf. case managers, Evans & Armstrong, 2002), supervisors, and local administrators. These FGCs were the single point of access to services, which were authorized by the FGC care coordinators and provided by private agencies that were funded through state contracts. Each FGC was designed to be flexible and responsive to the needs of their community, and care coordinators worked to facilitate coordinated service plans that incorporated services and supports that matched the strengths and needs of each identified youth.

Research suggests that a systems-of-care design is associated with increased access to services, increased length of service, the use of less restrictive services, and increased family satisfaction (Bickman, 1996; Bickman et al., 1995). Comprehensive, formal data collection procedures had not yet been established in Phase II to determine whether the effects of system design were consistent with what would be suggested by the system of care literature. Nevertheless, some basic data on access to services were available: in the years from 1996 to 1998, the number of youth registered in the system went from 1,938 to 8,343, representing an increase of 330%.

Family Partnerships

At the same time, continued work was done to develop partnerships with families to enhance and sustain the new developments in the state system. The Child and Adolescent Mental Health Division (CAMHD) developed a relationship with Hawaii Families As Allies (HFAA), a statewide family organization, to coordinate with state leadership at all levels of system design, management, implementation, and evaluation. At each FGC, the state also employed a parent of a youth with mental health needs. These "Parent Partners" made outreach presentations and distributed printed materials at schools, public and private agencies, and community organizations. They also conducted workshops, provided technical assistance to families and professional services providers, and made outreach contacts with families and service providers. As noted above, this inclusion of parents as leaders in programmatic aspects of the system ensured a commitment to values that were critical to the success of system change and accelerated this change by increasing the credibility and openness of the change agent (Rogers, 1995).

In addition, HFAA staff participated in a state-led initiative to transition children and adolescent from residential and out-of-state placements to live in family and community settings, by helping families prepare for the return of their children and adolescents through one-on-one technical assistance and by administering follow-up. HFAA has also provided assistance in the development of a transition curriculum for training professional and family members.

Array of Services

The service array during Phase II included emergency or crisis services of mobile outreach, and crisis stabilization placements. These allowed for service providers to travel to a youth in an emergency situation and, if necessary, to secure a temporary safe residence for that youth. Outpatient services included mental health assessment, as well as individual, group, and family therapy. Other services included (1) day treatment programs, (2) therapeutic aides based in homes or classrooms, (3) intensive home- and community-based services, which allowed for the provision of psychological services to the youth in the home with no limit on the amount of hours, (4) therapeutic foster homes (Chamberlain & Reid, 1991, 1998), (5) group homes, which were therapeutic residential settings for up to four youth who attended school in their communities, (6) community residential programs, which accommodated multiple youth (up to the limits of licensing standards) and provided educational services within the residence, and (7) secure, hospital-based residential services. In addition, the state established flexible funding to support informal community services and programs. This continuity of services came directly from the structures outlined in the systems-of-care literature (e.g., Friedman, 1994), and most were not in place prior to the consent decree.

Consequences of the Innovation

The initiative to change the structure of the mental health delivery as a related service to education under the consent decree was both rapid and comprehensive. In this sense, the change was a success. As described above, the available data suggested that access to services had increased significantly, and at the end of 1999, the upward trend was continuing.

Nevertheless, as has been illustrated elsewhere in the literature on innovation (e.g., Rogers & Shoemaker, 1971), change is often achieved without a full awareness of its consequences. History is replete with examples of innovations whose consequences were ultimately harmful, and in Hawaii's history even more so. Given the controversial literature regarding systems of care and their effects on child functioning and symptoms (e.g., Bickman, 1996), it became clear that hard questions needed to be asked. At the same time, the presence of the courts made it clear that there was no turning back. Whatever problems arose with the system of care would have to be addressed with a second major initiative.

STAGE III (1999–2002): DIFFUSION OF EVIDENCED-BASED PRACTICE WHILE PRESERVING THE SYSTEM OF CARE

Early in calendar year 1999, it became clear that the cost was dramatically increasing with questionable results and outcomes for children and families. Approximately 4 years into implementation, costs were escalating rapidly, and yet the system did not appear to be fully meeting the needs of children and families. These findings were not entirely surprising, given evidence that systems of care are expensive and do not show increased benefits for child functioning (e.g., Bickman et al., 1995; Weisz, Han, & Valeri, 1997). This pattern of development is consistent more broadly with the literature on pro-innovation bias and unintended consequences of innovation (Rogers, 1995). Indeed, the implementation of the system of care was successful, but not surprisingly, costs were high, and there was no evidence that functional outcomes were improved. Further, there was limited evidence to suggest that Hawaii youth were being served at less restrictive levels of care. Expenditures climbed from $30.6 million in fiscal year 1995 to $81.5 million in 1999. In January 1999, 84 youth were still receiving services out of the state, suggesting that insufficient capacity had been developed in Hawaii, despite the massive infusion of funding. Just as the federal courts were the stimulus for change that catalyzed the development of the system of care, the state legislature, motivated by concerns about clinical outcomes and cost-effectiveness, provided the stimulus for the next big change to face the system.

The Empirical Basis to Services (EBS) Task Force

In October 1999, CAMHD executed a strategic leadership decision to evaluate the empirical basis for the services being provided within the system. In accordance with he principles outlined by the Surgeon General (U.S. Department of Health and Human Services, 1999) and the American Psychological Association (APA), this task force evaluated the relative effectiveness of treatments in children's mental health and developed strategies for how to apply these interventions within the system. The primary goal of the task force was to identify the most promising treatments using methodology similar to that used by national review committees (e.g., Lonigan, Elbert, & Bennett Johnson, 1998; Task Force on Promotion and

Dissemination of Psychological Procedures, 1995); the ultimate goal for the group was to change clinical child practice in Hawaii. This required establishing partnerships with administrators, families, and multiple mental health disciplines, and further meant that a scientific review of treatment literature and subsequent development of practice guidelines would need to be both practical and expedient. Participants in this review process included department of health administrators, parents of children with mental health needs, clinical service providers, and academicians from the areas of psychology, psychiatry, nursing, and social work. Clinical supervisors in the practice network were included from the outset, so as to keep the process from remaining purely theoretical and to help anticipate and minimize real-world obstacles related to implementation of empirically based services. These strategies were consistent with the literature on innovation, which suggests that the following strategies are important catalysts in the implementation process: (1) involvement of opinion leaders, (2) incorporation of multiple perspectives, and (3) adaptation or "reinvention" of the technology or practice (Rogers, 1995).

Along those lines, one of the first steps taken by the task force was to adapt the nationally sanctioned definition of efficacy to fit local needs. While the national guidelines proposed by APA, designated interventions as either "Well Established," or "Probably Efficacious" (see Chambless & Hollon, 1998; Task Force on Promotion and Dissemination of Psychological Procedures, 1995 for criteria), the EBS Task Force chose to establish five levels of empirical support. Because the APA criteria left entire parts of the Hawaii youth population (e.g., Autism) without recommendations for services, the EBS Task Force added a third level of evidence, representing a relaxation of the original Division 12 category of "Probably Efficacious." Another adaptation deemed important was to add levels representing "Not supported" and "Known Risks." Thus, all treatments could be placed within one of the five categories, with highest-ranking treatments to be considered first. Those treatments identified as possessing "Known Risks" would be eliminated from practice as quickly as possible or implemented with strong warnings about potential negative side effects (e.g., group treatment for externalizing disorders; Dishion, McCord, & Poulin, 1999).

A second "reinvention" of the practice definitions occurred through the coding and inclusion of contextual parameters into treatment decisions. Until that time, most existing reviews of treatments were largely based on the degree to which those treatments had worked in carefully controlled clinical research trials (e.g., Weisz, Donenberg, Han, & Weiss, 1995). A strong reaction from case managers, practitioners, and families was that such trials were not applicable to children in Hawaii, whose diversity in culture, background, and emotional needs far exceeded those represented in most clinical trials. Thus, it was the consensus of the EBS Task Force that the mere distribution of existing lists of such treatments to mental health providers and administrators would be insufficient to ensure that the most promising treatments would ultimately be delivered to children. An emphasis on evaluating the potential relevance or irrelevance of research findings was needed. The Hawaii EBS review therefore involved not

Evidence-Based Child and Adolescent Psychosocial Interventions. This tool has been developed to guide teams (inclusive of youth, family, educators and mental health practitioners) in developing appropriate plans using psychosocial interventions. Teams should use this information to prioritize promising options. For specific details about these interventions and their applications (e.g., age setting, gender) see the most recent Evidence-Based Services Committee Biennial Report (http://www.state.hi.us/doh/camhd/index.html).

Problem Area	Level 1—Best Support	Level 2—Good Support	Level 3—Moderate Support	Level 4—Minimal Support	Level 5—Known Risks
Anxious or avoidant behaviors	Cognitive behavior therapy (CBT); exposure; modeling	CBT with parents; group cognitive behavior therapy; CBT for child and parent; educational support	None	Eye movement desensitization and reprocessing (EMDR), play therapy, individual (supportive) therapy; group (supportive) therapy	None
Attention and hyperactivity behaviors	Behavior therapy	None	None	Biofeedback; play therapy, individual or group (supportive) therapy, social skills training; "parents are teacher," parent effectiveness training, self-control training	None
Autistic spectrum disorders	None	None	Applied behavior analysis; functional communication training; caregiver psychoeducation program	Auditory integration training; play therapy, individual or group (supportive) therapy	None
Bipolar disorder	None	Interpersonal and social rhythm therapy*	Family psychoeducational interventions*	All other psychosocial therapies	None
Depressive or withdrawn behaviors	CBT	CBT with parents; interpersonal therapy (manualized IPT-A); relaxation	None	Behavioral problem solving, family therapy, self-control training, self-modeling, and individual (supportive) therapy	None

	Parent and teacher training; parent child Interaction therapy	Anger coping therapy; assertiveness training; problem-solving skills training, rational emotive therapy, AC-SIT, PATHS, and FAST track programs	Social relations training; project achieve	Client-centered therapy, communication skills, goal setting, human relations therapy, relationship therapy, relaxation, stress inoculation, supportive attention.	Group therapy
Disruptive and oppositional behaviors					
Eating disorders	CBT* (bulimia only)	Family therapy (anorexia only)	None	Individual (supportive) therapy	Some group therapy
Juvenile sex offenders	None	None	Multisystemic therapy***	Individual or group (supportive) therapy	Group therapy***
Delinquency and willful misconduct behavior	None	Multisystemic therapy	Multidimensional treatment foster care, wrap-around foster care	Individual therapy, juvenile justice system	Group therapy
Schizophrenia	None	None	Behavioral family management*; family-based intervention*; personal therapy*; social interventions*	Supportive family management*; applied family management*	None
Substance use	CBT**	Behavior therapy; Purdue Brief Family Therapy	None	Individual or group (supportive) therapy, interactional therapy, family drug education, conjoint family therapy, strategic structural systems engagement	Group therapy

*Based on findings with adults only.
**Appropriate only if child is already in inpatient setting, otherwise consider Level 2.
***If delinquency and willful misconduct are present.

Figure 1. Evidence-Based Services Committee "Blue Menu."
Note: This matrix is updated quarterly, and the present example was issued on 7-03-03.

only the classification of treatments into their five different levels of efficacy, but also a cataloguing of as much information as possible about the context (e.g., level of therapist training, ethnicity of participants, duration of treatment, effect size). In a manner consistent with the work of the APA Task Force on Psychological Intervention Guidelines (1995), the EBS Task Force coded and catalogued all treatment studies for adherence rate, acceptability of interventions, gender, age and ethnicity of participants, effect size, cost, training of therapists, and similar variables. Treatments could therefore be selected based not only on their efficacy data, but also in the context of what was known about them and to whom and under what conditions they were applied. In August of 2000, the EBS Task Force published and disseminated its findings statewide, and a detailed version of the review itself was also disseminated nationally (Chorpita et al., 2002).

Blue Menu

Rogers (1995) points out that in research on innovation, the simplicity of initiatives or technologies is associated with more rapid diffusion into a system. Summarizing the complexity of the EBS findings was therefore an important challenge to ensure that the results of the review would not remain simply an academic exercise. To meet that goal, the results were simplified into a usable, single-page matrix of interventions and child problems, known locally as the "Blue Menu" (printed on blue paper), whose function is to summarize the efficacy review by the EBS Task Force (see Figure 1). Often in the context of training, the menu has been distributed statewide to all case managers in health centers and public schools as a tool to facilitate procurement of the most promising interventions. Supervisors and therapists have been provided with the menu as well to assist in the review and selection of techniques and interventions.

Research on diffusion often speaks of the "KAP" chain (knowledge, attitude, practice; see Rogers, 1995). This model, which originates in the cognitive and social psychology literatures, states that knowledge of an innovation precedes attitude change toward the innovation, which precedes change in practice (i.e., adoption or implementation of the innovation). The blue menu was itself an interesting indicator of one's position in the chain. Anecdotal evidence showed that those who possessed the blue menu had knowledge of the new practice initiative. Those who taped it to the wall above their desk had a positive attitude toward the initiative. Finally, those who taped one copy to their wall and kept a second copy in their briefcase or backpack to use for treatment planning had demonstrated true practice change. As the initiative to prioritize evidence-based services moved forward, the blue menu was both a strategic instrument and a barometer for change.

Training Initiative

Of course, it was important to move beyond mere knowledge of how to identify or select interventions. It was also necessary that CAMHD-contracted providers knew how to deliver those interventions. To that end, several individuals—all doctoral-level psychology staff—were hired to provide training and consultation in evidence-based approaches. One state position was dedicated to the full-time development of training curricula and provision of training workshops that featured the local adaptations of evidence-based approaches. Other positions offered clinical consultation available upon request for challenging cases. These positions were in part designed to reinforce or refine implementation of the most promising approaches. Not all training was developed internally. In fall of 1999, the state chose to implement one of the identified evidence-based approaches, Multisystemic Therapy (e.g., Henggeler, Melton, & Smith, 1992), by purchasing the training from the developer.

Hawaii's state-funded trainers and consultants were part of a larger network of trainers who more generally fostered and trained on the values of using evidence to make decisions. The logic of these decisions is outlined in Figure 2. Generally, the "evidence-based decision making" model prioritizes immediate local evidence as being of the highest order. Thus, if there are objective data showing clinical progress and lack of significant concerns, there is no need for further review. At this time, the state initiated quarterly administration of objective measures of symptoms and functioning (Achenbach System of Empirically Based Assessment; Achenbach & Rescorla, 2001; Child and Adolescent Functional Assessment Scale; Hodges & Wong, 1996) to meet these objectives. In the absence of documented progress, one needs to ask whether the intervention is appropriate, for which the blue menu is a potential tool, and if so, whether that intervention is being delivered with integrity. Consultants and regional clinical directors in the system often served the function of making such determinations.

Utilization Management

While the diffusion of evidence-based services was underway, further mechanisms were developed to capitalize on existing gains regarding the system of care. Rogers (1995) describes the "confirmation stage" of innovation as involving integration of the new practices into the usual work routine, such that they are no longer perceived as new. Thus, while carrying the evidence-based initiative forward, Stage III also focused on solidifying the infrastructure related to the system of care and its values. One of the most important activities in that regard was the functioning of the state's utilization management program. This body designed and distributed regular reports summarizing the patterns of service utilization. Because the literature on systems of care suggests that children should be served in more home-like environments and should have rapid access to care, such indicators as the number of hospital and mainland facility placements and the number of youth with unmet service needs were tracked. When goals were not met, interventions were crafted using FGC staff, trainers, and consultants to effect change. Such procedures included the implementation of concurrent authorization reviews for restrictive services and

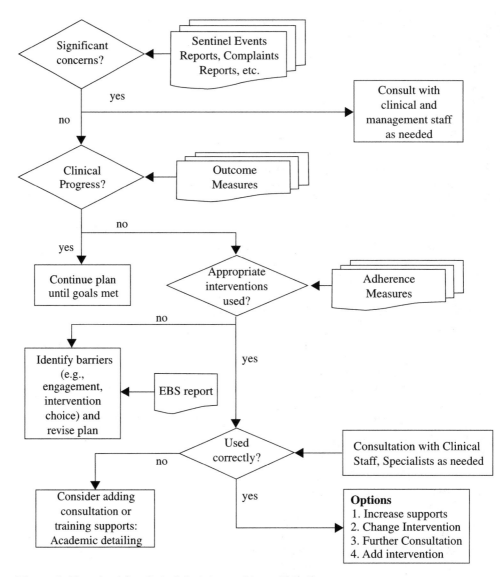

Figure 2. Flowchart for clinical decision making within the CAMHD.
Note: "EBS" = evidence-based services.

critical service planning for youth with unmet needs. From 2000 to 2002, the number of youth receiving services on the mainland dropped from 69 to 10, the number of youth hospitalized dropped from 47 to 15, and the number of youth with unmet or mismatched service needs for a period longer than 30 days dropped from 176 to 11. Most importantly, review of system performance against CASSP standards had become part of routine operations.

STAGE IV (2003–2004): QUALITY IMPROVEMENT
AND ADDRESSING "MANDATE DRIFT"

In July 2002, the Federal Court Monitor determined that the state had substantially met the requirement of the Felix Consent Decree, and in September 2002, the federal court determined that the state was in substantial compliance with the requirements of the Felix Consent Decree. The sustainability period was scheduled to end in December of 2003, after which the state would be evaluated to allow the federal court to determine whether to exit the consent decree or to extend the sustainability period further. At the time of writing, five youth received services out of state, eight received services in a hospital setting, eight youth were without appropriate services for greater than 30 days, and 64% of the youth served demonstrated improvements on objective outcome measures. These numbers represent a significant positive change. The Departments of Health and Education together continue to serve over 9,000 youth.

The system of care appears to be functioning as designed, with access to services roughly 4 times higher than at the outset, and the vast majority of youth (approximately 96% of youth served jointly by Departments of Health and Education) receiving services in home or in school. Meanwhile, the evidence-based practice initiative is itself moving into the confirmation phase (Rogers, 1995). This has meant a variety of new developments in incorporating evidence-based principles into everyday fiscal, clinical, and management operations. For example, the EBS Task Force has now become a standing committee of the CAMHD, and its operations are documented in both the Division's State Strategic Plan and its Quality Assurance Improvement Plan. Although there are significant advances in the awareness of and attitudes toward evidence-based approaches, only time will tell the full impact of these advances on practice and child outcomes.

Meanwhile, some of the developments in Stage IV have involved increased emphasis on system research and evaluation, performance measures, quality improvement, and improved measurement strategies for clinical practice (cf. Bickman & Noser, 1999). An example of the latter has involved the development and refinement of a clinical supervision module in the Child and Adolescent Mental Health Management Information System. This module allows for customized review of clinical progress on a variety of multiinformant, objective outcome measures (Daleiden & Chorpita, 2003). Scores can be examined for trends over time, or compared within and across caseloads to allow for improved clinical decision making in accord with the logic model outlined in Figure 1. In particular, the information module provides a wealth of current and historical data to address the question of whether a youth demonstrates clinical progress. The supervision module has been incorporated into ongoing supervision within the family guidance centers.

Another development just underway involves the detailed measurement of adherence to evidence-based approaches systemwide. A newly developed Provider Monthly Summary involves a monthly checklist of intervention targets (e.g., depressed mood, aggression, anxious avoidance) and clinical strategies (e.g., use of rewards, relaxation training, cognitive restructuring). These have been operationalized in a detailed codebook that allows the routine monitoring of intervention targets and content, and their completion is part of all Department of Health service contracts. This protocol allows for regular review of provider adherence to evidence-based approaches as identified by the EBS Committee. The hope is that such procedures may point to gaps in adherence to evidence-based approaches that will ultimately facilitate the development of new strategies for practice development in the provider network. In general, the most important aspects of Stage IV have been the efforts to build the evidence-based initiative into routine operations and to build internal capacity to test for the effects of nearly 10 years of innovation. This work is largely completed.

SUMMARY AND CONSIDERATIONS

The efforts to settle the Felix Consent Decree on the part of the CAMHD of Hawaii's Department of Health have essentially involved two major innovations. The first was to build a system of care to allow access to services and to define the values that would guide service delivery. The second initiative was to infuse that system with specific recommendations for clinical practice through attention to the evidence base. Each initiative was characterized by a powerful external stimulus for change. The system of care was propelled by concerns at the federal level; evidence-based practice was a response to the resulting concerns of the state. Both innovations involved significant amounts of consensus building, reinvention or adaptation of strategies, and formation of partnerships prior to implementation. Both innovations were followed by periods of confirmation, during which new practices were integrated into routine operations. Most importantly, both innovations took significant amounts of time. It was several years before the CASSP principles and values showed their full effect on practice in Hawaii, and the full impact of the EBS initiative in Hawaii still awaits further investigation.

One question that has been raised in the recent past as the system has developed is whether these two major initiatives in fact needed to be staged. The evidence-based initiative was a reaction to an unintended consequence of the system of care initiative; it was not a planned design feature from the outset. Given that those early consequences should not have been fully unexpected based on the literature, it is possible to imagine that a wiser choice would have been to build an evidence-based system of care all at once. It is an idea that challenges the imagination and possibly even the limits of systems to handle change, but it also makes for an excellent empirical question. Perhaps the next mandate to develop such a system—wherever that may be—will incorporate both sets of values and principles from the outset. It will be interesting to see what happens.

REFERENCES

Achenbach, T. M., & Rescorla, L. A. (2001). *Manual for ASEBA school-age forms & profiles*. Burlington, VT: University of Vermont, Research Center for Children, Youth, & Families.

Bickman L. (1996). A continuum of care: More is not always better. *American Psychologist, 51*, 689–701.

Bickman, L., Guthrie, P. R., Foster, E. M., Lambert, E. W., Summerfelt, W. T., Breda, C. S. et al. (1995). *Evaluating managed mental health services: The Fort Bragg experiment*. New York: Plenum.

Bickman, L., & Noser, K. (1999). Meeting the challenges in the delivery of child and adolescent mental health services in the next millennium: The continuous quality improvement approach. *Applied and Preventive Psychology, 8*, 247–255.

Chamberlain, P., & Reid, J. B. (1991). Using a specialized foster care community treatment model for children and adolescents leaving the state mental hospital. *Journal of Community Psychology, 19*, 266–276.

Chamberlain, P., & Reid, J. B. (1998). Comparison of two community alternatives to incarceration for chronic juvenile offenders. *Journal of Consulting and Clinical Psychology, 66*, 624–633.

Chambless, D. L., & Hollon, S. D. (1998). Defining empirically supported therapies. *Journal of Consulting and Clinical Psychology, 66*, 7–18.

Chorpita, B. F., Yim, L. M., Donkervoet, J. C., Arensdorf, A., Amundsen, M. J., McGee, C. et al. (2002). Toward large-scale implementation of empirically supported treatments for children: A review and observations by the Hawaii Empirical Basis to Services Task Force. *Clinical Psychology: Science and Practice, 9*, 165–190.

Daleiden, E. L., & Chorpita, B. F. (2003, March). The evaluation framework of the Hawaii child and adolescent system of care. In H. Ringeisen (Chair), *Integrating CASSP, evidence-based services, and evaluation in the Hawaii system of care*. Symposium conducted at the annual Research Conference of the Research and Training Center for Children's Mental Health, Tampa, FL.

Dishion, T. J., McCord, J. Poulin, F. (1999). When interventions harm: Peer groups and problem behavior. *American Psychologist, 9*, 755–764.

Evans, M. E. & Armstrong, M. I. (2002). What is case management? In B. J. Burns & K. Hoagwood (Eds.), *Community treatment for youth* (pp. 39–68). New York: Oxford University Press.

Friedman, R. M. (1994). Restructuring of systems to emphasize prevention and family support. *Journal of Clinical Child Psychology, 23*, 40–47.

Hawaii Department of Health. (2002). *Hawaii Health Survey 2001*. Honolulu, HI: Office of Health Status Monitoring, Hawaii Department of Health.

Henggeler, S. W., Melton, G. B., & Smith, L. A. (1992). Family preservation using Multisystemic Therapy: An effective alternative to incarcerating serious juvenile offenders. *Journal of Consulting and Clinical Psychology, 60*, 953–961.

Hodges, K., & Wong, M. M. (1996). Psychometric characteristics of a multidimensional measure to assess impairment: The Child and Adolescent Functional Assessment Scale. *Journal of Child and Family Studies, 5*, 445–467.

Lonigan, C. J., Elbert, J. C., & Bennett Johnson, S. (1998). Empirically supported psychosocial interventions for children: An overview. *Journal of Clinical Child Psychology, 27*, 138–145.

Pelto, P. J. (1973). *The snowmobile revolution: Technology and social change in the arctic*. Menlo Park, CA: Cummings.

Rogers, E. M. (1995). *Diffusion of innovations* (4th ed.). New York: The Free Press.

Rogers, E. M., & Shoemaker, F. F. (1971). *Communication of innovations: A cross-cultural approach* (2nd ed.). New York, Free Press.

Stroul, B. A., & Friedman, R. (1986). *A system of care for children and youth with severe emotional disturbances* (Revised ed.). Washington, DC: Georgetown University Child Development Center, CASSP Technical Assistance Center.

Task Force on Promotion and Dissemination of Psychological Procedures, Division of Clinical Psychology, American Psychological Association. (1995). Training in and dissemination of empirically-validated psychological treatments: Report and recommendations. *The Clinical Psychologist, 48,* 3–23.

Task Force on Psychological Intervention Guidelines, American Psychological Association. (1995). *Template for developing guidelines: Interventions for mental disorders and psychosocial aspects of physical disorders.* Washington, DC: American Psychological Association.

U.S. Department of Health and Human Services. (1999). *Mental health: A report of the Surgeon General.* Rockville, MD: U.S. Department of Health and Human Services, Substance Abuse and Mental Health Services Administration, Center for Mental Health Services, National Institutes of Health, National Institute of Mental Health.

Weisz, J. R., Donenberg, G. R., Han, S. S., & Weiss, B. (1995). Bridging the gap between laboratory and clinic in child and adolescent psychotherapy. *Journal of Consulting and Clinical Psychology, 63,* 688–701.

Weisz, J. R., Han, S. S., & Valeri, S. M. (1997). More of what? Issues raised by the Fort Bragg study. *American Psychologist, 52,* 541–545.

Weisz, J. R., Walter, B. R., Weiss, B., Fernandez, G. A. et al. (1990). Arrests among emotionally disturbed violent and assaultive individuals following minimal versus lengthy intervention through North Carolina's Willie M Program. *Journal of Consulting and Clinical Psychology, 58,* 720–728.

22

Children's Services in Disasters and Other Emergencies

GILBERT REYES, TRISHA T. MILLER, MERRITT D. SCHREIBER, and BETH TODD-BAZEMORE

The present chapter focuses on the psychological and social impact of disasters on children and the services targeting children's needs in post-disaster reconstruction. The relevant literature is reviewed to establish a reliable basis for predicting children's reactions to disasters, the approaches to coping and adaptation that children and families will most likely employ, and the types of mental health needs that are likely to emerge. Particular emphasis is placed on the importance of identifying children who are at heightened risk or are particularly vulnerable to the disruptions in development that can result from exposure to the acutely stressful aspects of mass casualty events. Because children's mental health needs can best be understood and served in the contexts of their communities and families, emphasis is placed upon the need to integrate psychosocial services into existing social structures and institutions. Moreover, since disaster-affected populations vary along dimensions of race, class, affluence, religion, and other demographic indices of social status, this chapter highlights the importance of culturally sensitive assessment of children's needs and contextually appropriate modes of intervention. The commonly available services offered to meet children's psychosocial needs are described and service gaps or other areas of inadequacy are identified. Finally, recent initiatives are described and recommendations

GILBERT REYES, TRISHA T. MILLER, and BETH TODD-BAZEMORE • Disaster Mental Health Institute, University of South Dakota, Vermillion, South Dakota 57069. MERRITT D. SCHREIBER • Terrorism and Disaster Branch, National Center for Child Traumatic Stress, David Geffen School of Medicine at UCLA, Los Angeles, California.

for further development of children's mental health services in disasters are proposed.

PSYCHOSOCIAL IMPACT OF DISASTERS ON CHILDREN

Until recently the psychosocial impact of disasters was often overlooked or underestimated, perhaps because the cost in lives and property was much more salient, immediate, and compelling. The recent shift toward incorporating disaster mental health services as part of the compassionate response to people affected by disasters, however, signifies a widening recognition of the emotional toll such events may exact and their potential for damaging long-term psychological adjustment. An extensive review of the disaster mental health literature reports that the most commonly expressed symptoms found among disaster survivors are those of posttraumatic stress disorder (PSTD), depression, anxiety, somatic complaints, substance abuse, and nonspecific distress (Norris et al., 2002).

Studies of children's reactions in the aftermath of natural disasters and intentional acts of mass violence reveal a more or less consistent set of findings. A thorough review (Vogel & Vernberg, 1993) described a wide range of reactions among children exposed to disasters, including common reactions of sleep problems, separation anxiety, increased dependency on parents, specific fears associated with stimulus characteristics of the disaster, and symptoms of posttraumatic stress. The authors also distinguished between these more common reactions and clinical levels of disturbance such as depression, anxiety, and diagnosable PTSD, which are frequently found and are associated with more severe levels of disaster exposure and more extensive loss and bereavement. The normal course of these symptoms is to rapidly decrease in concert with a decreasing level of threat, a rebound toward relatively normal routines, and an accommodation of any enduring negative consequences. Those children and adolescents who demonstrate long-term symptoms and deficits in functioning are likely to have experienced either an extreme degree of survival threat or to have incurred substantial losses with an enduring deleterious impact. In particular, preexisting or emergent deficits in family functioning have been identified as risk factors for delayed or problematic post-disaster adjustment (Green et al., 1991).

Several subsequent studies examining children's reactions to high-magnitude disasters have both supported and extended these findings. La Greca and her colleagues conducted a series of studies focusing on predictors of children's reactions and recovery in the wake of Hurricane Andrew (La Greca, Silverman, Vernberg, & Prinstein, 1996; Vernberg, La Greca, & Silverman, 1996). Comparisons of children's pre- and post-disaster characteristics revealed that children who exhibited higher anxiety, poorer academic performance, or were less attentive in school prior to the hurricane were more likely to report significant levels of posttraumatic stress symptoms in the month following the disaster (La Greca, Silverman, & Wasserstein, 1998). These findings not only support the need to provide psychosocial services to disaster-affected children, but also suggest risk factors that could be incorporated to screen for children at heightened risk.

Intentional acts of human violence convey a very different set of meanings than those that are likely to be inferred from acts of nature, and studies of disasters are often categorized in terms of whether they are intentional or unintentional in origin. A series of studies documenting children's psychosocial adaptation following the Oklahoma City Bombing (Pfefferbaum et al., 1999a, 1999b, 2000) provide remarkable insight. Significant posttraumatic stress symptoms were found among children and adolescents across a broad range of exposure levels and demographic variables. The authors noted that even children who were geographically distant and knew no one who was either killed or injured exhibited symptoms associated with posttraumatic stress. Several of these studies also suggest that intensive and persistent television coverage of the terrorist attack in Oklahoma City may help explain the emergence of PTS symptoms in adolescents who were not otherwise exposed to that tragic event (Pfefferbaum et al., 2001). This supports concerns that media coverage of high profile disasters may serve as a vector for disseminating psychosocial harm to children who might otherwise be relatively insulated from such events. As a result, it has become common for mental health experts and organizations to recommend that parents and schools monitor and limit children's exposure to media coverage of potentially traumatic events (Gurwitch, Silovsky, Schultz, Kees, & Burlingame, 2001; Hamblen, 2001).

Examinations of the long-term developmental impact of disasters have suggested that, while most symptoms have abated for most of the exposed children within the first few years, some children continue to exhibit symptoms far longer (Vogel & Vernberg, 1993). Among the most frequently detected long-term psychopathology is PTSD (e.g., Yule et al., 2000), which has been shown in some cases to persist for several years. Evidence from long-term follow-up studies conducted 17–33 years later (Green et al., 1994; Morgan, Scourfield, & Williams, 2003), suggests that most children affected by disasters rebound within the first 3 years and demonstrate remarkable resilience, but that some children will manifest enduring symptoms of posttraumatic stress persisting long into their adult lives.

DEVELOPMENTAL CONSIDERATIONS

The psychological reactions of children and adolescents to disasters and emergencies are known to differ depending on their stage of development (McDermott & Palmer, 2002). Some responses are more likely within particular age groups and it is important to note that children's reactions can also vary greatly within a given age group. Infants and toddlers lack words to describe stressful events or their feelings about their experiences, but may associate particular stimuli with an aversive event and react accordingly. Infants reacting to trauma may signal irritability by crying or wanting to be held and needing to be soothed by familiar caregivers.

Beginning with toddlers, children may enact elements or themes of the traumatic event in their play.

Younger children may not yet cognitively grasp the permanency of some losses and sometimes view destruction and even death as reversible (McConville, Boag, & Purohit, 1970). Children who have begun developing a sense of control over events may feel helpless and powerless when facing the chaotic nature of disasters. They may exhibit intense fears and insecurities related to their inability to protect themselves or others and to be protected by others. Beginning in middle childhood, children may increasingly compare themselves to others and wonder if what happens to them is either fair or normal. These children may especially seek reassurance of being normal or acceptable having experienced traumatic events or exhibiting unpleasant reactions.

Adolescent responses to disaster resemble adult reactions, but under sufficient stress youth may exhibit combinations of childlike and more mature reactions. Teenagers who equate surviving disasters with a sense of immortality may engage in risky behaviors (e.g., reckless driving, substance use, etc). For others the disaster may confirm that the world is dangerous and unpredictable, and they may feel overwhelmed by intense emotions and insecurity. Children of any age, but especially adolescents, may be reluctant to discuss these feelings with family members or other adults. If disaster mental health services are to be effective, developmental aspects of children's reactions, perceptions, needs, and capabilities must be given proper consideration.

FAMILY AND PARENTAL ASPECTS

Prominent among children's reactions to disaster are separation anxiety, developmental regression, and temporary elevation of dependency (Shelby & Tredinnick, 1995). Moreover, the impact of a disaster may include rendering normally reliable sources of support less available, and children may then be required to cope by moderating their stress until conditions improve. Following reunion with an emotionally available caregiver, most children will adapt in a resilient manner and exhibit few signs of residual distress. Considerable research on children's post-disaster adaptations indicates that parental and family functioning are among the strongest predictors of the child's resilience in the face of traumatic stress and chronic adversity (e.g., Scheeringa & Zeanah, 2001). To promote resilience, disaster mental health services provide support for parents and children to bolster family functioning, avoid stigmatization, and promote effective utilization of community and civic resources.

COMMUNITY AND CULTURAL ASPECTS

The psychosocial impact of disasters upon children is related to the broader effects on their communities (McFarlane & van der Kolk, 1996).

Children and their families share ties with adjacent systems, such as neighborhoods and schools, which also strongly influence children's immediate and developmental responses to crises and their utilization of available services (Clauss-Ehlers, 2003). Family and community finances, employment, religious affiliations, ethnicity, and other cultural connections may also affect the supportive resources available to a child. For instance, lower socioeconomic status has been consistently associated with greater post-disaster distress and the effect is strengthened as severity of exposure increases (Norris et al., 2002). Accurate assessment and response to the impact of disasters on children must account for the magnifying effects that poverty and other social disadvantages may have on children's reactions and upon their ability to access and benefit from interventions.

Cultural systems of meaning influence how disasters are interpreted, how reactions are expressed, and what is likely to be embraced as a healing response (Chemtob, 1996). For ethnic minority groups, cultural differences are sometimes accompanied by historical legacies of oppression, racism, and trauma. Racism affects the lives of many ethnic minority children, creating social environments afflicted by alienation, frustration, powerlessness, stress, and demoralization (Rivers & Morrow, 1995). These experiences can in turn serve as additional risk factors in dealing with the effects of a disaster. Similarly, a collective history of oppression and the legacy of traumatic events may result in a cumulative emotional and psychological wounding that seriously compromises resilience to subsequent disasters for ethnic minority children (Brave Heart, 2003). Aspects of the disaster and the response may aggravate preexisting wounds or intensify conflicts. Culturally responsive interventions that take these sociocultural issues into account may assess and serve children's needs more accurately and effectively. To be effective, service providers must confront the challenge of responding to disasters in a manner that is congruent with the cultural context of those they seek to help (deVries, 1996). Successful interventions may include efforts to strengthen extended family and community connections and encouraging the use of cultural knowledge that has sustained communities for generations (Dudley-Grant, Comas-Diaz, Todd-Bazemore, & Hueston, 2003).

PHASIC ASPECTS OF THE DISASTERS

Disasters are often described as unfolding in a series of phases, with each phase defined by its characteristic challenges and needs. Psychosocial services for children in disasters can therefore be understood to require a corresponding design that fits the particular phase of implementation. The earliest phase is the pre-disaster period during which preparedness is the major goal. Disaster mental health preparations mainly consist of educating, training, consulting, and strategic planning. The desired outcomes include reducing the psychosocial impact of potentially traumatic events, efficiently and effectively deploying mental health resources, and providing adequate care under severely limited conditions.

Once disaster strikes, the emergency phase unfolds. If preparations in the pre-disaster phase have been effective, the community response network has been sensitized to respect the emotional and psychological impact of the situation and is likely to be receptive and supportive of psychosocial activities. Mental health services for children are routed toward medical facilities, evacuation centers, and other places where people who are most acutely affected by the disaster are likely to congregate. The immediate goals will include triage to assess levels of exposure and other risk factors that predict the corresponding need for psychological support and deployment of providers who are well matched to the perceived needs.

By the third phase, the sense of immediate crisis has passed, most children will have been reunited with their caregivers, and for others substitute custodial arrangements have been made. Many children and families may still be living in shelters, with relatives or friends, or in other temporary housing, and some will still be hospitalized for their injuries. Disaster mental health professionals will be engaged in activities designed to serve the needs of both the majority of children and those who are at high risk or are already exhibiting signs of acute stress or trauma. Others will begin working with schools and other institutions to assess and serve the needs of children and adolescents across a wide variety of settings and neighborhoods. The higher-risk youth will be referred for more intensive and extensive services fitted to their particular needs and circumstances.

By the fourth phase, emotions are no longer as raw as before and most of the affected population have gradually recovered in a resilient fashion. For many others this will be a period of episodic growth and relapse, as anniversaries and developmental transitions stimulate a series of successive adaptations. An additional vulnerability to daily hassles and stressful life events may also emerge, rendering some survivors less able to tolerate and resolve their frustrations.

MODES OF SERVICE DELIVERY

Post-disaster psychosocial services include a flexible array of interventions delivered in a variety of forms. Interventions either directly or indirectly target children's needs and range from community-wide services for families to school-based crisis intervention services. Referrals to grief-focused and trauma-focused therapy are reserved for the most severely affected children and adolescents. The following descriptions of services are derived both from published sources and from recorded interviews conducted with representatives of several disaster relief organizations[1] who

---

[1]The organizations interviewed included the American Red Cross, Church of the Brethren, International Critical Incident Stress Foundation, National Association of School Psychologists, National Association of Social Workers, National Crime Victims Research and Treatment Center Salvation Army, and Southern Baptist Convention.

provided information on the services they normally provide to assist youth affected by disasters.

Public Education

Educational information is a common component of disaster service plans. These efforts can be divided into two parts: (1) pre-disaster preparedness and (2) post-disaster reactive education efforts. Preparedness education efforts are based on anticipating general aspects of disasters and bolstering the ability of those who might be affected to respond effectively. These efforts strive to equip the public with knowledge of various types of disasters or emergencies, the impact of various events on communities, what youth and their families can do before the event occurs to avoid complications at the time of the event, and what the normal reactions to such events usually are. Brochures, coloring books, and other reading material may also be created and distributed to children and caregivers explaining how to set up a family disaster plan, to locate the nearest emergency shelters, and other important information. These materials may be provided for children through schools to ensure that a maximum number of youth are reached. The secondary benefits of these methods may include providing children with a measure of control and self-efficacy if an analogous event should actually transpire.

Relief agencies and organizations have created materials for educating youth about disasters with the intention of fostering mastery and understanding. For instance, the Federal Emergency Management Agency (FEMA) has created a website[2] for children that offers activities, information, and free materials about disasters. The American Red Cross (ARC) has designed courses known as the *Masters of Disaster* curriculum to prepare children for various disasters through activities that are both fun and educational, with distinct sets of materials for youth in grades K-2, 3-5, and 6-8. No training is required to employ the curriculum and it is designed for use by families, schools, or other groups aiming to prepare children for disasters.

Reactive education efforts differ in that they are more specifically tailored to the distinctive aspects of the existing situation. The electronic media may be utilized to a larger extent for reactive education efforts due to their ability to rapidly and widely disseminate timely information. Messages most often include up-to-date information about the disaster itself, but may also address psychological reactions, adaptive coping strategies, more alarming symptoms that may indicate a need for services, and local locations and contact information for disaster response agencies and service providers. Humanitarian relief organizations, faith-based organizations, and many others use websites to communicate supportive information and recommended links assist people with finding useful information.

---

[2]http://www.fema.gov/kids/

Disaster Mental Health Services

The American Red Cross (ARC), a mainstay of disaster relief operations, mobilizes licensed mental health professionals as part of its Disaster Services response. These Disaster Mental Health Services (DMHS) volunteers are deployed to a variety of locations where a need for psychological support is anticipated, such as emergency shelters and distribution sites where ARC volunteers and large numbers of disaster victims can be expected to congregate under conditions of elevated stress. Children are plentiful in disasters relief facilities, often showing signs of agitation and fatigue after long hours without either sufficient sleep or nourishment. For parents seeking assistance, caring for children can be an additional burden of stress at a time when capacity is low and tempers are short. Under these conditions, DMHS volunteers can provide a supportive presence for beleaguered parents and can defuse tensions that might otherwise lead to anger, punishment, and even abusive discipline (Curtis, Miller, & Berry, 2000).

Crisis Intervention

Formal models of crisis intervention identify optimal goals and tasks to pursue in a logical sequence to assist adults with the reduction of arousal and confusion while facilitating effective coping strategies, marshaling of supportive resources, and collaborative problem solving (Roberts, 2000). Developmentally appropriate crisis intervention models for use with children are less established, tend to define crises more broadly and mostly emphasize intervention in systems that affect the child (e.g., school, family, social service agencies). Common elements, however, include ensuring safety, rapid deescalation of arousal, coping assistance, and enhancing parent–child relational functioning. This may include obtaining information about aspects of situational exposure, the child's appraisal of the situation and ensuing reactions, available social supports, cultural variables, extent of loss, and other critical aspects surrounding the event. The central goals include assessing the need for further services, making appropriate referrals, and following up at a planned interval to reevaluate the effectiveness of the procedure.

The follow-up step, which affords the opportunity to detect unanticipated changes in the child's needs, is one that is easily neglected as attention is shifted to more pressing issues. As a result, errors in the assessment and referral processes go undetected and corrections are less likely to be made. The resulting assessment can be a flawed or inadequate continuity of care. For example, researchers reviewing the mental health services provided to children after the Oklahoma City bombing suggested that the emphasis and reliance on crisis intervention was too brief in duration and too narrowly focused (Gurwitch, Sitterle, Young, & Pfefferbaum, 2002), and thus failed to adequately detect and respond to the different phases of psychological responses that the victims experienced over time.

Crisis intervention employs a wide array of methods, and several differently named techniques share similar characteristics. For this reason, psychological first aid, crisis hotlines, and debriefing are also described in this section.

Psychological First Aid

Psychological first aid describes the use of many common elements of crisis intervention, such as establishing rapport, providing protection and reassurance, mobilizing support, restoring connection with significant others, and following up. Pynoos and Nader (1988) offer developmentally sensitive guidelines for responding to children's reactions in a manner that helps to relieve immediate distress while scaffolding early assimilation of the experience. This approach has been widely embraced and has become an established element of crisis management plans in schools and other child-focused settings (Center for Mental Health in Schools at UCLA, 2000).

Toll-Free Crisis Hotlines

Following disasters and emergencies, children and their caregivers may have any number of questions or concerns, but feel reticent to seek professional help for a variety of reasons, not the least of which have to do with the ongoing strains of disaster itself. Expense, travel, embarrassment, and many other barriers to care can interfere with identifying and responding to children's mental health needs. To facilitate opportunities for children or their caregivers to speak with professionals about troubling events, toll-free crisis hotlines are often employed. The benefits of this tool include the ability to extend the reach of the disaster response far beyond the immediate geographical area in which the event occurred. Examples such as the Oklahoma City bombing and the September 11 attacks demonstrate the importance of reaching out to children from distant communities who are also feeling anxious and confused.

Psychological Debriefing

Debriefing methods have received widespread acceptance in recent years and are employed in almost every type of crisis with people of all ages and occupations. The most popular form, Critical Incident Stress Debriefing (CISD; Mitchell, & Everly, 1995), was originally developed for use with emergency responders but more recently has been applied to work with children of emergency responders as well as children directly affected by disasters and emergencies (Wraith, 2000). No controlled studies were found evaluating the use of CISD with children or adolescents, but empirical studies of the effectiveness of CISD and psychological debriefing in general have produced mixed results and fueled an ongoing controversy regarding its use (Rose, Bisson, & Wessely, 2002). Reviews of the debriefing literature (e.g., Litz, Gray, Bryant, & Adler, 2002) have generally discouraged the use of these methods, but debriefing techniques continue to be employed with children and adolescents across numerous crisis settings.

Caregiver Support

Support for caregivers is a crucial component of disaster mental health and is employed as an indirect means of providing psychosocial support to youth. Children are influenced by family models of emotional expression, grief, and coping strategies. Caregivers who have coping support may in turn provide better support to their children. Coping support can help the caregiver recognize the importance of balancing awareness and responsiveness to their own reactions and needs with those of their children. Moreover, caregivers who are averse to accepting assistance for themselves, may be more accepting of support if the purpose is to enhance their children's care (Speier, 2000). The modes of support for caregivers are diffused across most of the psychosocial services to adult disaster survivors with children, and often take the form of identifying and responding to caregiver concerns about their children. Caregivers in such instances are provided with informational support regarding children's reactions to traumatic events and advice on effective coping as well as referral information when that is applicable. One very tangible form of support for caregivers, a type of respite care, is described below.

Temporary Childcare

Disaster relief facilities typically contain crowds of people who must stand in long lines and encounter repeated frustrations as they seek emergency assistance for themselves and their children. In these situations, caregivers may feel overwhelmed by the challenges of meeting basic needs while also caring for children who are often tired, bored, and restless. The Church of the Brethren, for example, provides two child care programs for families affected by disasters. *Disaster Childcare* refers to a temporary facility set up by the Church of the Brethren volunteers in the immediate stages of a disaster or emergency situation, usually by request from another organization such as the ARC or FEMA. The second program, *Critical Response Childcare* (CRC), began as a specialized version of Disaster Childcare exclusively for implementation in aviation disasters, but has been extended to include terrorist attacks and other mass casualty disasters. Disaster Childcare and the CRC each serve children between 2 and 6 years of age, but younger and older children may be served if staff numbers permit. Background checks are required for all child care volunteers and a photo ID system is used to control who can remove children from the care center. The emergency child care center is typically set up in sections to give children the opportunity to participate in a variety of activities. For instance, it may include a quiet section where children can play with puppets, read, or do puzzles; a creative section allowing children to draw, paint, color, or sculpt; a physical activity section for jumping rope or playing ball; or a sensual section containing pillows, blankets, and stuffed animals. Although these temporary childcare centers do not directly serve in a "mental health" role, their assistance can reduce the potentially overwhelming strain on children and families during the early phases of disasters.

COMMUNITY OUTREACH

Responding to disasters at the community level has several advantages, not the least of which is that communities provide neighbors with a sense of connection and shared interests. Also, disaster relief efforts are temporary fixes and the affected communities will be working on the recovery effort long after the dust has settled and the outside resources have withdrawn. Perhaps most importantly, even devastated communities retain knowledge and other resources that are necessary, if not sufficient, in the endeavor to relieve suffering and facilitate resilient recovery. Children and their parents are likely to be more comfortable receiving psychological support from people who have already worked with the local youth and who are familiar with local values, customs, and institutions (Jackson & Cook, 1999). The most effective roles for mental health professionals from outside the affected community are often found in forming alliances with local leaders and helpers whose influence is vital in obtaining community acceptance and support for services that would otherwise be wasted.

GROUP INTERVENTIONS

To normalize children's reactions to a disaster or emergency, interventions are sometimes employed involving a classroom or other group of youths with shared or similar traumatic experiences. Dependent on the developmental context of youth in the group, various activities can be used in group settings. For younger children, the use of drawings, stories, coloring books, and other forms of play can be helpful in processing the event and reactions ensuing from it (Frederick, 1985). Together, classroom teachers and mental health professionals may facilitate disaster debriefing sessions for older students in which students are given the chance to process emotional reactions to the event (Pynoos, Goenjian, & Steinberg, 1998). These sessions can allow a chance for facilitators to address typical reactions, adaptive coping strategies, provide facts about the event, as well as allow students to address fears of similar future events. Depending on the extent of loss ensuing from a disaster or emergency, grief groups may also be utilized for children who have experienced the death of a significant other (e.g., parent, sibling). Stubenport, Donnelly, and Cohen (2001) offer a session-by-session outline of grief group therapy conducted with youth after an aviation disaster.

PROGRESSIVE INITIATIVES

Recent historical events have challenged the emergency mental health resources of the United States and raised questions about what changes might need to be made. The Institute of Medicine (IOM, 2003) recently produced a persuasive and influential monograph addressing the need for nationwide preparation for the psychological consequences of mass casualty terrorist attacks. That report addressed various gaps in knowledge, planning, preparedness, and policies, as well as in the infrastructure of the public health and mental health systems. Although the IOM report repeatedly addressed the impact that terrorism could be expected to have on children, it lacked substantial recommendations regarding services for children and adolescents. By comparison, the report from a consensus conference addressing the national level of preparedness of pediatric services for responding to disasters and terrorism more pointedly addressed children's mental health needs (Markenson & Redlener, 2003), and recommended that mental health concerns should be integral to preparations and services at every level. Clearly, there is evidence of an existing need to improve emergency systems of care for our children affected by disasters and other major public health emergencies. The goals, means, time frame, and funding, however, remain undefined. The following description of a federally funded nationwide network of trauma centers illustrates recent progress toward improving services for traumatized children.

Development of a National Child Traumatic Stress Network

In response to several high profile crises, a national initiative was undertaken in 2001 to develop a National Child Traumatic Stress Network (NCTSN). The ambitious mission of the NCTSN includes raising standards of care and improving access to services for traumatized children, their families and communities. The network, comprising over 50 centers from around the United States, is coordinated by the National Center for Child Traumatic Stress (NCCTS[3]), jointly located at UCLA and Duke University. Based on their primary functions, the network members are classified either as *Intervention Development and Evaluation Centers* or *Community Treatment and Service Centers*. Whereas the breadth of the NCTSN and its mission extend far beyond emergency and disaster relief services for children, this initiative has the potential to develop and test models of service delivery that could greatly improve the efficiency and effectiveness of existing services.

The terrorist attacks on September 11, 2001 amplified the need to revise existing disaster mental health service plans in light of the potential for mass casualty events that would exceed the magnitude of anything previously anticipated. The monumental challenges of marshaling and coordinating the deployment and allocation of children's mental health resources during a national emergency exceed the capacity of the existing paradigm. The NCTSN responded by establishing a Terrorism and Disaster Branch (TDB) specifically focusing on the unique effects of mass casualty events. In an effort to strengthen nationwide preparedness to respond to disasters and terrorism, The TDB developed a Rapid Response Support Team (RRST) to provide consultation to local, state, and federal agencies

[3]http://www.nctsnet.org

regarding preparedness, acute phase response, and long-term recovery strategies. Additional initiatives include developing a seamless model of triage, screening, and surveillance following mass casualty events that incorporates developmentally sensitive psychological first aid.

Given that most disaster response agencies focus primarily on preserving life, protecting property, and maintaining social order it is not surprising that children's psychosocial needs are seldom among the foremost considerations in planning and executing disaster relief operations. In this regard, the NCTSN represents a substantial step toward raising awareness of children's psychosocial needs across a spectrum of disasters and other potentially traumatic events.

Toward a National Public Health Model for Disaster Mental Health

The impact on children, families, schools and other child-serving agencies following a weapons of mass destruction (WMD) attack could include an unparalleled surge of demand upon the medical, public health, and mental health systems of the nation. But in such an event, the central public health priorities would almost certainly emphasize "physical" survival and might then consign mental health concerns to a category of post-crisis peripheral interventions reserved for the most distinctly disturbed survivors. Pynoos et al. (1998) have long advocated adopting a "public mental health" approach to the needs of children. A related suggestion is to enlist primary care physicians in detecting signs of mental health conditions related to disasters and trauma (Taubman-Ben-Ari, Rabinowitz, & Feldman, 2001). The benefits of such approaches to disaster mental health could include improving public awareness regarding traumatic stress and positive coping strategies, enhancing the integration of mental and physical health services, improving the probability of detecting otherwise obscure psychosocial needs, and decreasing the stigma attached to utilizing mental health services. Efforts to develop and test public mental health models for confronting the unique challenges of terrorism, WMD, and other mass casualty disasters have begun and the initial results appear to be promising (Pynoos, Schreiber, Steinberg, & Pfefferbaum, in press-a; Pynoos, Steinberg, Schreiber, & Brymer, in press-b).

Disaster Systems of Care

Without a systematic method of rapid triage and tracking, many children with acute mental health needs may not be located or linked with care until after clinical levels of distress and impairment have become entrenched. A study of children following the Northridge Earthquake revealed that many children with the worst event exposures were not identified until months or years later (Asarnow, Glynn, & Pynoos, 1999). Another study looking at children's mental health care in New York City following the World Trade Center disaster found that 27% of children with severe or very severe posttraumatic reactions only received mental health care 4–5 months later (Stuber et al., 2002). To improve these conditions, a model referred to as the "disaster systems of care" was developed (Schreiber, 2002). This approach creates an interactive linkage among numerous systems (e.g., medical, mental health, schools, etc.) that typically have contact with children in times of disaster but do not typically coordinate, communicate, or collaborate on their activities. A rapid triage system allows local communities to access a network of mental health resources through the National Incident Management System (NIMS). The strengths of this model (psySTART; Weedn et al., 2004) include a set of shared definitions of risk factors for use across its collaborative network, which can identify, triage, and route cases toward a provider who offers an appropriate type and level of care. The importance of such a system might be most salient during a high surge of pediatric cases that exceeds the capacity of local systems of care. The goal is to enable synchronized and integrated services for children across a continuum of mental health-related services and providers. This system may decrease the problem of gaps in traditional service delivery and referral systems in a manner similar to existing medical tracking systems, but with the added advantages of a triage component and multisystemic integration.

CONCLUSIONS AND RECOMMENDATIONS

Substantial research evidence exists to support the need to provide mental health services for children affected by disasters and other emergency situations. Whereas many of these children will have received adequate support through family and other systems, some are likely to require supportive interventions that foster resilient adaptations. The major goals of disaster mental health interventions include reducing exposure to stressful circumstances, providing information about psychological reactions, promoting effective coping strategies, detecting problematic reactions, and connecting children and adolescents with long-term mental health needs with local resources and providers. Disaster mental health services are mostly designed to reduce short-term stress for the affected population and are often not targeted specifically for children or for those with the greatest needs.

This approach is reasonably congruent with a community-focused, public health model of service and does not emphasize diagnostic assessment or clinical interventions. Instead, public education and crisis intervention techniques are preferred and more severe needs are handled mostly by referral. Services are almost always provided in nonclinical community settings and schools are often preferred for their superior potential to gain access and acceptance from children, adolescents, and caregivers. The targets of services are sometimes indirectly helpful to children; for example, supportive services for caregivers, child care services at relief facilities, and educational consultations with schools and other institutions to improve their responsiveness to children's psychosocial needs.

A challenge that is particularly salient in disasters is that of providing culturally sensitive and effective assistance. The impact range of a major disaster is likely to cut across a variety of distinct and subtle civic, community, neighborhood, and economic zones containing a great deal of cultural and ethnic diversity. Providers who travel to the affected region are likely to encounter values, beliefs, customs, and expectations that differ from those with which they are familiar and comfortable. Even providers living nearby may discover that there are local cultural differences that become much more salient in the context of a disaster relief operation. Therefore, it is important to collaborate with culturally competent local providers when adapting "general" models of mental health services to match the needs and preferences of the community being served.

Schools are often among the public systems that are most affected by disasters. Not only do disasters directly strike in school-related settings, but the impact of disasters affecting children anywhere in the community is likely to be felt and processed at school. Because schools provide locations where children can most conveniently receive a variety of services, the disaster mental health response also relies heavily upon schools as a means of reaching children and families. In response, schools have begun to develop disaster plans that include mental health concerns and strategies for detecting and responding to children's psychosocial needs. Thus, psychologists and counselors in K-12 grades have become a major national mental health resource, not only in times of crises, but on a daily basis as well. Therefore, a fuller integration and collaboration between the educational and mental health systems at all stages (e.g., preparatory planning, policy development, implementation of services, follow-up and evaluation) are recommended to improve children's mental health services in emergencies.

The recent history of increasingly lethal and destructive events coupled with fears of terrorist attacks involving weapons of mass destruction have led to questions regarding the adequacy of the present paradigm of disaster mental health response. New initiatives have begun to improve the availability and coordination of trauma services, both in conventional disasters and in mass casualty events of the highest magnitude. These models and projects are laudable and promising, but they are not intended and will not serve as a panacea for gaps in the existing capacity of mental health resources for children and families. The existing mental health infrastructure is the foundation upon which an emergency mental health response is built. Weaknesses in that foundation can be temporarily buttressed by a massive influx of resources, but the inevitable withdrawal of these assets usually means that the preexisting mental health resource base must deliver more services without a corresponding increase in capacity. Moreover, it is widely recognized that children who are symptomatic following a disaster often had preexisting mental health needs that may not have been adequately served. Thus, whereas improvements in services directed at the needs of traumatized children are helpful, what must also be considered is a meaningful improvement in the existing capacity to serve the mental health needs of children and adolescents both before and after disasters.

REFERENCES

Asarnow, J., Glynn, S., & Pynoos R. S. (1999). When the earth stops shaking: Earthquake sequelae among children diagnosed for pre-earthquake psychopathology. *Journal of the American Academy of Child and Adolescent Psychiatry, 38*, 1016–1023.

Brave Heart, M. Y. H. (2003). The historical trauma response among Natives and its relationship with substance abuse: A Lakota illustration. *Journal of Psychoactive Drugs, 35*, 7–13.

Center for Mental Health in Schools at UCLA. (2000). *A resource aid packet on responding to a crisis at a school.* Los Angeles: Author.

Chemtob, C. M. (1996). Posttraumatic stress disorder, trauma, & culture. *International Review of Psychiatry, 2*, 257–292.

Clauss-Ehlers, C. C. C. (2003). Promoting ecologic health resilience for minority youth: Enhancing health care access through the school health center. *Psychology in the Schools, 40*, 265–278.

Curtis, T., Miller, B. C., & Berry, E. H. (2000). Changes in reports and incidence of child abuse following natural disasters. *Child Abuse & Neglect, 24*, 1151–1162.

deVries, M. W. (1996). Trauma in cultural perspective. In van der Kolk, B. A., McFarlane, A. C., & Weisaeth, L. (Eds.), *Traumatic stress* (pp. 398–413). New York: Guilford.

Dudley-Grant, G. R., Comas-Diaz, L., Todd-Bazemore, B., & Hueston, J. D. (2003). Fostering resilience: A fact sheet for psychologists working with people of color. In the *Fostering Resilience* series of the APA Task Force on Resilience in Response to Terrorism, R. Levant & L. Barbanel, co-chairs. Washington, DC: American Psychological Association.

Frederick, C. (1985). Children traumatized by catastrophic events. In S. Eth & R. S. Pynoos (Eds.), *Post-traumatic stress disorder in children* (pp. 71–100). Washington, DC: American Psychiatric Press.

Green, B., Grace, M., Vary, M., Kramer, T., Gleser, G., & Leonard, A. (1994). Children of disaster in the second decade: A 17-year follow-up of Buffalo Creek survivors. *Journal of the American Academy of Child and Adolescent Psychiatry, 33*, 71–79.

Green, B. L., Korol, M., Grace, M. C., Vary, M., Leonard, A., Gleser, G. et al. (1991). Children and disaster: Age gender and parental effects on PTSD symptoms. *Journal of the American Academy of Child and Adolescent Psychiatry, 30*, 945–951.

Gurwitch, R. H., Silovsky, J. F., Schultz, S., Kees, M., & Burlingame, S. (2001). *Reactions and guidelines for children following trauma/disaster.* Retrieved May 17, 2004, from http://www.apa.org/practice/ptguidelines.html

Gurwitch, R. H., Sitterle, K. S., Young, B. H., & Pfefferbaum, B. (2002). The aftermath of terrorism. In A. M. La Greca, W. K. Silverman, E. M. Vernberg, & M. C. Roberts (Eds.), *Helping children cope with disasters and terrorism* (pp. 327–357). Washington, DC: American Psychological Association.

Hamblen, J. (2001). How the community may be affected by media coverage of the terrorist attack: A National Center for PTSD fact sheet. Retrieved May 17, 2004, from http://www.ncptsd.org/facts/disasters/fs_media_disaster.html

Institute of Medicine (IOM). (2003). Butler, A. S., Panzer, A. M., & Goldfrank, L. R. (Eds.), *Preparing for the psychological consequences of terrorism: A public health strategy.* Washington, DC: National Academies Press.

Jackson, G., & Cook, C.G. (1999). *Disaster mental health: Crisis counseling programs for the rural community* (DHHS Publication No. SMA 99-3378). Washington, DC: Government Printing Office.

La Greca, A. M., Silverman, W. S., Vernberg, E. M., & Prinstein, M. J. (1996). Posttraumatic stress symptoms in children after Hurricane Andrew: A prospective study. *Journal of Consulting and Clinical Psychology, 64*, 712–723.

La Greca, A. M., Silverman, W. K., & Wasserstein, S. B. (1998). Children's predisaster functioning as a predictor of posttraumatic stress following Hurricane Andrew. *Journal of Consulting and Clinical Psychology, 66*, 883–892.

Litz, B., Gray, M., Bryant, R., & Adler, A. (2002). Early interventions for trauma: Current status and future directions. *Clinical Psychology: Science and Practice, 9*, 112–134.

Markenson, D., & Redlener, I. (2003). *Pediatric preparedness for disasters and terrorism: A national consensus conference: Executive summary.* Retrieved May 20, 2004, from www.childrenshealthfund.org/CHF2286VFinal_adj.2.pdf

McConville, B. J., Boag, L. C., & Purohit, A. P. (1970). Mourning processes in children of varying ages. *Canadian Psychiatric Association Journal, 15,* 253–255.

McDermott, B. M., & Palmer, L. J. (2002). Postdisaster emotional distress, depression, and event-related variables: Findings across child and adolescent developmental stages. *Australian and New Zealand Journal of Psychiatry, 36,* 754–761

McFarlane, A. C., & van der Kolk, B. A. (1996). Trauma and its challenge to society. In B. A. van der Kolk, A. C. McFarlane, & L. Weisaeth (Eds.), *Traumatic stress* (pp. 24–46). New York: Guilford.

Mitchell, J. T., & Everly, G. S., Jr. (1995). *Critical incident stress debriefing: An operations manual for the prevention of traumatic stress among emergency and disaster workers* (2nd ed.). Ellicott City, MD: Chevron.

Morgan, L., Scourfield, J., & Williams, D. (2003). The Aberfan disaster: 33-year follow-up of survivors. *British Journal of Psychiatry, 182,* 532–536.

Norris, F. H., Friedman, M. J., Watson, P. J., Byrne, C. M., Diaz, E., & Kaniasty, K. (2002). 60,000 disaster victims speak: Part I: An empirical review of the empirical literature, 1981–2001. *Psychiatry: Interpersonal and Biological Processes, 65,* 207–239.

Pfefferbaum, B., Nixon, S. J., Krug, R. S., Tivis, R. D., Moore, V. L., Brown, J. M. et al. (1999a). Clinical needs assessment of middle and high school students following the 1995 Oklahoma City bombing. *American Journal of Psychiatry, 156,* 1069–1074.

Pfefferbaum, B., Nixon, S. J., Tivis, R. D., Doughty, D. E., Pynoos, R. S., Gurwitch, R. H. et al. (2001). Television exposure in children after a terrorist incident. *Psychiatry, 64,* 202–211.

Pfefferbaum, B., Nixon, S. J., Tucker, P. M., Tivis, R. D., Moore, V. L., Gurwitch, R. H. et al. (1999b). Posttraumatic stress responses in bereaved children after the Oklahoma City bombing. *Journal of the American Academy of Child and Adolescent Psychiatry, 38,* 1372–1379.

Pfefferbaum, B., Seale, T. W., McDonald, N. B., Brandt, E. N., Jr., Rainwater, S. M., Maynard, B. T. et al. (2000). Posttraumatic stress two years after the Oklahoma City bombing in youths geographically distant from the explosion. *Psychiatry, 63,* 358–370.

Pynoos, R. S., Goenjian, A. K., & Steinburg, A. M. (1998). A public mental health approach to the postdisaster treatment of children and adolescents. *Child and Adolescent Psychiatric Clinics of North America, 7,* 195–210.

Pynoos, R. S., & Nader, K. (1988). Psychological first aid and treatment approach to children exposed to community violence: Research implications. *Journal of Traumatic Stress, 1,* 445–473.

Pynoos, R. S., Schreiber, M. D., Steinberg, A. M., & Pfefferbaum, B. (in press-a). Children and terrorism. In B. Saddock & S. Saddock (Eds.), *Comprehensive textbook of psychiatry* (5th ed.). New York: Williams and Witkins.

Pynoos, R. S., Steinberg, A. M., Schreiber, M. D., & Brymer, M. J. (in press-b). Children and families: A new framework for preparedness and response to danger, terrorism, and trauma. In L. A. Schein, H. I. Spitz, G. M. Burlingame, & P. R. Mushkin (Eds.), *Group approaches for the psychological effects of terrorist disasters.* New York: Haworth.

Rivers, R. Y., & Morrow, C. A. (1995). Understanding and treating ethnic minority children. In J. F. Aponte & R. Y. Rivers (Eds.), *Psychological interventions and cultural diversity* (pp. 164–180). Needham Heights, MA: Allyn & Bacon.

Roberts, A. R. (2000). An overview of crisis theory and crisis intervention. In A. R. Roberts (Ed.), *Crisis intervention handbook: Assessment, treatment, and research* (2nd ed., pp. 3–30). New York: Oxford University Press.

Rose, S., Bisson, J., & Wessely, S. (2002). Psychological debriefing for preventing post traumatic stress disorder (PTSD) (Cochrane review). In: *The Cochrane library* (p. 3). Oxford: Update Software.

Scheeringa, M. S., & Zeanah, C. H. (2001). A relational perspective on PTSD in early childhood. *Journal of Traumatic Stress, 14,* 799–815.

Schreiber, M. D. (2002). *Children's emergencies in weapons of mass destruction and terrorism: Disaster system of care, rapid triage, and consequence management*. Presented at the 16th Annual California Injury Prevention Conference, Sacramento, CA.

Shelby, J. S., & Tredinnick, M. G. (1995). Crisis intervention with survivors of natural disaster: Lessons from Hurricane Andrew. *Journal of Counseling and Development, 73*, 491–497.

Speier, A. H. (2000). *Psychosocial issues for children and adolescents in disasters* (DHHS Publication No. ADM86-1070R). Washington, DC: Government Printing Office.

Stubenport, K., Donnelly, G. R., & Cohen, J. A. (2001). Cognitive-behavioral group therapy for bereaved adults and children following an air disaster. *Group Dynamics: Theory, Research, and Practice, 5*, 261–276.

Stuber, J., Fairbrother, G., Galea, S., Pfefferbaum, B., Wilson-Genderson, M., & Vlahov, D. (2002). Determinants of counseling for children in Manhattan after the September 11 attacks. *Psychiatric Services, 3*, 815–822.

Taubman-Ben-Ari, O., Rabinowitz, J., & Feldman, D. (2001). Post-traumatic stress disorder in primary-care settings: Prevalence and physicians' detection. *Psychological Medicine, 31*, 555–560.

Vernberg, E. M., La Greca, A. M., & Silverman, W. K. (1996). Prediction of posttraumatic stress symptoms in children after Hurricane Andrew. *Journal of Abnormal Psychology, 105*, 237–248.

Vogel, J. M., & Vernberg, E. M. (1993). Task force report part I: Children's psychological responses to disasters. *Journal of Clinical Child Psychology, 22*, 464–484.

Weedn, V. W., McDonald, M. D., Locke, S. E., Schreiber, M., Friedman, R. H., Newell, R. G. et al. (2004). Managing the community response to bioterrorist threats: Crisis health risk self-assessment tools to triage the patient surge. *Engineering In Medicine and Biology Magazine, 23*, 162–170.

Wraith, R. (2000). Children and debriefing: Theory, interventions, and outcomes. In B. Raphael & J. P. Wilson (Eds.), *Psychological debriefing: Theory, practice, and evidence* (pp. 195–212). New York: Cambridge University Press.

Yule, W., Bolton, D., Udwin, O., Boyle, S., O'Ryan, D., & Nurrish, J. (2000). The long-term psychological effects of a disaster experienced in adolescence. I: The incidence and course of PTSD. *Journal of Child Psychology and Psychiatry, 41*, 503–511.

23

Program Evaluation Approaches to Service Delivery in Child and Family Mental Health[†]

MICHAEL C. ROBERTS and RIC G. STEELE

Mental health services for children have existed in a variety of forms and organizational frameworks for many years. Unfortunately, decisions to start, maintain, or discontinue a mental health service program all too frequently have been based on ideological, political, philosophical, and financial considerations and a bit too infrequently on empirical evidence of what works or does not. Additionally, when evaluation of programmatic efforts in mental health services has been made, it is often not integrated with clinical applications. As a result, many programs in child and family mental health have been implemented with either no plan to evaluate from the outset or the evaluation is considered an added-on, unimportant, and interfering component. Accordingly, programs are not evaluated or are evaluated in a haphazard manner. The current era of increased accountability may lead to more evaluation of mental health programs and interventions; however, the need to know what works, for whom, and under what circumstances has been evident for many decades (Roberts, Vernberg, & Jackson, 2002; Steele & Roberts, 2003). In sum, if something is considered worth doing with expenditures of effort, time, and money, it is worth evaluating whether the outcomes justified the expenditures.

MICHAEL C. ROBERTS and RIC G. STEELE • Clinical Child Psychology Program, University of Kansas, Lawrence, Kansas 66045.

[†]The first author was supported by a grant from the U.S. Department of Education (R305T010147) during the preparation of this chapter. The views expressed are those of the authors.

In their outline of strong programs in child and family mental health, Roberts and Hinton-Nelson (1996) noted that such programs respond to a need for accountability and provide documentation of effectiveness:

> Program developers recognize the need to know whether or not their programs are doing any good, for whom services were effective, and what sorts of changes might be made to improve acceptance and efficacy of services. All too often, what might be excellent programs lose credibility and funding because they are unable to document success. Service delivery should be able to monitor their effectiveness in serving the needs of their target populations and their progress toward meeting their own organizational goals (p. 13).

Similarly, Harinck, Smit, and Knorth (1997) noted that program evaluation systematically examines the function of program activities as well as "the manner in which these are carried out and how they are geared to each other (process evaluation). In other cases, it concerns the results or outcome of the program (product evaluation)" (p. 370). Harinck et al. emphasized the feedback function of program evaluation, identifying six specific goals: (a) to clarify the identity of a program; (b) to adjust or improve the program components; (c) to check that services meet quality standards; (d) to increase rationality and organization in the system of service delivery; (e) to transfer or initiate interventions; and (f) to provide information to the funding source and in determining decisions about the program.

Program evaluation as an empirical research approach has developed into its own field of identity in recent years (Chelimsky & Shadish, 1997; Shadish, Cook, & Leviton, 1991) as distinguished from other activities designed to determine the more precise effects associated with psychotherapy research (e.g., the movement toward empirically supported or evidence-based practice).[1] Although there is a possibility of considerable overlap between the two, the goal of psychotherapy outcome research is to validate or disconfirm a specific psychotherapy technique or intervention, whereas program evaluation is designed to provide information regarding how and how well services are being delivered.

To distinguish these different research purposes, the Clinical Treatment and Services Research Workgroup of the National Institute of Mental Health (1998) categorized four domains of treatment or interventions research: (1) efficacy, (2) effectiveness, (3) practice, and (4) service system research (as an iterative continuum; Street, Niederehe, & Lebowitz, 2000). Efficacy and effectiveness research are intended to examine well-specified interventions with specific disorders or populations in a lab-based clinic (for efficacy research) or moving to a broader population and more naturalistic clinical service setting (for effectiveness research), although methodological rigor and careful controls remain strong. Practice research

---

[1]Harinck, Smit, and Knorth (1997) defined a program as a "coherent system of activities with which one wants to provide specific services or bring about specific effects" (p. 369). Thus, program activities are coherent, clustered, and organized as opposed to psychotherapy treatment outcome studies that are oriented to specific techniques and psychological change.

examines "how and which treatments or services are provided to individuals within service systems and evaluates how to improve treatment or service delivery" (Clinical Treatment and Services Research Workgroup, 1998, p. 11). Service system research examines how quality of care and treatment effects might be influenced by differing characteristics and structures of mental health service systems. These latter two domains, practice research and service system research, are more related to what is considered program evaluation, although as will be seen in this chapter, some effectiveness studies might border on evaluating programmatic aspects of service delivery.

To some degree, the level of specificity of focus or the magnitude of the mental health intervention or the size of the evaluation may be larger for program evaluation. Nonetheless, program evaluation in children's mental health can range from relatively small or local intervention projects to much larger projects of regional or national examinations of services. For example, a program evaluation might focus on a smaller unit providing a program of interventions such as a city-wide project run by hospital volunteers to decrease medical fears through a "Let's Pretend Hospital" (Elkins & Roberts, 1984). Similarly, a narrowly focused evaluation might examine decision making and outcomes in using a hospital-based sick child day center (Alexander, Roberts, & Prentice-Dunn, 1989) or the services in an outpatient behavioral pediatrics clinic (Sobel, Roberts, Rayfield, Bernard, & Rapoff, 2001). At a different level, program evaluation might conduct large-scale, multisite investigation, with alternative program interventions for comparison, such as the Fort Bragg demonstration project or the Comprehensive Community Mental Health Services for Children and Their Families Program. Both of these large-scale programs are described in this volume (Bickman & Mulvaney, this volume; Holden et al., 2002).

Often, the organization of program evaluation (a pattern often discerned after the fact) may move from efficacy and effectiveness research at a smaller focus of studies to those of implementation on a larger scale in the iterative process suggested by the Clinical Treatment and Services Research Workgroup. For example, the development and continual evaluation of the Multisystemic Family Therapy programmatic approach to serving delinquent youth (Henggeler, Schoenwald, Borduin, Rowland, & Cunningham, 1998; see Smith-Boydston, this volume) moved from tests in small implementations to large state and national evaluations. Similarly, the empirical base of the approach exemplified by *Project 12-Ways* to prevent child abuse and neglect has been established through clinical data reports, single-case experiments, group designs, and epidemiological studies (Lutzker, 1996). Of course, as represented by these cited projects, different research methodologies and statistical techniques were appropriately incorporated into different forms of the program evaluation: There is no one "gold standard" for program evaluation of services. As Schorr (2003) noted, although there is a certainty with experimental findings using random assignment, for example, sometimes experimental methodology may not be the most appropriate evaluation: "it is the very nature of the most promising responses to persistent social problems that makes them almost impossible to evaluate by the methodologically elegant ways in which we evaluate drugs or electric toothbrushes" (p. 6). The critical considerations are what questions are being asked and what data are needed to draw appropriate conclusions. Of course, any program evaluation relies on both explicit and implicit values and is not value free (Cook & Shadish, 1986). Choices inevitably are made based on judgments about what is important, what standards should be applied, what information is considered and analyzed, as well as how these are integrated into a conclusion about a program.

Evaluation might work best when it is integrated into ongoing program activities, not separated by different staff, different data collected, or different purposes. This aspect is exemplified by the program evaluation activities conducted on the Intensive Mental Health Program (see Jacobs et al., this volume) in which information collected for ongoing clinical decision making was aggregated to measure overall outcomes of the program itself (Vernberg, Roberts, & Nyre, 2002). Similarly, the Multisystemic Family Therapy programs integrated clinically important information with their outcomes evaluation. In contrast, some program evaluations may require information that is not regularly gathered in a mental health service program and an external research staff is devoted to collecting and analyzing data (e.g., see Bickman and Mulvaney, this volume, for a description of the very large-scale Fort Bragg demonstration project). Bickman and Mulvaney argue for keeping separate the clinical activities and personnel from that of the program evaluation. In any program evaluation, the data collected should be prioritized to provide analysis and feedback for accountability and improvement without upsetting the program's implementation.

Different aspects of program evaluation have been outlined depending on the purpose and stage of implementation (Schalock, 2001; Thompson & McClintock, 2000). *Formative evaluation* begins with the planning of a program to insure that continual feedback about potential functioning, problems, and modifications is received as it develops. This stage allows for an examination of all aspects before implementation and during its early stages or when an existing program is being transported and implemented in another setting or with a different population than originally designed. *Process evaluation* tests whether and how the program is affecting the people or behavior that it is intended to change. The process may include how the program is being implemented, what are the obstacles the population may encounter in accessing the program, as well as the characteristics of the population served. *Impact evaluation* assesses whether the program is moving adequately toward its immediate goals. Impact may be measured on proxy variables or intervening variables related to eventual outcome variables. *Outcome evaluation* measures whether the program goals are achieved, often considered longer term, and of the most interest when a program is implemented. For example, whereas *impact* evaluation may assess whether children improved psychological functioning in a therapeutic milieu, the *outcome* evaluation examines whether the children achieve satisfactory functioning in a more naturalistic setting such as schools or playgroups (if that is the goal of the program). Similarly, an educational program about substance abuse may measure the participants' immediate knowledge gain about drug dangers as an impact evaluation, whereas the outcomes evaluation of the program would assess whether the participants eventually use drugs or are arrested for possession of illegal substances.

MODELS OF PROGRAM EVALUATION

As illustrated by the range of activities and settings or venues for mental health services presented in other chapters in this volume, from camps, to schools, to hospitals, to outpatient clinics and others, the questions and evidentiary data can be diverse. To help organize program evaluation conceptualizations and activities, a number of models or approaches to issues related to program evaluation have been articulated.

Outcome-Based Evaluation

Schalock (2001) presented a model of evaluation and analysis that examines how well a program achieves its outlined goals and objectives for performance. This model of outcome-based evaluation attempts to "(1) compare the program's goals with its achieved outcomes; (2) report the program's performance and value outcomes, and (3) provide formative feedback information to program change and continuous improvement" (p. 42). He outlined a comprehensive list of potential outcomes and their indicators such as service coordination, person-referenced outcome data, expenditure data, recipient characteristics, service intensity levels, access to services, staff characteristics, health status, and wellness indicators. This model is generically applicable to physical health, mental health, and educational programs. Comparing stated goals with actual outcomes is exemplified by Koontz (2001) and Bickman et al. (1995).

COMPREHENSIVE CONCEPTUAL MODEL FOR OUTCOMES OF MENTAL HEALTH CARE FOR CHILDREN AND ADOLESCENTS

Hoagwood, Jensen, Petti, and Burns (1996) described five domains in a model for evaluating outcomes of mental health care for children and adolescents. They proposed that these outcome domains comprise the variables of interest in program evaluation (such as for practice and service system research).

Symptoms are the behavioral or emotional symptoms exhibited by the child. These may warrant a DSM or ICD diagnosis, but may be organized differently. Included here may be type, number, and frequency of these exhibited problems in different settings.

Functioning captures how children adapt to various settings and situational demands. This domain also involves the degree of impairment of a symptoms in interfering with children's functioning, such as in schools, family, or community activities appropriate to the child's development.

Consumer perspectives include the assessment of a child's symptoms and functioning by the child and family including perceptions of services and quality of life.

Environmental contexts are features of home, school, and community that might have been affected by the symptoms and interventions.

Systems refers to the different components of mental health services or care. Systems might include schools or the community services. System outcomes can be further subdivided into service-related (e.g., outcomes, in terms of service utilization) and organizational or cost-related (e.g., interactions between service providers, financial issues for organizations and provision of services).

This SFCES model (i.e., Symptoms, Functioning, Consumer Perspectives, Environmental Context, Systems) is fairly generic in categorization, by providing a set of categories for evaluating services to improve accountability. Jensen, Hoagwood, and Petti (1996) applied this SFCES model to review the literature in traditional child and adolescent mental health.

CATEGORICAL VARIABLES OF PROGRAM EVALUATION IN CHILD AND FAMILY MENTAL HEALTH

Roberts, Brown, and Puddy (2002) presented a longer series of categories of variables for comprehensive and consistent evaluation of programs intended for psychological or behavioral change. The categories were presented as flexible for programs, personnel, settings, problem behaviors targeted, and outcomes, as well as different stages of program contact. (The categories or variables can be distributed into the SFCES model of Hoagwood et al., 1996, but have greater specificity suggesting the variables to be considered.) Roberts et al. reviewed the literature to illustrate these categories of program evaluation, specifically in pediatric psychology services as a subset of children' mental health services.

In the next section, we present these variables of interest in program evaluation with more general applicability to child and family mental health similar to that outlined by Roberts et al. (2002). These program evaluation variables will be defined and illustrated by the program evaluation literature in clinical child, pediatric, and school psychology and social work.

VARIABLES OF INTEREST IN PROGRAM EVALUATION IN CHILD AND FAMILY MENTAL HEALTH SERVICES

Demographic and Basic Variables

As we have noted elsewhere (Steele & Roberts, 2003), the provision of demographic and other descriptive data regarding study samples is necessary for the appropriate evaluation of the generalizability of study results.

This is especially true for program evaluations, where descriptive data may take on greater importance because such information also provides some indication of who utilizes the programs, and whether the programs are actually serving the intended populations. For example, Alexander, Roberts, and Prentice-Dunn (1989) examined the characteristics of families utilizing a "sick-child day care center" relative to nonusers of the facility, with the intent of describing the degree to which the hospital-based program was meeting the needs of working parents and their families. Similarly, Martin, Barbee, Antle, and Sar (2002) examined the demographic characteristics of children served by a federally funded project designed to enhance and expedite advanced permanency planning for children at risk for removal from their biological parent(s). By carefully reporting demographic and descriptive data of children included in the Kentucky Adoptions Opportunities Program (KAOP) Martin et al. were able to demonstrate that the demographic characteristics of children served by the KAOP were consistent with the state gender and ethnic breakdowns of children in foster care, but (as intended by program developers) were significantly younger than the state foster care population. Among intervention studies presented in the clinical child and pediatric psychology literatures, the frequency of reporting on demographic or descriptive data varies.

Diagnostic Information

Similarly, reporting participant diagnostic information may be essential to the adequate evaluation of a program. This consideration is particularly true for programs that involve differential treatment settings for varying conditions or severity of conditions. For example, Arcelus, Bellerby, and Vostanis (1990) evaluated the mental health services utilized by youth under the care of the social services department in Birmingham, UK. One of the goals of the evaluation was to determine and to improve upon the service's system of care (i.e., formative evaluation). Thus, the referral problem (e.g., difficult behaviors, abuse) and diagnostic considerations (i.e., ICD-10 diagnosis) were necessary for appropriate tracking of mental health services and outcomes.

In some cases, reports of program evaluations that include child or adolescent diagnostic data may represent an advantage in terms of program applicability and generalizability. As will be discussed in more detail below, the presence of comorbid or co-occurring conditions may moderate the effectiveness of intervention programs, even introducing iatrogenic effects. For example, as commented on by Dishion, McCord, and Poulin (1999), the presence of primary or comorbid conduct disorder among adolescent boys may actually *increase* the likelihood of negative developmental outcomes following peer-based interventions for delinquency.

However, one of the challenges to program evaluation research is that the diagnostic status of program participants may be unavailable or difficult to ascertain. Unlike clinical trials, in which participants are routinely given comprehensive diagnostic evaluations (e.g., Antshel & Remer, 2003), program evaluations may be more likely to serve a large number of children who may or may not have clinical conditions. For example, participants of the Alvin Ailey Dance Camp (described by Brown, this volume) included children identified as being "at risk" by community leaders and educators, but did not necessarily carry a clinical diagnosis. In this case, inclusion of structured or clinical interviews to ascertain diagnostic information may have elevated the cost of the program evaluation to an unacceptably high level and would have altered the evaluation of the program's mission. Thus, the purposes of the evaluation and the intended effects of the evaluation may necessitate differential collection and use of participant diagnostic information.

Program Description or Characteristics

Beyond information regarding what populations are served, program evaluations can also supply valuable information regarding the characteristics of programs, and how services are delivered. The value of such description lies in the ability of individuals or organizations to implement similar programs in new settings, to apply components of effective programs or methods to new populations, or to provide further evaluation of the program. The description of the PREVENT (Prevention and Evaluation of Early Neglect and Trauma) program by Malik, Lederman, Crowson, and Osofsky (2002) provides an excellent example. The PREVENT program was designed to provide a structured evaluation of young children's development at their entry into the foster care system, and to systematically use that evaluation to make service referrals for the children. The published description includes background information and goals of the program, as well as the framework in which assessments are conducted. Specific assessment instruments and procedures are discussed at length, and the expected outcomes of the program are provided. Outcome dates are forthcoming, and will address whether and how the PREVENT program has impacted the quality of care for children in the foster care system.

Valuable information can also be provided when program evaluators outline changes in program procedures across settings or populations. Cardemil, Reivich, and Seligman (2002) reported on the implementation among minority samples of the Penn Resiliency Program (PRP), a school-based prevention program for children thought to be at risk for depression due to their low-income status. Cardemil et al. described the implementation of the program among primarily African American and Hispanic students of low-income families, including changes in the program to address specific cultural needs, and hypothesized mechanisms of prevention. Differences in outcome across the two cultural or ethnic groups were also discussed in terms of different mechanisms for change.

Processes of Change

In addition to studies of the components of programs, some program evaluations provide an insight into the processes responsible for change. Roth and Brooks-Gunn (2003) conducted a review of the theoretical elements of change of youth development programs[2] (i.e., competence, confidence, connections, character, and caring) and examined the degree to which 48 specific programs reported in the literature addressed these theoretical elements. Rather than a strict meta-analysis of program efficacy or effectiveness, Roth and Brooks-Gunn provided a qualitative overview of program atmosphere, activities, and mechanisms of change. Further, the report detailed the degree to which youth development programs evaluated the five elements of change, and the percentage of programs that reported significant participant improvement across the elements. As such, Roth and Brooks-Gunn provided valuable information regarding both the processes of interventions and the range of expected outcomes for this genre of program.

Similarly, Holden et al. (2002) reported on the evaluation of the Connecticut Title IV-E Waiver Program, a large-scale randomized trial of a continuum-of-care (COC) approach to mental health service provision versus treatment as usual (TAU) within that state's system. One of the components of this program evaluation was an examination of the degree to which service providers in the two conditions (COC vs. TAU) were adherent to the underlying program theory and design. As noted by Holden et al., such information is vital to (1) identify threats to internal validity of the program evaluation, (2) provide information relevant to cost of the program, and (3) inform subsequent replications of the program evaluation.

Outcome Variables

Arguably, the most important variables for examination in program evaluations have to do with the outcomes that the programs produce. These may include health, behavioral or psychological, and educational outcomes for the participants. However, they may also include larger macrosystemic changes (i.e., changes in legal or policy conditions or parameters), as well as unintended negative (iatrogenic) effects. Regardless of the specific outcome in question, Huffman et al. (2002) recommended a number of principles that may guide decision making regarding outcome measures. These recommendations included careful selection of valid and treatment-sensitive measures that are theoretically and functionally related to the processes eliciting therapeutic change.

Behavioral or Psychological Outcomes

Behavioral or psychological variables are most relevant when the program is expected to exert its primary interest on the individual or the family. Such evaluations may require some indication of the individual or family's

---

[2]Youth development programs were defined as those programs designed to either reduce specific negative outcomes such as substance abuse, violence, and mental disorders, or to promote positive developmental outcomes, such as school completion, academic achievement, or social skills development.

behavior or psychological state prior to participation in the program. For example, as noted above, Cardemil et al. (2002) examined the efficacy of the Penn Resiliency Program (PRP) in terms of its ability to prevent symptoms of depression. Children were administered self-report measures of current psychological states and behaviors (e.g., depressive symptoms, attributional style, perceived self-confidence) both before and after treatment in order to examine changes in risk for depression. Similarly, Holden et al. (2002) reported that their Connecticut Title-IV-E program evaluation included multiple assessments of child and parent functioning, at program intake and at 6, 12, and 24 months post-intake. These assessments included both child and parent report of multiple relevant constructs, including psychological symptoms, risk behaviors, caregiver strain, and vocational arrangements of the child. As illustrated by this example, outcome variables serve a program evaluation best when they are directly linked to specific goals of the program.

In some cases, program evaluations may not be able to directly assess *change* in the target outcome variable, and must instead rely on other means to assess the efficacy or effectiveness of a program. This may be particularly true for certain types of prevention programs. For example, although the child sexual abuse prevention program *Keeping Ourselves Safe* (Briggs & Hawkins, 1994), has demonstrated that children's ability to recognize and respond to potentially unsafe situations improves as a result of the program, whether the participants actually *experience* fewer incidents of sexual abuse is not as clear. In these types of cases, evidence of program effectiveness may come from archival or epidemiological data, or from comparisons of self-report data drawn from program participants and nonparticipants. For example, Gibson and Leitenberg (2000) found that 8% of a sample of college women that had participated in a prevention program as children also reported having experienced sexual abuse as a child, whereas 14% of the women who had not participated in a prevention program reported childhood sexual abuse. The use of proxy variables may be important when a link has been established between the substitute variable and the eventual variable of interest. For example, measurement of dental plaque can be substituted for dental decay (Knapp, 1991) and seat belt use can be a proxy for injuries (Roberts, Layfield, & Fanurik, 1992) in evaluating outcomes of interventions where the outcomes may be long term or difficult to obtain. Similar methods of assessing program efficacy or effectiveness may be necessary for programs designed to reduce the risk of child abuse, adolescent drug abuse, adolescent risky sexual behaviors, and delinquency.

Educational Outcomes

In addition to psychological or behavioral outcomes, educational outcomes may be of particular interest in the evaluation of programs that provide mental health services for children. Although the outcome variables in educational program evaluation may be relatively straightforward (i.e., improvement in educational achievement or performance), the methods of eliciting change and of determining outcomes may vary considerably. Bradley and Gilkey (2002), for example, conducted a longitudinal evaluation of the Home Instructional Program for Preschool Youngsters (HIPPY) in terms of behavioral, social, and educational outcomes. A matched design was used such that school suspensions, grades, classroom behavior, and achievement test scores of HIPPY participants were compared to those of children who participated in other school-readiness programs, and to nonparticipants from the same classrooms when the children were in grades 3 through 6. The inclusion of achievement scores, grades, and para-educational variables (e.g., conduct, disciplinary actions) provided the authors the ability to examine both the results of the program and the likely mechanisms (processes) by which children obtained the results.

Taking a different approach, Bagnato, Suen, Brickley, Smith-Jones, and Dettore (2002) reported on a program evaluation of the Early Childhood Initiative (ECI), conducted in high-risk communities in Pittsburgh (PA). Rather than focusing solely on school-related educational outcome data, Bragnato and colleagues examined pre- to postintervention changes in standardized scores on the Developmental Observation Checklist System (DOCS; Hresko, Miguel, Sherbenou, & Burton, 1994), which have demonstrated acceptably high correlations with teachable school readiness skills.

Few evaluations of programs that provide mental health services in school settings have also reported on educational or psychoeducational outcomes data. In one such program evaluation, Attkisson and Rosenblatt (1993) reported on the implementation of the California System of Care Model of mental health service provision in three counties in California. Results indicated that in two of the counties youth that received mental health care in the schools demonstrated improvements on standardized achievement scores. Given the increasing demands on schools to meet external expectations of success (e.g., *The No Child Left Behind Act of 2001*; U.S. PL 107-110), programs that can demonstrate positive effects on academic achievement may be better received than programs with no such outcome data.

Health Outcomes

Consistent with the range of educational outcome measures, health or health-related outcome measures may vary along a number of dimensions. These may include process-related outcomes, such as knowledge of a pediatric treatment regimen, health-related quality of life, or specific individual health outcomes, such as decreases in Body Mass Index or increased adherence to a treatment regimen. For example, González-Martín, Joo, and Sánchez (2002) evaluated a comprehensive asthma education and adherence counseling program in an outpatient pediatric clinic. Rather than a single indicator of outcome, program success was evaluated in terms of changes in children's quality of life, limitations in physical activity, specific symptoms of asthma (e.g., fatigue, cough, wheezing), and laboratory spirometry data. Such outcome measures were consistent with the stated purposes of the program evaluation (i.e., "Does the program impact the children's physical health?").

Perhaps assessing a broader range of health outcomes, Koniak-Griffin, Anderson, Verzemnieks, and Brecht (2000) evaluated an intervention program for pregnant adolescent women in comparison to standard public health nursing or no prenatal intervention. The early intervention program carried the specific mandate of improving mother–child interactions by providing counseling, education, and parent training from pregnancy through 6 weeks postpartum. Outcome measures included mother psychosocial variables (e.g., school dropout rates), mother–child psychosocial variables (e.g., relationship quality), and child health outcome variables (e.g., birthweight, number of hospitalizations).

In each of the above examples, the health outcomes that were measured were relatively distal to the processes that were likely responsible for them. That is, the outcome variables (e.g., spirometry or birthweight) are dependent upon mediating variables that may have been affected by the intervention (e.g., adherence to treatment, prenatal nutrition). Although this provides valuable information as to the overall outcome of the program (i.e., summative evaluation), such data may be less useful in terms of *formative* evaluation. Health outcome variables that lend themselves to process evaluation (e.g., adherence, nutrition, health education) may be more closely tied to program components, and thus add an additional dimension to the program evaluation.

Legal, Policy, or Philosophical Outcomes

Outcomes may be measured that indicate change according to a legal standard, a policy decree, or a philosophical approach. For example, placing children in educational settings that are the "least restrictive environments" appropriate for each child's needs is a legal requirement of Individuals with Disabilities Education Act (IDEA; see Rueda, Gallego, & Moll, 2000). If a program demonstrates that it does transition children from more restrictive to less restrictive environments, then the program may be evaluated on this legal standard as successful (e.g., the IHMP model described by Jacobs et al., this volume). Although not an evaluation of a program *per se*, Santilli and Roberts (1990) analyzed the impact of a state supreme court ruling regarding child custody following divorce by examining judges' decisions before and after the legal decisions were rendered. Similarly, a policy decision at some level (e.g., federal, state, local governmental unit or within a service unit) might be evaluated in terms of implementation and outcomes. Jacobs, Roberts, and Luchene (2002) evaluated several policy shifts outside and within a community mental health center in terms of types of referrals, census, and treatment program outcomes. To a large degree, the Fort Bragg demonstration project was an evaluation of the implementation of a philosophy of how mental health services should be organized and delivered (Behar et al., 1996). Bickman and Mulvaney (this volume) describe the evaluation of the approach known as "system of care."

Potential Iatrogenic or Nosocomial Outcomes

Beyond reporting on the specific expected outcomes associated with a program, the accurate reporting of unintended negative outcomes (iatrogenic effects) may provide an invaluable service for the mental health community. However, despite the usefulness of such reporting, a number of influences may reduce the likelihood of reporting on programs that demonstrate null or iatrogenic effects, or may reduce the likelihood of such results having an effect on public policy decisions. For example, Brown (2001) attributed the continued public support of objectively ineffective school-based drug and alcohol programs (e.g., DARE) to factors such as inadequate discourse between researchers and policy makers and the role of special interest political groups. Further, Donnermeyer (2000) noted that programs such as DARE continue to receive significant public support from parents. The perception that "doing anything (even if it does not work) is better than doing nothing at all," may contribute to the apparent disjoint between research findings and public policy.

Unfortunately, the data from program evaluations do seem to suggest that sometimes "doing anything" (if it is the wrong thing) may be *worse* than doing nothing at all. For example, at least two recent independent program evaluations found that participation in a "boot camp" for adolescent offenders was associated with an increased likelihood of recidivism, relative to standard incarceration (Benda, Toombs, & Peacock, 2002; Stinchcomb & Terry, 2001). Further, as noted by Dishion et al. (1999), a number of investigations have consistently demonstrated that delinquent youth may not benefit from group therapy encounters, and in fact, may incur nosocomial outcomes. Despite political or social pressure to the contrary, publication of program evaluations that indicate unintended negative side effects is, at some level, an ethical obligation.

Individual Differences in Responsivity to Programs

As noted above, the accurate reporting of demographic information regarding program participants carries a number of advantages, one of which is the identification of individual differences in outcome. Findings that a program is differentially effective across racial or ethnic groups, for example, may suggest differences in mechanisms by which change occurs across those groups (i.e., different mediators of change). These differences might include cultural beliefs or values, economic barriers to services, or institutional or programmatic deficits (see Cardemil et al., 2002). These mechanisms might then be the focus of further evaluation. For example, Ryan et al. (2002) examined the relative efficacy of a comprehensive child development program across families receiving AFDC and those not receiving AFDC. The program was designed to help parents implement specific developmental goals for their children. Results suggested that AFDC status moderated the efficacy of the program, even after controlling for individual families' incomes. However, of potentially greater importance, Ryan and colleagues reported that these differences were mediated by parents' choices of goals that they brought to the program. The examination of mediation provided results that suggested mechanisms for improving program delivery: Helping families to recognize and prioritize child-centered goals.

Costs and Benefits

Because of the competing demands on the resources of public and private organizations, particularly those that provide mental health services, evaluations that include estimations of the costs to initiate and maintain programs may be particularly useful. Such estimations may include the actual dollar figures that are required to implement a program (e.g., purchasing materials, compensating employees), but may also include the resource costs to the sponsoring institution (i.e., unavailability for other projects; training; supervision; space), as well as costs to individuals or stakeholders (Holden et al., 2002). As noted by Yates (2003), the costs to the individual may include economic costs as well as other expenditures, including "hassles," time away from other activities, or other difficulties associated with program participation.

Similarly, evaluations of the benefits of programs may include many of the objective outcome data discussed above (e.g., improvement on self-report measures of depression), client or stakeholder satisfaction, or decreases in the utilization of other services. In each of these cases, the relative benefit of a program may be expressed in terms of cost–benefit or cost-effectiveness data. Unfortunately, the inclusion of cost-related analyses is not standard practice in the clinical literature (Yates, 2003).

At the most straightforward level, inclusion of cost analysis may provide information regarding the feasibility of a program in a given setting. This type of analysis does not provide a ratio of cost to benefit, but simply estimates the various costs associated with a program. Foster, Dodge, and Jones (2003) divided these costs into two categories: explicit and implicit costs. In the explicit category are included labor and material costs, fixed costs (e.g., space), and out-of-pocket expenses borne by families. Implicit costs include time spent delivering the service (i.e., to both provider and consumer), time spent preparing for the service (or supervising the service), as well as nonexplicit space costs. The latter might include classroom space used in the evening for parent education classes, and thus represent "opportunity" costs—the intervention is removing the opportunity for other uses of the space.

Another method of evaluating the relative economic costs associated with a program is to estimate the cost of participation versus the costs of nonparticipation. For example, in their review of programs for service delivery of treatment for juvenile sexual abusers, Brown and Kolko (1998) reported on the potential economic costs associated with untreated sex offences relative to the costs of treatment programs. For untreated offenders, the costs included those of incarceration and the costs associated with victim rehabilitation.

Cost–benefit analyses may provide additional information when questions regarding the relative benefits of a program arise—"How much benefit can I expect to accomplish given the allocation of 'X' resources?" Such evaluations are not limited to questions surrounding dollar amounts (Holden et al., 2002; Yates, 2003). The question can be recast in terms of any outlay of resources, including time, space, effort, or financial resources. With regard to the evaluation of the Connecticut Title IV-E Waiver Program, Holden et al. (2002) noted that the multiple constituencies that are invested in the program (e.g., federal, state, and local governments; stakeholders; service providers) might necessarily benefit from different kinds of cost–benefits analyses.

Utilization of Other Services

An additional means of evaluating the relative costs and benefits of a program is an examination of the degree to which program participants utilize additional or subsequent services. Depending on the nature of the program, one might expect reductions in the need for other services. For example, one might expect participants of an adolescent sex offender program to evidence lower utilization of subsequent correctional facilities (see Murphy et al., this volume). In such a case, utilization of other services might serve as an outcome variable for a summative evaluation of the program. In other cases, however, utilization of additional or subsequent services may serve as a means of assessing benefits (not outcomes) of a program. For example, Malla et al. (1998) evaluated a comprehensive case management program for adults with psychotic disorders. Although outcome data were gathered to determine whether the program had a noticeable impact on individual symptoms, data were also collected to determine the extent to which program participation reduced the need for other medical and psychosocial services (e.g., emergency room visits, inpatient treatment) over the subsequent 3 years.

Assessment of Satisfaction

With the increasing level of consumer sophistication and media attention surrounding treatment issues has come increased attention on the part of providers to client and stakeholder satisfaction. Depending on the scope of the program involved, a number of different parties may be appropriate sources of satisfaction assessment, including the clients themselves, their parents or caregivers, members of their immediate ecosystems (e.g., teachers), their referring party or other stakeholders (e.g., social worker), and program staff.

The assessment of client and parent satisfaction appears to be the most widespread method of evaluating perceptions about programs that deliver mental health services. Numerous examples of evaluations of consumer satisfaction can be found in the clinical child and pediatric psychology literatures, many of which employ self-report instruments as the primary source of satisfaction data from parents and caregivers, and occasionally, the children and adolescents themselves (e.g., Greenfield & Attkisson, 1999; Palisin, Cecil, Gumbardo, & Varley, 1997; Plante, Couchman, & Hoffman, 1998; Shapiro, Welker, & Jacobson, 1997).

What appears to be less common in the program evaluation literature is assessment of other interested parties' satisfaction with services provided. Roberts et al. (2002) noted a handful of studies in which referral sources were given the opportunity to provide their level of general satisfaction, perceptions of client or patient gains, and likelihood of referring clients to the program in the future. Such information may provide a useful means of evaluating outcome, and may well have a bearing on the sustainability of a program in a given context.

Similarly, few program evaluations have tapped the rich sources of information that can be provided by members of the child's ecosystem (e.g., teachers). Two notable exceptions deserve mention. The first is the Intensive Mental Health Program (IMHP; Vernberg et al., 2002; and described by Jacobs et al., this volume), which has been designed to obtain teacher and staff satisfaction regarding the IMHP. Such data are likely to provide valuable information regarding client performance in a more natural environment, and thus, contribute to a better understanding of program outcome.

The second exception was provided by Naar-King, Siegel, and Smyth (2002) in their evaluation of an interdisciplinary health care program for children with special needs. In addition to parent and child satisfaction, this program evaluation included a measure of staff or provider satisfaction as a means of assessing program acceptability. As with measures of referral source satisfaction, data regarding staff or provider satisfaction may provide useful information that may bear upon program sustainability, as well as the degree to which services are meeting the needs of the clients.

CONCLUDING COMMENTS

As presented in this chapter and evidenced by other chapters in this volume, program evaluation of service delivery might consider a variety of variables at different points. The variety of methods and measures may be daunting, but demonstrates the range of evaluation tools for the investigator. As noted by Greene (2003), the issues to be evaluated should "drive" the methodology, not choosing a methodology independent of the program aspects. Evaluating programs from a variety of perspectives is important for effective development, modification for improvement, engendering support for continuation, and simply justifying the program's existence. Indeed, the absence of evaluation may be more telling about a program and its implementers than the constellation of specific evaluative components.

REFERENCES

Alexander, K., Roberts, M. C., & Prentice-Dunn, S. (1989). A program evaluation of a sick child day care facility. *Children's Health Care, 18*, 225–231.

Antshel, K. M., & Remer, R. (2003). Social skills training in children with attention deficit hyperactivity disorder: A randomized-controlled clinical trial. *Journal of Clinical Child and Adolescent Psychology, 32*, 153–165.

Arcelus, J., Bellerby, T., & Vostanis, P. (1999). A mental-health service for young people in the care of the local authority. *Clinical Child Psychology and Psychiatry, 4,* 233–245.

Attkisson, C. C., & Rosenblatt, A. (1993). Enhancing school performance of youth with severe emotional disorder: Initial results from system of care research in three California counties. *School Psychology Quarterly, 8,* 277–290.

Bagnato, S. J., Suen, H. K., Brickley, D., Smith-Jones, J., & Dettore, E. (2002). Child developmental impact of Pittsburgh's Early Childhood Initiative (ECI) in high-risk communities: First phase authentic evaluation research. *Early Childhood Research Quarterly, 17,* 559–580.

Behar, L., Bickman, L., Lane, T., Keeton, W. P., Schwartz, M., & Brannock, J. E. (1996). The Fort Bragg Child and Adolescent Mental Health Demonstration Project. In M. C. Roberts (Ed.), *Model programs in child and family mental health* (pp. 351–372). Mahwah, NJ: Lawrence Erlbaum.

Benda, B. B., Toombs, N. J., & Peacock, M. (2002). Ecological factors in recidivism: A survival analysis of boot camp graduates after three years. *Journal of Offender Rehabilitation, 35,* 63–85.

Bickman, L., Gunthrie, P. R., Foster, E. M., Lambert, E. W., Summerfelt, W. T., Breda, C. S., & Helfilinger, C. A. (1995). *Evaluating managed mental health services: The Fort Bragg experiment.* New York: Plenum.

Bradley, R. H., & Gilkey, B. (2002). The impact of the Home Instructional Program for Preschool Youngsters (HIPPY) on school performance in 3rd and 6th grades. *Early Education and Development, 13,* 301–311.

Briggs, F., & Hawkins, R. M. F. (1994). Follow-up data on the effectiveness of New Zealand's national school based child protection program. *Child Abuse and Neglect, 18,* 635–643.

Brown, J. H. (2001). Youth, drugs and resilience education. *Journal of Drug Education, 31,* 83–122.

Brown, E. J., & Kolko, D. J. (1998). Treatment efficacy and program evaluation with juvenile sexual abusers: A critique with directions for service delivery and research. *Child Maltreatment, 3,* 362–373.

Cardemil, E. V., Reivich, K. J., & Seligman, M. E. P. (2002). The prevention of depressive symptoms in low-income minority middle school students. *Prevention and Treatment, 5,* article 8. Retrieved August 8, 2003, from www.journals.apa.org/prevention/volume5/pre0050008a.html

Chelimsky, E., & Shadish, W. R. (1997). *Evaluation for the 21st century: A handbook.* Thousand Oaks, CA: Sage.

Clinical Treatment and Services Research Workgroup of the National Institute of Mental Health, National Advisory Mental Health Council. (1998). *Bridging science and service.* Bethesda, MD: National Institutes of Health. Retrieved July 8, 2003, from http://www.nimh.nih.gov/research/bridge.htm

Cook, T. D., & Shadish, W. R. (1986). Program evaluation: The worldly science. *Annual Review of Psychology, 37,* 193–232.

Dishion, T. J., McCord, J., & Poulin, F. (1999). When interventions harm: Peer groups and problem behaviors. *American Psychologist, 54,* 755–764.

Donnermeyer, J. F. (2000). Parents' perceptions of a school-based prevention education program. *Journal of Drug Education, 30,* 325–342.

Elkins, P. D., & Roberts, M. C. (1984). A preliminary evaluation of hospital preparation for nonpatient children: Primary prevention in a "Let's Pretend Hospital." *Children's Health Care, 13,* 31–36.

Foster, E. M., Dodge, K. A., & Jones, D. (2003). Issues in the economic evaluation of prevention programs. *Applied Developmental Science, 7,* 76–86.

Gibson, L. E., & Leitenberg, H. (2000). Child sexual abuse prevention programs: Do they decrease the occurrence of child sexual abuse? *Child Abuse and Neglect, 24,* 1115–1125.

González-Martín, G., Joo, I., & Sánchez, I. (2002). Evaluation of the impact of a pharmaceutical care program in children with asthma. *Patient Education and Counseling, 49,* 13–18.

Greene, M. M. (2003). Program evaluation. In J. C. Thomas & M. Hersen (Eds.), *Understanding research in clinical and counseling psychology* (pp. 209–242). Mahwah, NJ: Lawrence Erlbaum.

Greenfield, T. K., & Attkisson, C. C. (1999). The UCSF Client Satisfaction Scales: II. The Service Satisfaction Scale-30. In M. E. Maruish (Ed.), *The use of psychological testing for treatment planning and outcomes assessment* (2nd ed., pp. 1347–1367). Mahwah, NJ: Lawrence Erlbaum.

Harinck, F. J. H., Smit, M., & Knorth, E. J. (1997). Evaluating child and youth care programs. *Child & Youth Care Forum, 26*, 369–383.

Henggeler, S. W., Schoenwald, S. K., Borduin, C. M., Rowland, M. D., & Cunningham, P. B. (1998). *Multisystemic treatment of antisocial behavior in children and adolescents.* New York: Guilford.

Hoagwood, K., Jensen, P. S., Petti, T., & Burns, B. J. (1996). Outcomes of mental health care for children and adolescents: I. A comprehensive conceptual model. *Journal of the American Academy of Child and Adolescent Psychiatry, 35*, 1055–1063.

Holden, E. W., O'Connell, S. R., Connor, T., Brannan, A. M., Foster, E. M., Blau, G. et al.. (2002). Evaluation of the Connecticut Title IV-E Waiver Program: Assessing the effectiveness, implementation fidelity, and cost/benefits of a continuum of care. *Child and Youth Services Review, 24*, 409–430.

Hresko, W., Miguel, S., Sherbenuo, R., & Burton, S. (1994). *Developmental observation checklist system (DOCS).* Austin, TX: Pro-Ed.

Huffman, L., Koopman, C., Blasey, C., Botcheva, L., Hill, K. E., Marks, A. S. K. et al. (2002). A program evaluation strategy in a community-based behavioral health and education services agency for children and families. *The Journal of Applied Behavioral Science, 38*, 191–215.

Jacobs, N. J., Roberts, M. C., & Luchene, L. (2002, October). *A program evaluation assessing outcomes of youth admitted to a psychiatric community facility: A study of the impact of policy changes over time.* Paper presented at the Kansas Conference in Clinical Child and Adolescent Psychology, Lawrence, KS.

Jensen, P. S., Hoagwood, K., & Petti, T. (1996). Outcomes of mental health care for children and adolescents: II. Literature review and application of a comprehensive model. *Journal of the American Academy of Child and Adolescent Psychiatry, 35*, 1064–1077.

Knapp, L. G. (1991). Effects of type of value appealed to and valence of appeal on children's dental health behavior. *Journal of Pediatric Psychology, 16*, 675–686.

Koniak-Griffin, D., Anderson, N. L. R., Verzemnieks, I., & Brecht, M. L. (2000). A public health nursing early intervention program for adolescent mothers: Outcomes from pregnancy through 6 weeks postpartum. *Nursing Research, 49*, 130–138.

Koontz, A. D. (2001). *A mission-based program evaluation and outcome study of a diabetes camp.* Unpublished doctoral dissertation, University of Kansas, Lawrence, KS.

Lutzker, J. R. (1996). An ecobehavioral model for serious family disorders: Child abuse and neglect; Developmental disabilities. In M. C. Roberts (Ed.), *Model programs in child and family mental health* (pp. 33–46). Mahwah, NJ: Lawrence Erlbaum.

Malik, N. M., Lederman, C. S., Crowson, M. M., & Osofsky, J. D. (2002). Evaluating maltreated infants, toddlers, and preschoolers in dependency court. *Infant Mental Health Journal, 23*, 576–592.

Malla, A. K., Norman, R. M. G., McLean, T. S., Cheng, S., Rickwood, A., McIntosh, E. et al. (1998). An integrated medical and psychosocial treatment program for psychotic disorders: Patient characteristics and outcome. *Canadian Journal of Psychiatry, 43*, 698–705.

Martin, M. H., Barbee, A. P., Antle, B. F., & Sar, B. (2002). Expedited permanency planning: Evaluation of the Kentucky Adoptions Opportunities Project. *Child Welfare, 81*, 203–224.

Naar-King, S., Siegel, P. T., & Smyth, M. (2002). Consumer satisfaction with a collaborative, interdisciplinary health care program for children with special needs. *Children's Services: Social Policy, Research, and Practice, 5*, 189–200.

Palisin, H., Cecil, J. Gumbardo, D., & Varley, C. (1997). A survey of parents' satisfaction with their children's hospitalization on a psychiatric unit. *Children's Health Care, 26*, 233–240.

Plante, T. G., Couchman, C. E., & Hoffman, C. A. (1998). Measuring treatment outcome and client satisfaction among children and families: A case report. *Professional psychology: Research and Practice, 29*, 52–55.

Roberts, M. C., Brown, K. J., & Puddy, R. W. (2002). Service delivery issues and program evaluation in pediatric psychology. *Journal of Clinical Psychology in Medical Settings, 9*, 3–13.

Roberts, M. C., & Hinton-Nelson, M. (1996). Models for service delivery in child and family mental health. In M. C. Roberts (Ed.), *Model programs in child and family mental health* (pp. 1–21). Mahwah, NJ: Lawrence Erlbaum.

Roberts, M. C., Layfield, D. A., & Fanurik, D. (1992). Motivating children's use of car safety devices. In M. Wolraich & D. Routh (Eds.), *Advances in developmental and behavioral pediatrics* (Vol. 10, pp. 61–87). London: Jessica Kingsley.

Roberts, M. C., Vernberg, E. M., & Jackson, Y. (2000). Psychotherapy with children and families. In C. R. Snyder & R. Ingram (Eds.), *Handbook of psychological change* (pp. 500–519). New York: Wiley.

Roth, J. L., & Brooks-Gunn, J. (2003). Youth development programs: Risk, prevention, and policy. *Journal of Adolescent Health, 32*, 170–182.

Rueda, R., Gallego, M. A., & Moll, L. C. (2000). The least restrictive environment: A place or context? *Remedial and Special Education, 21*, 70–78.

Ryan, C. S., McCall, R. B., Robinson, D. R., Groark, C. J., Mulvey, L., & Plemons, B. W. (2002). Benefits of the Comprehensive Child Development Program as a function of AFDC receipt and SES. *Child Development, 73*, 315–328.

Santilli, L., & Roberts, M. C. (1990). Custody decisions in Alabama before and after the abolition of the tender years doctrine. *Law and Human Behavior, 14*, 123–137.

Schalock, R. L. (2001). *Outcome-based evaluation* (2nd ed.). New York: Kluwer/Plenum.

Schorr, L. B. (2003, February). *Determining "what works" in social programs and social policies: Toward a more inclusive knowledge basis*. Washington, DC: The Brookings Institution. Retrieved July 8, 2003, from http://www.brook.edu/views/papers/sawhill/20030226.htm

Shadish, W. R., Cook, T. D., & Leviton, L. C. (1991). *Foundations of program evaluation: Theories of practice*. Thousand Oaks, CA: Sage.

Shapiro, J. P., Welker, C. J., & Jacobson, B. J. (1997). The Youth Client Satisfaction Questionnaire: Development, construct validation, and factor structure. *Journal of Clinical Child Psychology, 26*, 87–98.

Sobel, A. B., Roberts, M. C., Rayfield, A., Bernard, M. U., & Rapoff, M. (2001). Evaluating outpatient pediatric psychology services in a primary care setting. *Journal of Pediatric Psychology, 26*, 395–405.

Steele, R. G., & Roberts, M. C. (2003). Therapy and interventions research with children and adolescents. In M. C. Roberts & S. S. Ilardi (Eds.), *Handbook of research methods in clinical psychology* (pp. 307–326). London: Blackwell.

Stinchcomb, J. B., & Terry, W. C. (2001). Predicting the likelihood of rearrest among shock incarceration graduates: Moving beyond another nail in the boot camp coffin. *Crime and Delinquency, 47*, 221–242.

Street, L., Niederehe, G., & Lebowitz, B. D. (2000). Toward a greater public health relevance for psychotherapeutic intervention research: An NIMH workshop report. *Clinical Psychology: Science and Practice, 7*, 127–137.

Thompson, N. J., & McClintock, H. O. (2000). *Demonstrating your program's worth: A primer on evaluation for programs to prevent unintentional injury*. Atlanta: National Center for Injury Prevention and Control.

Vernberg, E. M., Roberts, M. C., & Nyre, J. (2002). School-based intensive mental health treatment. In D. T. Marsh & M. A. Fristad (Eds.), *Handbook of serious emotional disturbance in children and adolescents* (pp. 412–427). New York: Wiley.

Yates, B. T. (2003). Toward the incorporation of costs, cost-effectiveness analysis, and cost–benefit analysis into clinical research. In A. E. Kazdin (Ed.), *Methodological issues and strategies in clinical research* (3rd ed., pp. 711–727). Washington, DC: American Psychological Association.

24

Large-Scale Evaluations of Children's Mental Health Services

The Ft. Bragg and Stark County Studies

LEONARD BICKMAN and SHELAGH MULVANEY

What is large? Large can be defined in several ways. We can describe evaluations as large because they cost a great deal of money, include a large number of participants, include multiple sites or because they evaluate large programs. Our perspective is that the amount of funding can be used as a simple index of size. Dollars allocated is an estimate of the amount of investment and interest that an agency or foundation has in seeing evaluation questions answered. When a million dollars or more is spent on an evaluation the justification is usually based on the importance of the evaluation question. However, dollars or size do not always correlate with quality or impact.

Some aspects of large evaluations are unique and some are simply upward extensions of smaller evaluation projects. On the whole, one can assume that most aspects of the evaluation will be more complicated in large-scale projects. One example is budgeting and expenditures. Expenditures for an evaluation are correlated with the number of project staff, the length of the evaluation, the number of study sites, the number of data collection points, and the method of data collection (Bickman, 1992). The largest category of expense is typically personnel so it is to be expected that staff size is related to total expenditures. Each additional evaluation site, be it comparison or treatment site, contributes additional costs to an

LEONARD BICKMAN and SHELAGH MULVANEY • Department of Psychology, Peabody College, Vanderbilt University, Nashville, Tennessee 37212.

evaluation. Typically, this means that offices have to be maintained and support staff are needed for each office. Unless the evaluation data are archival (i.e., electronic records) most of the personnel costs are spent on collecting data. The number of waves or time periods of data collection greatly influences the budget. Finally, the type of data collected affects costs. In-person interviews are more expensive than telephone interviews and those are more expensive than mailed questionnaires. There are, of course, other costs that are correlated with size such as data preparation and analysis, and the number of project management staff. Large data sets can also pose other difficulties such avoiding violations of confidentiality and simultaneously tracking each participant's data over time.

One difference between smaller evaluations and larger projects is the form and degree of scrutiny and public debate that surrounds them. Large evaluations are typically of national interest and thus should be very visible. By "visible" we mean that the processes of design, implementation, analyses, and evaluation should be as open as possible to stakeholders. Because of the large investment and interest, evaluators on large-scale projects have a responsibility to produce timely results. The results will, and should, be scrutinized in these circumstances.

Paradoxically, large evaluations should be focused on important questions, but not on questions that are too important. If the topic is too "hot" then it is likely that a careful large-scale evaluation cannot be completed in the time frame necessary to answer a pressing question. On the other hand, a "cold" issue, or one that poses immediate demands for information, will not be seen as appropriate for large evaluation. Thus the focus should be on lukewarm issues. It also helps if the issue is one of long-standing interest so that no matter when the evaluation is completed it will still be relevant. It is a cheerless experience to spend years conducting a study for which there is no longer any interest when completed.

Ultimately, an evaluation should be no larger than it needs to be. Considerations of statistical power, feasibility, longitudinal performance, and generalizability are all important aspects of making decisions about size. The incremental utility or validity of the project does not necessarily increase with size alone.

IMPORTANT CHARACTERISTICS OF THE FT. BRAGG AND STARK COUNTY EVALUATIONS

The Ft. Bragg evaluation describes the implementation, quality, costs, and outcomes of a $94 million demonstration project designed to improve the mental health outcomes for children and adolescents who received mental health treatment funded by CHAMPUS, the Department of Defense's insurance program for civilian dependents of military personnel (Bickman et al., 1995). The demonstration provided a full continuum of mental health services in civilian facilities near Ft. Bragg, North Carolina, including outpatient therapy, day treatment, in-home counseling, therapeutic foster homes, specialized group homes, 24-hour crisis management services, and acute hospitalization. The comparison sites were also civilian facilities near similar army posts at Ft. Campbell, Kentucky, and Ft. Stewart, Georgia, where services to children were limited to outpatient, residential, and hospital care. The comparison sites provided no formal coordination among services or other systems such as education and juvenile justice as in the demonstration other than what would normally occur. The evaluation was a quasi-experiment with close to 1,000 families followed over 5 years. Extensive mental health, service use, and cost data were collected on children and their families over seven waves to evaluate the relative effectiveness of the demonstration. A random regression longitudinal model was used to analyze 10 key outcome variables. The findings were surprising and upsetting to many. Whereas *both* groups of children showed significant improvement, clinical outcomes in demonstration children were no better than those in the comparison sites. Moreover, although it was anticipated that the demonstration would be less expensive it was more expensive and there was no medical cost offset of the additional costs (Foster & Bickman, 2000).

The Stark County Ohio evaluation examined an established exemplary system of care designed to provide comprehensive mental health services to children and adolescents. Similar to the goals of the Fr. Brag Demonstration, it was believed that the Stark County system would lead to more improvement in the functioning and symptoms of clients compared to those receiving care as usual. The project employed a randomized experimental five-wave longitudinal design with 350 families. The results replicated the Ft. Bragg findings (Bickman, Noser, & Summerfelt, 1999). There was better access to care, more care, more types of services, but unfortunately greater costs, and no differences in clinical outcomes compared to treatment as usual. In addition, children who did not receive any services, regardless of experimental condition, improved at the same rate as treated children.

In both studies, the effects of systems-of-care policies and approach were primarily limited to system-level outcomes such as access and cost, but did not appear to affect clinical outcomes such as child and family functioning and symptom severity.

CHALLENGES AND BENEFITS OF CONDUCTING LARGE-SCALE EVALUATION STUDIES

Funding

Large-scale proposals are typically highly scrutinized, often politically sensitive, slow to develop, and are not easily funded. It took several years and the efforts of Dr. Lenore Behar, former Director of Children's Services for the North Carolina Department of Human Services, Division of Mental Health Health, Developmental Disabilities, and Substance Abuse and assistance from the U.S. Congress to obtain funds for the Ft. Bragg Demonstration. The Ft. Bragg and Stark County evaluations both qualify as large-scale evaluations if we use the criterion of dollars spent. The basic evaluation cost less than 5% of the $94 million Ft. Bragg Demonstration service system; including all of the evaluation research efforts the cost was less than 11% of the cost of the demonstration. Experience indicates that serendipity and politics can play a large role in funding large projects. If dedicated, an evaluation team can successfully participate in the elaborate and sometimes difficult funding process and come out with a feasible, valid, and important large-scale project.

Complexity

Large evaluations usually include more than one geographical location. The logistics of setting up and maintaining remote offices is not something learned in graduate school. Such mundane activities as arranging for phones and other utilities, renting space, and obtaining furniture can take time, especially if a university has little experience in processing off-campus requests. There are also advantages of being at university. Cash flow for basic necessities is seldom a problem in an academic setting. The university paid the bills (mostly on time) regardless of whether the funds had arrived from the agencies. For the federal grants this was not a problem. But, because the evaluation was more expensive than anticipated, our contracts had to be increased several times. These events were always cliffhangers with many jobs in the balance because we were never completely sure that the funds would appear at all, much less on time.

Staffing

One of the biggest challenges in conducting large-scale projects is the hiring and supervision of many staff with remote sites offering particular challenges. In our opinion, an academic Principle Investigator (PI) will have difficulty managing large studies because he or she is rarely full time on the project and usually has to continue regular academic duties that include teaching, advising, and committee work. Moreover, even without other responsibilities academics may or may not have the managerial skills necessary for such large projects (Bickman, 1981). Thus, hiring the right staff and a lot of on-the-job training for the PI is critical to success. Because there is no traditional career path for a general project manager we filled those positions with psychologists, social workers, lawyers, and clinicians and did not find that any particular training mattered. Hiring someone who is well organized, can supervise others, and pay attention to details is critical. Another characteristic of large projects is the need for teamwork, especially an interdisciplinary team. Ensuring that the group works together is a key responsibility of the PI.

Large-scale studies are also an investment in the careers of the researchers conducting the studies. How does this intensive and lengthy involvement in a study affect them? There were six other authors of the book summarizing the Ft. Bragg evaluation (Bickman et al., 1995). Two continue as productive research associates at the Center for Mental Health

Policy, two have gone on to gain tenure at universities, one went from being a graduate student to an assistant professor, and one went back to her clinical practice. Because these studies do not usually produce publications for several years some argue that only established investigators should commit to them. The experience of these researchers would argue otherwise.

Research Generated

Large evaluation projects are typically comprehensive and thus can often be divided into several related but smaller studies. The Ft. Bragg evaluation had the following components: cost, service use, quality of services, clinical outcomes, and implementation. Each substudy was managed by a different staff member and was coordinated by the PI and the project manager. This division also results in the potential for different individuals to take the lead in publishing in each area.

One of the potential advantages of large evaluations is the ability to answer many research questions that are not evaluation questions. Additional funds from the National Institute of Mental Health (NIMH) allowed us, for example, to test a family empowerment intervention, study the long-term outcomes of services, and collect data about families. Additional funds from the Army were spent on studying the Demonstration's transformation into a managed care system. Some of the papers we published are relevant to understanding the results of the evaluation and others had little to do with the evaluation. We have published a comprehensive summary of the evaluation (Bickman et al., 1995) and papers on topics such as functioning (Bickman, Lambert, Karver, & Andrade, 1998; Lambert, Salzer, & Bickman, 1998), service use (Lambert, Brannan, Breda, Heflinger, & Bickman, 1998), quality of services (Bickman, Summerfelt, & Bryant, 1996), policy issues (Bickman, 2000), cost analysis (Bickman et al., 1998), developmental psychopathology (Lambert, Wahler, Andrade, & Bickman, 2001), parent empowerment (Bickman, Heflinger, Northrup, Sonnichsen, & Schilling, 1998; Heflinger, Bickman, Northrup, & Sonnichsen, 1997), satisfaction (Lambert et al., 1998) caregiver strain (Brannan, Heflinger, & Bickman, 1997), service termination (Breda & Bickman, 1997), and program implementation (Bickman & Heflinger, 1994).

A large-scale evaluation also has greater potential for discovering the reasons why an intervention may not have produced the expected effects. We were able to conduct additional analyses to examine one of the major assumptions underlying a system of care: that the clinicians could appropriately assign children to a level of care (e.g., hospital vs outpatient) given the children's problem and resources. When the results showed that the additional options for level of care had no clinical benefit we reasoned that this could be caused by some clinicians not assigning children to the "appropriate" level of care regardless of their training and the existence of a manual on level of assignment. After making sure that there was sufficient information to make an assignment we were surprised to find that there was essentially no agreement among clinicians on level of assignment.

Thus, it could be that continuum care did not "work" because assignment to care appeared to be less than consistent (Bickman, Karver, & Schut, 1997).

A second study involved another interpretation for the lack of significant findings. A key underlying assumption of the demonstration was that what was needed was a new system for the delivery of services that were assumed to be effective. Clearly, the null results could be obtained if the treatments delivered were ineffective. Thus, no matter what changes were made at the system level there would be no difference in clinical outcomes if the treatments did not work. But how could we test this notion because there was no control group consisting of children who did not receive treatment? We assumed that if treatment was effective then there should be a dose–response relationship. That is, the more treatment was received (controlling for severity), the more improvement should occur. In three separate studies, using the both Stark and Ft. Bragg data, we could not find any evidence of a dose–response thus weakening the assumption that the services were indeed effective (Andrade, Lambert, & Bickman, 2000; Bickman, Andrade, & Lambert, 2002; Salzer, Bickman, & Lambert, 1999).

We believed that the quality of the services is a major factor in determining program success. We looked at the quality of two components that we thought were critical—case management and intake. These components were the "glue" that held the program together. To study the quality of case management we had case mangers keep logs of their activities, analyzed charts, conducted interviews and reviewed documents, used a scale that measured program philosophy, interviewed parents, and did a network analysis. In addition, we developed a "case management evaluation data checklist" that was our measure of quality based on concept mapping and document reviews. The checklist included such items as parent involvement in treatment planning, client monitoring and follow-up, and linkage and coordination activities. Our evaluation of the quality of case management involved comparing the checklist to the evidence we had collected from multiple sources. Details about this procedure were published in a special issue of *Evaluation and Program Planning* on evaluation methodology and mental health services (Bickman, 1996) and the more general issues of measuring quality are expanded in a special issue of *Evaluation Review* (Bickman & Salzer, 1997).

Design and Analysis

There are certain key aspects of the evaluation that will determine its success. Good design is key to successful evaluation. Undoubtedly, a randomized experiment is the strongest design to use for inferring causal relationships. The scope of the Ft. Bragg demonstration made it impossible to randomly assign Army posts throughout the world. Thus, a quasi-experiment was conducted. The primary threat to the internal validity of this design is selection. One needs to be as certain as possible that the participants and their problems are similar in the comparison and treatment sites. We were very fortunate that the study was conducted at Army posts because one cannot ask for more similar settings and persons. This is not the case in comparing, for example, services in Youngstown, Ohio with Stark County, Ohio.

The second area of concern is measurement. Poor or insensitive measures can mask a program effect or even miss it entirely if the wrong constructs are measured. To have good construct validity the instruments used to measure outcomes needed to be valid. This was a problem in some areas because the quality of existing measures was low. In some cases we had to develop new measures. Regardless, the leaders of the demonstration vetted all the measures. The evaluators also had to present the case that the demonstration was, in fact, a good example of a continuum of care and that it was successfully implemented. Many evaluation resources were devoted to documenting the implementation fidelity and quality of the continuum of care. Basically, this involved documenting that access was high, the new services were available, and that they were well coordinated.

The third component of a successful evaluation design is the sample size. It is widely accepted now that statistical power should be ascertained in the design phase. All studies need to ensure that if a null effect is found it is truly a null effect and not the result of low statistical power. Our calculations indicated that we needed close to 1,000 subjects and the Army accepted this evaluation design. Obtaining the number of required subjects may be the biggest challenge to large evaluation projects. Even when pipeline studies (subject flow) are conducted, researchers still tend to underestimate the rate at which subjects will need to be recruited. In our case we were given some incorrect information about how to contact families receiving services in the comparison sites. We needed to interview the families within a few days of starting services. We were told that the Army would provide a computerized list. As it turned out, they could provide us with such a list but it would be about 6–9 months after services were started. We devised several methods to recruit families but the most successful and the most time consuming (costly) was to visit every mental health practice in the area each week to determine if any new eligible families were seen. This kind of post hoc change in data collection can have large and unexpected effects on planned analyses and cost.

Stark County provided an excellent opportunity to examine substantive and methodological issues that emerged from Ft. Bragg using a stronger randomized design. In selecting our site for this study we required that the service system have more children applying than who could be served. We felt that it was then ethical to assign children randomly to the system of care or treatment as usual. However, there were limitations on the selection of cases for the study. Because the random assignment took place after the baseline data were collected (to avoid any initial differential attrition) it sometimes took 2 weeks to interview a family after they had applied for services. Clearly, we could not use any very severe or emergency cases because of this delay. The Ft. Bragg study, in contrast, recruited families whose children were receiving any services including hospitalization. All studies require making tradeoffs. In this case we traded better external validity (generalizability) in Stark for better internal validity. However, the

Ft. Bragg and Stark County evaluations are powerful when considered together because they compensate for each other's weaknesses. It is rare that two large-scale evaluations can be conducted to address similar questions using complementary designs.

Another design aspect of both evaluations is their longitudinal nature. No large-scale evaluation of mental health services should be based on only two data points (Lambert, Doucette, & Bickman, 2001). Longitudinal designs provide better estimation of the pattern of change and greater statistical power than the pre-post design. However, longitudinal studies pose additional challenges for large evaluations. In a field as new as children's mental health the measurement is not as good as we would like. Thus, it is tempting take advantage of an improved or new instrument in the later phases of the study. Our recommendation is that one should introduce new measures during the study very judiciously. The logistics of changing an instrument in a large study can be complex and the interpretation of the results will be more difficult. However, sometimes the investigators have little choice when standardized measures are updated. In that case the best a researcher can do is "flag" the change in the analysis and determine if it makes a difference in the results.

Outcomes

There are predictable challenges related to conducting large-scale projects and challenges in the process of dealing with findings. In the Ft. Bragg study, we tried to design an evaluation that was as technically defensible as possible. We carefully studied the implementation of the demonstration, used the best available instruments, and made sure that we had sufficient statistical power to detect meaningful results. The worst outcome possible for the persons who designed the program, the clients, and for the persons who implemented the program would have been concluding that the program was harmful. Although the evaluator might not be pleased with this outcome, it is, nonetheless, an indicator that the evaluation performed an important function. Arguably, for the evaluator a null effect would be the worst outcome. When there are no meaningful differences found between the treatment and comparison groups there are three key attributions that can be made: (1) there really is no difference and thus the theory underlying the program was wrong; (2) there really was no difference but the program was poorly implemented and thus a poor test of the program theory; and (3) the evaluation was poorly designed or poorly implemented and no conclusions could be drawn. The field can learn something important based on reason 1 but the two others simply inform evaluators that either the conditions were not right for the program or the evaluation or that the staff were not competent. How can the evaluator help guard against outcomes 2 and 3? In the case of large-scale evaluations there is not much the evaluator can do about the quality of implementation because these evaluations tend to be summative, not formative (see Roberts & Steele, this volume). If formative evaluation is possible, systematic feedback from the evaluators may be provided to the program personnel on how to improve the program and improve implementation beforehand. For large-scale projects, a formative evaluation is not typically possible because it adds more expense and draws out the study longer. Regardless, the primary focus for the evaluator always has to be the quality of the evaluation and not post hoc redesign of the program itself.

Integrity and Controversy

Earlier we noted that there should be a correlation between the size of an evaluation and its visibility. The size of a project can present challenges for methods and design integrity. The Ft. Bragg research evaluation team struggled to keep the integrity of the design and the measures throughout the study while under considerable political pressure. For example, one of the few previous studies of children's mental health services (Burns, Thompson, & Goldman, 1993) could not collect clinical outcome data because the funder was only interested in cost reduction. Most importantly, however, throughout the project we felt that the Army questioned our integrity because we were closely associated with the program developer who had presented the Army with a package that included both the demonstration and the evaluation. They would have preferred to find and fund their own evaluator. However, the Army learned to trust our independence and our integrity after the results were delivered and even awarded us a contract to conduct additional analyses of the data at the termination of the evaluation.

REACTIONS TO THE STUDIES

For program evaluation, and most academic research, appraisal is a public process. Generally speaking, critique and interpretation are done initially by the program evaluators and program stakeholders, and then by the evaluation, research, or programmatic communities at large through publications and nonprint forums. Large-scale studies will receive large amounts of scrutiny and critical attention. In large-scale evaluations that attract widespread interest, the act of interpretation can be a complicated process that has the potential to become emotional and political in nature. In particular, when findings are not supportive of the prevailing thinking postevaluation criticisms may take on a life of their own.

Ideally, public scientific discourse resulting from a large project should focus on the meaning of data and not on questions about basic methodology. One might believe that if an evaluation is done well the results will speak for themselves. However, if findings are unpopular, no matter how well a large-scale evaluation has been conducted, or the extent of support for the design, both methods and data interpretation will be debated. One could argue that intense scrutiny *should* be directed at any large project spending lots of dollars. If the design or methods are truly flawed, discussion will be short-lived and critique will probably never reach the level of interpretation of the results. However, if the evaluation is well done, it will withstand detailed scrutiny and criticism. In planning the Ft. Bragg evaluation, possible criticisms were anticipated. Extensive data were collected on many different outcomes from many different sources. Subgroup analyses were conducted to test various hypotheses and explore extensively for possible effects. For example, we examined whether the continuum of care was more effective for children with different levels of severity and diagnoses (Bickman et al., 1995).

The Ft. Bragg demonstration and evaluation project was subjected to much scrutiny and debate over the course of several years. There was a wide range of responses to Ft. Bragg from many different types of professionals. In an interview with the first author about the Ft. Bragg and Stark evaluations published in the *American Journal of Evaluation,* Fitzpatrick (2002) states "... [they] have received more recognition in the field of evaluation than any study that I can recall in my 25 years of practice" (p. 69). Fitzpatrick also quotes several other evaluators from letters supporting the project for an award: "Tom Cook has cited the studies as "among the 10 or 20 best evaluation studies ever done in any field by anyone" (Fitzpatrick, 2002, p. 65). Carol Weiss called the evaluation "one of the landmark studies of the decade," noting not only its excellent research design, but also the integrity of the process and the courage in reporting unpopular results (in Fitzpatrick). Michael Patton noted "... the success of Bickman and his colleagues in disseminating the findings, engaging their critics in constructive discussion, and ultimately, achieving great import, influence, and utilization for the results." (cited in Fitzpatrick, p. 65). In reference to Ft. Bragg, Saxe and Cross (1997) stated: "It has generated unparalleled discussion of actual data on the effects of children's mental health services ... " (p. 555). The enduring and public nature of the critique and discussion about Ft. Bragg were a result of the cost of the project, the methodological rigor in which it was conducted, the dissemination efforts of the evaluation team, and the fact that the findings did not support the prevailing thinking. However, praise such as that described above was not found uniformly in the mental health community.

Although many reviewers found that Ft. Bragg was well done there were inevitable debates regarding basic qualities and even purpose of the evaluation. Criticism and discussion were directed at nearly every methodological and theoretical characteristic of the project. Although both demonstration and control sites showed substantial clinical improvement, the importance of efficacy and effectiveness of treatments used at the sites became a focus of discussion (Henggeler, Schoenwald, & Munger, 1996; Weisz, Han, & Valeri, 1997). DeLeon and Williams (1997) pointed out that approximately 80% of children improved at both demonstration and comparison sites, but also suggested that the results of Ft. Bragg should cause clinicians to question whether what they are doing has an impact. The question of effectiveness of the treatments was not an initial focus of the evaluation. The problem was that there was no *differential* effectiveness of the continuum-of-care model. Thus, although the discussion spawned by questions of treatment effectiveness did ultimately have a positive influence on children's mental health research (see below), maintaining focus on critical aspects of the project was difficult at times.

Some of the public discussion regarding Ft. Bragg surrounded implementation. Implementation studies are important for formative evaluation, as validity checks, and for satisfying later questions regarding null findings. Most authors commended the Ft. Bragg study for completing an implementation analysis. One limitation of the Ft. Bragg implementation study that emerged was that the evaluators conceptualized, or at least measured, implementation as a static event (Friedman & Burns, 1996). Although it is not always possible to continuously and validly measure implementation or fidelity, we now realize how important it is to try to do just that. Implementation and fidelity probably do evolve and change over time and need to be monitored continuously. We have also learned that the process of implementation should be guided by theory and planned to prevent failure, not simply analyzed post hoc. This is important in the implementation of empirically supported treatments (Bickman et al., in preparation) and has been highlighted in the continuous quality improvement approach.

One aspect of the project that received particular attention was the fact that it was conducted in a military setting. This was seen as a limitation in terms of the analysis of cost, the single agency in a "system" of care, and generalizability of the findings (Kingdon & Ichinose, 1996). Arguments regarding generalizability of evaluation findings are the easiest as well as the most difficult type of criticism to address. What makes defending generalizability easy is that the assertion of poor generalizability must have some specific concern or basis to be valid. Most often assertions regarding lack of generalizability are not associated with specific theoretical hypotheses. Given adequate scientific practices the onus, or burden of proof, falls on the critic to provide a reasonable explanation for why findings do not apply to the population at large. To successfully support this argument the critical dimensions upon which results are not generalizable need to be spelled out (Sechrest & Walsh, 1997). The difficult aspect of defending the generalizability of a study is that despite a lack of a logical or theoretical basis for the criticism beliefs surrounding it may persist.

Several special journal issues, prompted by the evaluators, were published to provide forums for Ft. Bragg debate. One of the most illuminating series of articles about Ft. Bragg appeared in a special issue of the *American Psychologist*. In this special issue Sechrest and Walsh (1997) were instrumental in directing the public debate back to the basics of research methods and practices. They reiterated the basic purpose and intent of the project, the types of validities necessary to judge a study, as well as how the Ft. Bragg study compared against those validities. The authors invoked the "principle of symmetry" (often ignored or forgotten in interpretation of research). They pointed out that, assuming that acceptable standards of scientific practice have been met, all reasonable interpretations of a valid scientific process need to be treated equally. One cannot dismiss the outcome of the research process simply because it does not conform to preexisting beliefs.

Potentially consequential evaluation projects benefit greatly from the practice of keeping the evaluators independent from the program they are evaluating. Several authors noted the importance of this in the Ft. Bragg discussions (Behar, 1997; Weisz et al. 1997). The importance of independent evaluators becomes even more crucial under circumstances when a majority of stakeholders see the results as unfavorable. Although program funders, developers, and staff should always be aware of the potential for null findings, the consequences and acceptance of findings (given proper methods and implementation) need to be discussed before summative evaluation begins. Independence and objectivity adds credibility and validity to evaluation findings regardless of the outcomes and cannot be stressed enough here.

RESPONSE TO THE REACTIONS

In response to some criticisms additional analyses were conducted. However, having a large data set at one's disposal can lead to over-analysis or over-interpretation. By this we mean the kind of minute analyses and post hoc explanations that were not part of the analysis plan and are typically carried out in the presence of null findings. The core Ft. Bragg analyses were planned *a priori* and relied on patterns of effects over time and clinical significance as a relatively more important indicator of differences between the demonstration and control sites (Evans & Banks, 1996). In program evaluation, the main hypotheses should be explicated, core measures examined, and all principal analyses completed before the data are taken apart in the process of addressing post hoc critiques. Although it may be difficult to defend not doing more and more analyses to satisfy many critics, the findings are rarely changed through that process, and are more likely to be obfuscated in details.

The relative focus on some null findings may overshadow other aspects of large projects and minor but positive results may be relatively ignored. Some authors did focus on positive findings in the Ft. Bragg evaluation. For example, there were benefits associated with the demonstration site: a significantly larger number of children were seen, client satisfaction was higher, children stayed in treatment longer, more of the less restrictive type of treatments was provided, and fewer subjects had only a single session in the demonstration site (DeLeon & Williams, 1997; Friedman & Burns, 1996; National Institute of Mental Health, 1998; Saxe & Cross, 1997). However, the evaluators noted that these positive features did not result in better clinical outcomes and increased the cost of services.

The Ft. Bragg evaluation generated many thoughtful ideas, comments, and concerns by a wide range of evaluators and mental health professionals. Although some issues had been put to rest, questions remained that could not be resolved through further data analyses or discussion. The

Stark County project was designed to address some of the issues raised in the discussion of Ft. Bragg (e.g., quasi-experiment, military families, single agency system). Stark County findings, although similar to Ft. Bragg, did not generate the same type of widespread scrutiny and response. This second evaluation served to provide additional data and some closure regarding several theoretical and methodological concerns surrounding Ft. Bragg. Together, the two projects addressed, as thoroughly as was possible, the questions that the evaluators set out to answer, the methodological concerns of critics, and moved the public discussion closer toward the implications of the findings.

What may have been the last official word on the Ft. Bragg and Stark County evaluations came from the Surgeon General's report on mental health (NIMH, 1998). Ultimately, the report provided a balanced summary of the positive findings, the null findings, and the impact that the evaluation had on children's mental health research. The report stated that a shift in focus from the organization of mental health services to the mental health interventions themselves was indicated for the field as a result of the Ft. Bragg and Stark County studies.

This review hopefully underscores the duration, range, and nature of public criticism that is possible in the process of conducting large-scale evaluations. Sechrest and Walsh (1997) pondered what the public discourse would or could have been if potential critics had been involved in the planning of the evaluation. Although this is not always feasible or advisable, this is a relevant idea to consider in planning large projects as they have the potential to affect many programs and individuals. However, if an evaluation is well done it should withstand criticisms. Most importantly, regardless if a general consensus is reached about the conclusions, large projects provide a spotlight and public forum for important issues and weaknesses in children's mental health to be debated.

CONSEQUENCES AND IMPLICATIONS

Thoughtful criticism of Ft. Bragg brought about attention to important problems that were not unique to Ft. Bragg, but that the entire field needed to deal with such as the limited measurement options in children's mental health, particularly the need for measures that are sensitive to change over time (Friedman & Burns, 1996), to the use of and importance of the theory of change in evaluation (Friedman & Burns), the importance of the effectiveness of community mental health interventions (Henggeler et al., 1996; Weisz et al., 1997), and the timing, nature, and utility of large evaluation projects. Interestingly, few critics explicitly called for further demonstration and evaluation projects (DeLeon & Williams, 1997; Evans & Banks, 1996). This seems to have indicated an immediate and collective step back from large-scale projects.

There are clearly unpredictable risks as well as benefits of large-scale evaluation projects. Scientific discovery, innovation, and change are reliably associated with both positive and negative unintended consequences. Ft. Bragg and Stark County undoubtedly resulted in both negative and positive unintended consequences. Although not unique to large-scale projects, one must be ready to "take the heat" for large-scale expenditures with null findings. One possible unintended consequence of large-scale studies is that the field may see the pendulum of science and policy swing far back in another direction. For example, the conclusion that any or all systems-level changes are ineffective was not warranted. Similarly, broad conclusions that large-scale studies are unjustifiable or unhelpful may be an example of this type of "overcorrection." Is there a time at which anyone can say a field of research is "ready" for a large-scale study? There are no simple answers to this question. Agency funding priorities do not always coincide with the evolution of a given scientific area. However, thoughtful public discussion related to the timing and appropriateness of large-scale studies for a particular field will bring about a more efficacious use of research dollars.

What does the future hold for large-scale evaluations? Having focused on system-level variables in these evaluations and finding no effect, it was time to reconsider other elements that could bring about change in clinical outcomes. What were the gaps that Ft. Bragg uncovered on which research should focus? First, investigators need to be able to measure outcomes in the real world. It was clear that few community-based services had the ability to determine if they were delivering effective services. Second, investigators need to look at the general process of care to determine those mediators that are important in affecting outcomes. For example, the adult literature is clear that therapeutic alliance, the relationship between the provider and the client, can be very important. Third, clinical investigators have recognized that the clinician is a key element in changing services. We have developed a comprehensive theory of change that could be applied to changing the behavior of the professionals and implementation of workplace innovations (Bickman et al., in preparation; Riemer & Bickman, submitted).

Larger studies do have a relatively greater potential to act as a catalyst for positive changes in the field. The most obvious effects of the Ft. Bragg and Stark evaluations was to shift the focus of the children's mental health research community, to influence how the field thinks about large-scale studies, society's propensity to fund them, and how evaluators interpret and use their results. Recommendations that we focus on efficacy and effectiveness of interventions and stay with small science until the time is "ripe" for large-scale evaluations seem to be the consensus. Post Ft. Bragg, it seems that there is more emphasis on and necessity for building bridges between the research and clinical worlds with the examination of services under real-world conditions a greater a priority. Finally, there is more attention being paid to evaluating treatments rather than systems, as evidenced by such efforts on empirically supported treatments and transportability of laboratory-developed service to the community.

REFERENCES

Andrade, A. R., Lambert, E. W., & Bickman, L. (2000). Dose effect in child psychotherapy: Outcomes associated with negligible treatment. *Journal of the American Academy of Child & Adolescent Psychiatry, 39,* 161–168.

Behar, L. B. (1997). The Fort Bragg evaluation: A snapshot in time. *American Psychologist, 52,* 557–559.

Bickman, L. (1981). Some distinctions between basic and applied social psychology. In L. Bickman (Ed.), *Applied social psychology annual* (Vol. 2, pp. 23–44). Beverly Hills: Sage.

Bickman, L. (1992). Resource planning for applied research. In F. Bryant, J. Edwards, L. Heath, E. Posavac, & R. Tindel (Eds.), *Methodological issues in applied social psychology* (pp. 1–24). New York: Plenum.

Bickman, L. (Ed.). (1996). Special Issue: Methodological issues in evaluating mental health services. *Evaluation and Program Planning, 19*(2).

Bickman, L. (2000). Improving Children's Mental Health: How no effects can affect policy. *Emotional and Behavioral Disorders in Youth, 1,* 3–4, 21–23.

Bickman, L., Andrade, A. R., & Lambert, E. W. (2002). Dose response in child and adolescent mental health services. *Mental Health Services Research, 4,* 57–70.

Bickman, L., & Fitzpatrick, J. L. (2002). Evaluation of the Ft. Bragg and Stark County systems of care for children and adolescents. *American Journal of Evaluation, 23,* 69–80.

Bickman, L., Guthrie, P. R., Foster, E. M., Lambert, E. W., Summerfelt, W. T., Breda, C. S. et al. (1995). *Evaluating managed mental health services: The Fort Bragg experiment.* New York: Plenum.

Bickman, L., & Heflinger, C. A. (1994). Seeking success by reducing implementation and evaluation failures. In L. Bickman & D. J. Rog (Eds.), *Children's mental health services: Research, policy and innovation* (pp. 171–205). Newberry Park, CA: Sage.

Bickman, L., Heflinger, C. A., Northrup, D., Sonnichsen, S., & Schilling, S. (1998). Long term outcomes to family caregiver empowerment. *Journal of Child and Family Studies, 7,* 269–282.

Bickman, L., Karver, M., & Schut, L. J. A. (1997). Clinician reliability and accuracy in judging appropriate level of care. *Journal of Consulting and Clinical Psychology, 65,* 515–520.

Bickman, L., Lambert, E. W., Karver, M. S., & Andrade, A. R. (1998). Two low-cost measures of child and adolescent functioning for services research. *Evaluation and Program Planning, 21,* 263–275.

Bickman, L., Noser, K., & Summerfelt, W. T. (1999). Long term effects of a system of care on children and adolescents. *The Journal of Behavioral Health Services and Research, 26,* 185–202.

Bickman, L., Riemer, M., & Mulvaney, S. (in preparation). Psychological factors that influence the implementation of empirically supported treatments.

Bickman, L., & Salzer, M. S. (Eds.). (1997). Special issue: Measuring quality in mental health services. *Evaluation Review.*

Bickman, L., Summerfelt, W. T., & Bryant, D. (1996). The quality of services in a children's mental health managed care demonstration. *The Journal of Mental Health Administration, 23,* 30–39.

Brannan, A. M., Heflinger, C. A., & Bickman, L. (1997). The caregiver strain questionnaire: Measuring the impact on the family of living with a child with serious emotional disturbance. *Journal of Emotional and Behavioral Disorders, 5,* 212–222.

Breda, C. S., & Bickman, L. (1997). Termination of mental health services for children. *Journal of Child and Family Studies, 6,* 69–87.

Burns, B. J., Thompson, J. W., & Goldman, H. H. (1993). Initial treatment decisions by level of care for youth in the Champus Tidewater Demonstration. *Administration and Policy in Mental Health, 20,* 231–246.

DeLeon, P., & Williams, J. (1997). Evaluation research and public policy formation: Are psychologists collectively willing to accept unpopular findings? *American Psychologist, 52,* 551–552.

Evans, M. E., & Banks, S. M. (1996). The Fort Bragg managed care experiment. *Journal of Child and Family Studies, 5*, 169–172.

Fitzpatrick, J. L. (2002). A conversation with Leonard Bickman on the evaluation of the Ft. Bragg and Stark County systems of care for children and adolescents. *American Journal of Evaluation, 23*, 69–80.

Friedman, R. M., & Burns, B. J. (1996). The evaluation of the Fort Bragg demonstration project: An alternative interpretation of the findings. *Journal of Mental Health Administration, 23*(1), 128–136.

Foster, E. M., & Bickman, L. (2000). Refining the cost analysis of the Fort Bragg evaluation: The impact of cost offset and cost shifting. *Mental Health Services Research, 2*, 13–25.

Heflinger, C. A., & Bickman, L. (1996). Family Empowerment: A theoretically driven intervention and evaluation. In C. A. Heflinger & C. Nixon (Eds.), *Families and mental health services for children and adolescents* (Vol. 2, pp. 96–116). Newbury Park, CA: Sage.

Henggeler, S., Schoenwald, S., & Munger, R. (1996). Families and therapists achieve clinical outcomes, systems of care mediate the process. *Journal of Child and Family Studies, 5*, 177–183.

Kingdon, D. W., & Ichinose, C. K. (1996). The Fort Bragg managed care experiment: What do the results mean for publicly funded systems of care? *Journal of Child and Family Studies, 5*, 191–195.

Lambert, E. W., Brannan, A. M., Breda, C., Heflinger, C. A., & Bickman, L. (1998). Common patterns of service use in children's mental health. *Evaluation and Program Planning, 21*, 47–57.

Lambert, E. W., Doucette, A., & Bickman, L. (2001). Measuring mental health outcomes with pre-post designs. *Journal of Behavioral Health Services Research, 28*, 273–286.

Lambert, W., Salzer, M. S., & Bickman, L. (1998). Clinical outcome, consumer satisfaction, and ad hoc ratings of improvement in children's mental health. *Journal of Consulting and Clinical Psychology, 66*, 270–279.

Lambert, E. W., Wahler, R. G., Andrade, A. R., & Bickman, L. (2001). Looking for the disorder in conduct disorder. *Journal of Abnormal Psychology, 110*, 110–123.

National Institute of Mental Health. (1998). *Bridging science and service: A report by the National Advisory Mental Health Council's Clinical Treatment and Services Research Workgroup* (pp. 99–4353). Rockville, MD: National Institutes of Health, National Institute of Mental Health.

Salzer, M. S., Bickman, L., & Lambert, E. W. (1999). Dose–effect relationship in children's psychotherapy. *Journal of Consulting and Clinical Psychology, 67*, 228–238.

Saxe, L., & Cross, T. P. (1997). Interpreting the Fort Bragg Children's Mental Health Demonstration Project: The cup is half full. *American Psychologist, 52*, 553–556.

Sechrest, L., & Walsh, M. (1997). Dogma or data: Bragging rights. *American Psychologist, 52*, 536–540.

Weisz, J. R., Han, S. S., & Valeri, S. M. (1997). More of what? Issues raised by the Fort Bragg study. *American Psychologist, 52*, 541–545.

25

Methodological Challenges in the National Evaluation of the Comprehensive Community Mental Health Services for Children and Their Families Program

E. WAYNE HOLDEN, ROBERT L. STEPHENS, and ROLANDO L. SANTIAGO

The Comprehensive Community Mental Health Services for Children and Their Families Program is the federal government's principal response to the service needs of the estimated 4.5–6.3 million children in the United States who have serious emotional disturbance (Friedman, Katz-Leavy,

E. WAYNE HOLDEN and ROBERT L. STEPHENS • Applied Research Division, ORC Macro, Atlanta, Georgia 30329.   ROLANDO L. SANTIAGO • Center for Mental Health Services, Substance Abuse and Mental Health Services Administration, Rockville, Maryland 20857.

Work on this chapter by the first two authors was supported by contracts 280-97-8014, 280-99-8023, and 280-00-8040 from the federal Center for Mental Health Services, Substance Abuse and Mental Health Services Administration, United States Department of Health and Human Services.

This chapter would not have been possible without the hard work and assistance of family members, service providers, evaluators, and project directors at the communities funded by the Comprehensive Community Mental Health Services for Children and Their Families Program. In addition, national evaluation team members at ORC Macro were instrumental in conducting the research and evaluation work that serves as a basis for this chapter.

Portions of this chapter were based upon a presentation made at the 110th annual meeting of the American Psychological Association, August 23, 2002, Chicago, IL.

Manderscheid, & Sondheimer, 1999). The program provides grants to states, communities, territories, and American Indian tribes to improve and expand their systems of care to meet the needs of children and adolescents with serious emotional disturbance and their families. These include children and youth with a serious emotional disturbance (SED) from birth to the age of 21 years who currently have, or at any time during the past year, had a mental, behavioral, or emotional disorder of sufficient duration to meet diagnostic criteria specified in the DSM-IV (American Psychiatric Association, 1994). In addition, this diagnosis must have resulted in functional impairment that substantially interferes with or limits one or more major life activities. The program is administered by the Child, Adolescent, and Family Branch within the Substance Abuse and Mental Health Services Administration's (SAMHSA) Center for Mental Health Services (CMHS).

This program is the translation of the systems-of-care approach first articulated by Stroul and Friedman in 1986 and now a major organizing force shaping the development of community-based children's mental health services in the United States. The model includes a comprehensive spectrum of mental health and other necessary services and supports that are guided by a specified set of principles (see Fig. 1). Whereas the actual

---

Definition of Systems-of-Care Principles

Family focused – The recognition that (a) the ecological context of the family is central to the care of all children; (b) families are important contributors to, and equal partners in, any effort to serve children; and (c) all system and service processes should be planned to maximize family involvement.

Culturally competent – Sensitivity and responsiveness to, and acknowledgment of, the inherent value of differences related to race, religion, language, national origin, gender, socioeconomic background, and community-specific characteristics.

Interagency – The involvement and partnership of core agencies in multiple child-serving sectors, including child welfare, health, juvenile justice, education, and mental health.

Community based – The provision of services within close geographical proximity to the targeted community.

Accessible – The minimizing of barriers to services in terms of physical location, convenience of scheduling, and financial constraints.

Coordination or collaboration – Professionals working together in a complimentary manner to avoid duplication of services, eliminate gaps in care, and facilitate the child's and family's movement through the service system.

Individualized – The provision of care that is expressly child centered, addresses the child's specific needs, and recognizes and incorporates the child's strengths.

Least restrictive – The priority that services should be delivered in settings that maximize freedom of choice and movement, and that present opportunities to interact in normative environments (e.g., school and family).

Figure 1. Definition of Systems-of-Care Principles.

components and organizational configurations of the system of care may differ from community to community, the key components of the model include *individualized*, *family-focused*, and *culturally competent* services and supports. These should be *community based* and *accessible*, and provided in the *least restrictive* environment possible through a *collaborative, coordinated interagency* network.

To explain how systems of care are intended to work, a *theory-based framework* was developed with input from program stakeholders across the country (Hernandez & Hodges, 2003). The framework articulates the underlying assumptions that guide service delivery strategies and are believed to be critical to producing change and improvement in children and families. It has three core elements—population, strategies, and outcome—as well as a mission statement, guiding principles, and an evaluation or feedback cycle. The mission statement addresses the need for intensive community-based services for children with SED and their families. The guiding principles provide a foundation upon which systems-of-care strategies are built. These strategies are grounded in a community ownership and planning process that engages multiple partners. Outcomes are organized into practice, child and family, and system outcomes. The framework includes an evaluation or feedback cycle making use of the best and most current research and incorporates concepts of internal evaluation, quality improvement, adaptation, and accountability.

This federal demonstration program has resulted in widespread implementation of the systems-of-care approach and principles. Since its inception, the potential for children and their families to receive mental health services and supports in their own communities has grown, as has the number of providers and stakeholders knowledgeable about and committed to delivering services using a systems-of-care approach. Grant-funded communities have actively expanded their service arrays, adding new services and tailoring others to meet the specific needs of their communities (Brannan, Baughman, Reed, & Katz-Leavy, 2002; Holden & Brannan, 2002; Holden, Friedman, & Santiago, 2001b; Holden et al., 2003; Vinson, Brannan, Baughman, Wilce, & Gawron, 2001). Breaking with the past, the norm in the grant communities is for families to be partners in service planning and provision and, in many grant communities, in evaluating services (Osher, van Kammen, & Zaro, 2001). There is growing recognition of the importance of natural support systems within culturally diverse communities and the advantage of adapting services to be congruent with them (Cross, Earle, Echo-Hawk Solie, & Manness, 2000; Running Wolf et al., 2002). In some cases, changes in policies at the state and federal levels have led to legislation that supports system change both within and beyond the grant communities (Holden, De Carolis, & Huff, 2002). Finally, systems-of-care proponents have been able, in some instances, to harness managed care technologies to further systems-of-care goals (Stroul, Pires, Armstrong, & Zaro, 2002).

A legislatively mandated national, cross-site evaluation of the Comprehensive Community Mental Health Services for Children and Their Families Program began in 1994. The evaluation responds to the legislation authorizing the program (Public Health Service Act 565), which requires an annual evaluation to (1) describe the children and families served by the systems-of-care initiative, (2) assess how systems of care develop and what factors impede or enhance development, (3) measure whether children served through the program experience improvement in clinical and functional outcomes and whether those improvements endure over time and why, (4) determine whether the consumers are satisfied with the services they receive, and (5) measure the costs associated with the implementation of a system of care and determine its cost effectiveness. Besides responding to the legislation, the evaluation serves as a laboratory for addressing many of the questions described above. Findings from the evaluation also provide information upon which to base future treatment, program, funding, and policy decisions (Holden et al., 2002, 2003).

Any mental health services evaluation must be undertaken with the recognition that a complex set of factors determines the outcomes for a particular child and family. Key questions often posited in mental health services research are: What works? For whom? And under what conditions? (Burns & Hoagwood, 2002). These questions are not easy or straightforward to answer. The service system is one critical factor, but others, such as child and family characteristics and the quality of treatment, must be taken into consideration as well (Friedman, 2001; Friedman & Hernandez, 2002). The national evaluation is designed to address many complex and related dimensions of effectiveness. It is longitudinal in nature; children and families are followed over time so that changes in outcomes can be understood from a developmental point of view. It includes a comprehensive assessment of outcomes across several domains. The service delivery systems are also assessed over time, so that their developmental trajectories can be better understood. This process includes identifying the ingredients necessary to sustain systems of care, whether system-level changes result in concomitant practice-level changes, and how families engage in systems of care. Other critical questions addressed by the evaluation include whether systems of care are more effective than traditional service systems in improving outcomes for children with SED and whether providing community-based mental health services and supports to this population are cost effective. This level of complexity is necessary to understand the relationships between system, practice, and individual outcomes, recognizing that changes at different levels can occur simultaneously. The evaluation is comprehensive and includes the 92 grantees, the children and families served by the programs, service providers, and partner agencies (Holden, Friedman, & Santiago, 2001a; Holden et al., 2003). It also includes information from nonfunded comparison communities. The number of grantees and participants, the number of components, and the variety of methodologies incorporated into the evaluation are extensive.

The two major goals of this large-scale program evaluation are (1) to obtain an overall program evaluation of the Comprehensive Community Mental Health Services for Children and Their Families Program that informs federal policy making and (2) to develop evaluation capacity locally within the funded communities. The second goal is directed toward improving quality assurance, management information systems, and sustainability of programs post-federal funding by informing local- and state-level policy development. In the conduct of a large-scale program evaluation, a significant amount of tension can exist between these two goals. This dynamic tension creates a unique contextual challenge that has implications for the overall design and successful implementation of evaluation strategies.

METHODOLOGICAL CHALLENGES

A program evaluation of this size and scope has not been without significant methodological challenges, some that were apparent at the beginning of the evaluation 10 years ago, and others that have become apparent as the evaluation and the services program itself have evolved over time. Key methodological challenges and their solutions are discussed below.

Conducting a Multisite Evaluation

Coordination of evaluation and research activities across multiple funded sites is a consistent challenge for large-scale program evaluations (Herrell & Straw, 2002). This evaluation simultaneously maintains a cross-site focus to obtain and utilize information at the federal program level and a within-site focus to obtain and utilize information at the individual grantee level. For the most part, data collection activities overlap with these dual and complementary purposes. Consistent implementation and quality monitoring of data collection require close partnering with site-level evaluation personnel (who are employed by the individual grantees) and national evaluation personnel. This coordination is accomplished through consistent communication via electronic media, including an Internet-based data collection and management system, multiple technical assistance and training visits to each funded community, national training meetings for site evaluation staff, quality monitoring protocols to track progress, and consistent national evaluation staff responsiveness to problems that are being encountered in the field. The provision of analyzed and interpreted information from the national evaluation for use in the field on a regular basis and the engagement of local evaluators in the analysis and interpretation of data at the national level have created a learning community of evaluators that heightens motivation to maintain quality in the field and overall coordination of evaluation activities.

Developing and Selecting Measures

Variables at multiple levels from the individual child to the family to the service system have been targeted for assessment as part of the evaluation. These levels of measurement have been dictated partially by the systems-of-care theoretical model (Hernandez & Hodges, 2003; Stroul,

1996; Stroul & Friedman, 1986) and partially by the emerging literature on the effectiveness of children's mental health services (Bickman et al., 1995; Burns & Hoagwood, 2002; Burns, Hoagwood, & Mrazek, 1999). Measures used to assess variables at the individual child and family level have been selected based upon strong psychometric characteristics and comparability of use within the children's mental health services field. Many of these measures have proven to be quite useful in evaluating individual and family change across time (CMHS, 1998, 1999, 2000, 2001, 2002; Manteuffel, Stephens, & Santiago, 2002).

Measures of more complex constructs such as systems development and services experiences have required a high level of investment to develop and implement. The systems-of-care theoretical model posits that implementation of a system of care within a community will produce system-level changes (e.g., increased interagency collaboration, a wider array of traditional and innovative services, flexible funding arrangements, increased involvement of consumers, culturally competent services, etc.) that will alter the care that is provided directly to children and families and result in positive outcomes. This major tenet of the model required the development of a measurement approach for evaluating systems-of-care implementation and development that did not previously exist in the children's mental health arena. To address this methodological challenge, the systems-of-care assessment protocol was developed (Brannan et al., 2002; Vinson et al., 2001). This protocol consists of a mixed quantitative and qualitative methodology with data collected through semistructured interviews conducted with multiple stakeholders during regular site visits to grant-funded communities. The data obtained are scored within a conceptual framework to evaluate the operationalization of the major systems-of-care principles across the infrastructure and service delivery dimensions of children's mental health services. These data are also analyzed qualitatively to evaluate factors influencing the development of child-serving systems. To complement this system-level measure, an individual case study protocol was developed to assess the experiences of services at the interface between providers and families (Hernandez et al., 2001). Scores from this measure have been significantly related to reductions in behavioral and emotional symptoms 12 months after entering services (Stephens, Holden, & Hernandez, 2004).

Ecological validity has been an important issue to be addressed within the measurement area. Some consumers and some providers within systems of care do not respond positively to deficit-oriented measures due to direct conflicts with the underlying strengths-based philosophy of the systems-of-care approach. The evaluation has responded by incorporating a measure of strengths that has shown greater positive change within the first 6 months of services within systems of care than symptom-oriented scales (CMHS, 2001, 2002) and has been widely accepted at the program level. Functional indicators, such as educational progress and juvenile justice involvement, have also received greater acceptance from consumers, service providers, and policy makers than measures of symptoms and impairment.

Integrating Quantitative and Qualitative Data Collection and Analysis

As discussed previously, measurement approaches have been developed for this evaluation that use mixed methodologies to comprehensively capture complex systems constructs. For the most part, these data collection methodologies rely on qualitative methods for obtaining data through semistructured or open-ended interview protocols. These data have been directly analyzed using qualitative software or more basic content analysis approaches. In addition, scoring systems have been used to derive quantitative information from these qualitative data. Interrater reliability and internal consistency of these scoring systems have been within the acceptable range and have been monitored closely across time (Brannan et al., 2002; Vinson et al., 2001).

The integration of qualitative and quantitative data within analyses is currently ongoing. This has involved clustering sites based on characteristics of their systems of care and concurrently analyzing differences in their descriptive and longitudinal outcome data. These complex analyses must take into account the substantial variability in demographics, target populations, services array, and overall structure of grant-funded programs. The actual array of services and procedures for service provision are embedded within individual communities and the cultural context influencing the development of systems of care. With the continuing accumulation of system-level data from the currently funded programs, multilevel analyses (Brannan et al., 2002) that relate the degree of community- and system-level change directly to child and family outcomes are possible. For example, a recent analysis of these data using hierarchical linear modeling revealed that the level of collaborative or coordinated care in grant-funded communities at their initial systems-of-care assessment was related to behavioral and emotional outcomes, with higher levels of care predicting greater positive change across time (Gilford, Stephens, & Foster, 2003). Furthermore, the extent to which a system had implemented the principle of collaborative or coordinated care differentiated the influence that race had on rates of change in clinical symptoms across systems. These results suggest that the racial disparities present in other areas of the health care delivery system are also present in systems of care.

Study Design and Analysis Challenges

Since its inception, the national evaluation has attempted to address the overall question of the effectiveness of systems of care. Because it was not feasible to randomly assign children to service delivery systems, the national evaluation has employed quasi-experimental matched comparison group designs that match federally funded systems of care to service delivery systems without federal funding for the development of a system of care. A complex set of issues is involved in conducting and analyzing the results of these studies. These comparatively weak designs lack the power to detect effects within community settings where sources of error variance are much more difficult to control than in university settings where efficacy trials are typically conducted. Lack of assessment of the specific types of treatments delivered within outpatient settings and interactions at the service provider–family level have hampered the ability to determine who benefits most from what treatment. This is compounded by the heterogeneity of presenting problems for the samples that are being treated within community settings making it difficult in quasi-experimental designs to identify differential change vectors.

These contextual factors have had a significant impact on data analysis approaches within the national evaluation. Statistical approaches for analyzing change have advanced significantly over the last decade. These more sophisticated analyses of change strategies have proven to be useful in addressing hypotheses about variables that may be significantly related to change rates in systems of care. Although many questions continue about the effectiveness of systems of care at the clinical outcome level (Burns & Hoagwood, 2002; U.S. Department of Health and Human Services [USDHHS], 1999), data exist to support continued work on the implementation of the approach within community settings.

Results from these comparison studies have documented differences in systems development (Brannan et al., 2002) and services experiences (Hernandez et al., 2001), with federally funded programs displaying greater operationalization of key systems-of-care principles at the community and services experience levels, and appropriately matched subsets of children displaying more positive outcomes in systems-of-care programs (Greenbaum & Brown, 2002). Although spending within the mental health sector is higher within federally funded communities, cost offsets occur within juvenile justice, child welfare, and education that result in near-equal community expenditures for the care of children with serious emotional disturbance (Foster & Connor, 2004). Differential outcomes using symptom-based and functional impairment measures continue to be difficult to clearly detect within these large, weakly powered quasi-experimental designs.

Maintaining a Utilization Focus and Stakeholder Involvement

The national evaluation has consistently maintained stakeholder involvement and a utilization focus (Patton, 1997) since its inception. Multiple stakeholders, including family members, service delivery personnel, program administrators, policy makers, and researchers, were involved in the initial design of the evaluation and have continued to provide advisory input and feedback as the evaluation has evolved over the last 9 years. This has been accomplished through yearly advisory board meetings and regular, ongoing input through workgroup participation on specific tasks that were being implemented within this large-scale program evaluation. Satisfying the needs of the multiple stakeholder groups for evaluation information can be a daunting task. Conflicts occur between groups with respect to priorities for the evaluation, and many of these conflicts have not been easy to resolve. For example, family members' concerns lie with the acceptability of the data that are collected and the direct relevance of the information for continued service provision for their children. Researchers, on the other hand, are more concerned with methodologic and analytic rigor and the utility of the results within the scientific community (e.g., peer-reviewed publications). Reconciling these differences requires educating the different stakeholder groups about the various needs and priorities and creating common concerns across groups.

Taking a utilization approach and heavily involving stakeholders in evaluation is not without controversy. Many professional researchers maintain that objectivity and methodologic rigor may be sacrificed from too extensive involvement of stakeholder groups in the evaluation process. Alternatively, stakeholder groups are concerned about the relevance of information, especially when the results of methodologically elegant and analytically sophisticated studies are not made available to consumers and the general public outside of the peer-reviewed literature or presentations within the professional research community. National evaluators of large service delivery programs such as the Comprehensive Community Mental Health Services for Children and Their Families Program often find themselves in the role of translators of information between stakeholder groups and facilitators of collaborative relationships between groups that may on the surface appear to have conflicting goals and priorities.

Addressing the Evolution of Research Questions Across Time

A number of issues arise as a result of conducting large-scale community-level effectiveness studies over a lengthy period of time. The general context of the research literature may shift and change, directly affecting the relevance of the questions that are being addressed. New measures or restandardization of existing measures may occur, which require consideration of shifting measurement strategies midstream within longitudinal designs. There are advantages and disadvantages to decisions that are made to address these issues within the context of longitudinal research with children and families within community settings (Black & Holden, 1995).

The questions of critical importance throughout the evaluation have revolved around effectiveness defined on a broad scale. At the initiation of the evaluation, the initial results of the Fort Bragg Evaluation Project (Bickman et al., 1995) indicated that continuum-of-care services had a negligible effect on clinical outcomes when compared to services as usual for military dependents, with increased costs for children receiving these enhanced mental health services. Access to services and satisfaction were higher for the group that participated in the continuum of care. A smaller follow-up study in Ohio using a randomized design (Bickman, Noser, & Summerfelt, 1999), further emphasized the lack of differences in clinical outcomes between children participating in a system of care versus those receiving other community-based services. Despite the disadvantages of the design, the national evaluation initiated quasi-experimental comparison studies to provide a more controlled test of the effectiveness of the systems-of-care approach. As noted previously, initial analyses of these complex data have provided support for the development of systems of care at the program or community level (Brannan et al., 2002) and documentation of service delivery experiences that are consistent with systems-of-care principles (Hernandez et al., 2001; Stephens et al., 2004). For small, selected samples of children on specific measures, improved outcomes appear to be obtained (Greenbaum & Brown, 2002), and medication effects, when closely monitored, appear to produce greater reductions in functional impairment for children and adolescents participating in systems of care (Holden, 2002). As expected, more financial resources are devoted to mental health services within funded communities, although a broader costs perspective across child-serving agencies suggests that this investment in communities with federally funded programs may offset increased costs within juvenile justice, inpatient or residential placements, child welfare, and education (Foster & Connor, 2004, Foster, Qaseem, & Connor, 2004). Although more information has been derived from these studies about the overall effectiveness of systems of care, incontrovertible evidence indicating a main effect for effectiveness at the level of differential clinical outcomes for all children and families has not emerged. Further analyses of these data that focus more on functional rather than clinical outcomes are currently underway that should continue to shed light on who benefits most from specific services within community settings.

The Surgeon General's Report on Mental Health (USDHHS, 1999) and the evidence-based treatment movement within children's mental health (Burns & Hoagwood, 2002) have affected the evolution of research questions and the direction of the evaluation. Systems of care are an area in need of further study, especially with respect to the integration of evidence-based interventions within these community-based programs. More recent special studies within the national evaluation are employing randomized clinical trial designs specifically to measure the effects of evidence-based interventions and survey methods to ascertain the degree to which evidence-based interventions are being implemented naturalistically and the variables affecting their implementation. These studies will not only assess the effectiveness of evidence-based interventions within systems of care on clinical outcomes, but also will collect both quantitative and qualitative information to identify facilitators and barriers to the faithful implementation of evidence-based interventions within community settings.

Administrative Oversight and Control

The data coordinating center for this federally funded program is under separate contract to the Center for Mental Health Services to conduct the national evaluation. On the one hand, national evaluation personnel are directly responsible to the Center for Mental Health Services for the design and conduct of the national evaluation protocol. On the other hand, site-level evaluation personnel are direct employees of the service grants and are responsible to the project directors and principal investigators of the community-based programs. Their responsibilities include both national evaluation data collection and other specific evaluation activities determined locally. Although central control of the service grants rests with the Center for Mental Health Services, the authority of the data coordinating center to conduct training, maintain quality control, and obtain data from the sites rests upon a complex collaborative relationship involving federal personnel, national evaluation personnel, grant program administrative personnel, and grant program evaluation staff. In summary, the coordinating center does not fund the service grants, but evaluates the programs when the federal government has direct oversight.

This complex set of relationships, which is not unusual in large-scale evaluations of federal programs (Herrell & Straw, 2002), presents a number of challenges. Selection of evaluation personnel at the grant programs is determined by a number of local-level factors that may conflict with the needs dictated by the national evaluation protocol. Capacity and competence to conduct a rigorous evaluation at the site level varies, especially in rural or remote areas where it is difficult to recruit and retain staff. This can have a significant impact on the quality of the data that are obtained. A finite level of resources at the data coordinating center level places limits on the degree of collaboration and control that can be exerted centrally on sites with lower levels of evaluation capacity or higher personnel turnover. Clarity of direction at the federal level can assist with bolstering the relationships between the data coordinating center and programs that are struggling to meet evaluation demands. Local political factors may also dictate the degree to which resources are directed toward supporting the national evaluation protocol relative to local evaluation and more pressing service delivery needs.

This set of dynamics creates an organizational context in which the types of collaborative relationships and level of control vary tremendously across the funded programs and in many instances change significantly over the course of conducting the evaluation. Despite devoting significant resources to training and monitoring of site activities across all funded programs, almost constant demands are placed on the data coordinating center staff for addressing the appropriate titration of collaboration and control at multiple sites for effectively conducting the evaluation. The degree to which these factors periodically affect the quality of data collection can have a significant impact on the integrity of the evaluation process. A recent study conducted by the Judge David L. Bazelon Center for Mental Health Law (2003), however, suggested that the integration of federal data collection and reporting requirements across funding streams may assist with the development of local evaluation capacity that can lead to the sustainability and expansion of services initiatives.

CONCLUSIONS AND FUTURE DIRECTIONS

The methodological challenges associated with conducting national evaluations of large-scale federal demonstration programs, such as the

Comprehensive Community Mental Health Services for Children and Their Families Program, are important to consider as we move into the future. Many of these challenges parallel those encountered in efforts to evaluate the effects of other socially complex services delivered in community settings (Herrell & Straw, 2002; Wolff, 2000). These include the difficulties encountered in measuring complex and innovative approaches that are being implemented in community-based service delivery settings whose structure and boundaries differ significantly from research settings. Conducting evaluations in these service delivery settings is also complicated by political, organizational, and financial parameters that shift continually across time. Without comprehensive evaluation information, however, the level of implementation of programs cannot be monitored effectively and the aggregate outcomes expected from these programs may be impossible to detect. Information on community-level effectiveness is critical for shaping and influencing program and policy development at the federal, state, and local levels.

Expansion of this information base in the future will benefit from a broad approach to program evaluation that spans the disciplines and methodologies that apply to public health concerns. Continued use of traditional experimental and quasi-experimental methodologies is a critical feature for understanding the transportability and effectiveness of evidence-based practice in community settings. Formative evaluation strategies that rely more on qualitative data collection and analysis to address emerging issues and innovative approaches developed in the field are equally as important. Undergirding the evaluation of children's mental health services within a public health conceptual framework, however, is perhaps the most important challenge that lies ahead for the field. Recent recommendations have been made for applying public health models such as diffusion of innovations into the dissemination of evidence-based practice (Schoenwald & Hoagwood, 2001), using broad public health constructs for understanding the relationships between evaluation and public policy (Friedman, 2003; Rosenblatt & Woodbridge, 2003) and more firmly integrating concepts from developmental epidemiology into the study of child and adolescent mental health (Mason, 2003; Tu, 2003). Public health models raise additional questions for evaluation such as penetrance of service delivery systems, the monitoring and surveillance of not only child and adolescent mental health but also the services that are being provided, and efficiency as well as equity of services provision in community settings.

The future of children's mental health services evaluation clearly will be contextualized by recent concerns raised by the international public health community and emerging policy initiatives. The publication of the World Health Report *Mental Health: New Understanding, New Hope* (World Health Organization [WHO], 2001) indicated that on an international level, increases of 15% in mental illness overall and 50% in childhood neuropsychiatric disorders are predicted by 2020, with the overall burden of mental health currently the leading cause of disability in the United States and Western Europe. In the United States, the President's New Freedom

Commission on Mental Health has completed studying and reviewing the federal government's role in promoting a more effective mental health service delivery system. The final report, *Achieving the Promise: Transforming Mental Health Care in America* (NFC, 2003), contains specific recommendations for improving community-based care for children with serious emotional disturbance. This report suggests that screening assessment and treatment in multiple community settings, consumer- and family-centered care, evidence-based practices, improved and expanded information infrastructure, and the elimination of disparities in care are critical to transforming the mental health system in the United States. The implementation of these recommendations will have direct implications for defining the questions that will be addressed in future evaluations of community-based children's mental health services.

REFERENCES

American Psychiatric Association. (1994). *Diagnostic and statistical manual of mental disorders* (4th ed.) Washington, DC: Author.

Bickman, L., Guthrie, P. R., Foster, E. M., Lambert, W., Summerfelt, W. T., Breda, C. S. et al. (1995). *Evaluating managed mental health services: The Fort Bragg experiment.* New York: Plenum.

Bickman, L., Noser, K., & Summerfelt, W. M. (1999). Long-term effects of a system of care on children and adolescents. *The Journal of Behavioral Health Services & Research, 26,* 185–202.

Black, M. M., & Holden, E. W. (1995). Longitudinal strategies for intervention research. *Journal of Clinical Child Psychology, 24,* 163–172.

Brannan, A. M., Baughman, L., Reed, E., & Katz-Leavy, J. (2002). System-of-care assessment: Cross-site comparison of findings. *Children's Services: Social Policy, Research, and Practice, 5,* 37–56.

Burns, B. J., & Hoagwood, K. (Eds.). (2002). *Community treatment for youth: Evidence-based interventions for severe emotional and behavioral disorders.* New York: Oxford University Press.

Burns, B. J., Hoagwood, K., & Mrazek, P. J. (1999). Effective treatment for mental disorders in children and adolescents. *Clinical Child and Family Psychology Review, 2,* 199–254.

Center for Mental Health Services. (1998). *Annual report to Congress on the evaluation of the Comprehensive Community Mental Health Services for Children and Their Families Program, 1998.* Atlanta, GA: Macro International.

Center for Mental Health Services. (1999). *Annual report to Congress on the evaluation of the Comprehensive Community Mental Health Services for Children and Their Families Program, 1999.* Atlanta, GA: ORC Macro.

Center for Mental Health Services. (2000). *Annual report to Congress on the evaluation of the Comprehensive Community Mental Health Services for Children and Their Families Program, 2000.* Manuscript under review, U.S. Department of Health and Human Services.

Center for Mental Health Services. (2001). *Annual report to Congress on the evaluation of the Comprehensive Community Mental Health Services for Children and Their Families Program, 2001.* Manuscript under review, U.S. Department of Health and Human Services.

Center for Mental Health Services. (2002). *Annual report to Congress on the evaluation of the Comprehensive Community Mental Health Services for Children and Their Families Program, 2002.* Manuscript under review, U.S. Department of Health and Human Services.

Cross, T., Earle, K., Echo-Hawk Solie, H., & Manness, K. (2000). Cultural strengths and challenges in implementing a system of care model in American Indian communities. *Systems of care: Promising practices in children's mental health, 2000 series* (Vol. I).

Washington, DC: Center for Effective Collaboration and Practice, American Institutes for Research.

Foster, E. M., & Connor, T. (2004). *The public costs of better mental health services for children and adolescents. Psychiatric Services.*

Foster, E. M., Qaseem, A., & Connor, T. (2004). Can better mental health services reduce juvenile justice involvement? *American Journal of Public Health, 94(5)*, 859–865.

Friedman, R. M. (2001). The practice of psychology with children, adolescents, and their families. In J. N. Hughes, A. M. La Greca, & J. C. Conoley (Eds.), *Handbook of psychological services for children and adolescents* (pp. 3–23). New York: Oxford University Press.

Friedman, R. M. (2003). A conceptual framework for developing and implementing effective policy in children's mental health. *Journal of Emotional and Behavioral Disorders, 11*, 11–18.

Friedman, R. M., & Hernandez, M. (2002). The national evaluation of the Comprehensive Community Mental Health Services for Children and Their Families Program: A commentary. *Children's Services: Social Policy, Research, and Practice, 5*, 67–74.

Friedman, R. M., Katz-Leavy, J. W., Manderscheid, R. W., & Sondheimer, D. L. (1999). Prevalence of serious emotional disturbance: An update. In R. W. Manderscheid & M. J. Henderson (Eds.), *Mental health, United States, 1998* (pp. 110–112). Rockville, MD: U.S. Department of Health and Human Services.

Gilford, J. W., Jr., Stephens, R. L., & Foster, E. M. (2003, March). *The influence of system-of-care implementation on clinical outcomes.* Presentation at the 16th Annual Research Conference, A System of Care for Children's Mental Health: Expanding the Research Base, Tampa, FL.

Greenbaum, P. E., & Brown, E. C. (2002, May). *Growth mixture modeling and propensity analysis: Evaluating an integrated services program for children with serious emotional disorders.* Paper presented at the annual meeting of the Society for Prevention Research, Seattle, WA.

Hernandez, M., Gomez, A., Lipien, L., Greenbaum, P. E., Armstrong, K., & Gonzalez, P. (2001). Use of the system-of-care practice review in the national evaluation: Evaluating the fidelity of practice to system-of-care principles. *Journal of Emotional and Behavioral Disorders, 9*, 43–52.

Hernandez, M., & Hodges, S. (2003). *Crafting logic models for systems of care; Ideas into action.* Tampa, FL: University of South Florida, Department of Child and Family Studies, Louis de la Parte Florida Mental Health Institute.

Herrell, J. M., & Straw, R. B. (Eds.). (2002). Conducting multiple site evaluations in real world settings. *New Directions for Evaluation, 94*, 1–100.

Holden, E. W. (2002, March). *Medication use for children in systems of care.* Presentation at the Annual Meeting of the American Psychiatric Association, Philadelphia, PA.

Holden, E. W., & Brannan, A. M. (Eds.). (2002). Special Issue: Evaluating Systems of Care: The National Evaluation of the Comprehensive Community Mental Health Services for Children and Their Families Program. *Children's Services: Social Policy, Research and Practice, 5*, 1–74.

Holden, E. W., De Carolis, G., & Huff, B. (2002). Policy implications of the national evaluation of the Comprehensive Community Mental Health Services for Children and Their Families Program. *Children's Services: Social Policy, Research, and Practice, 5*, 57–66.

Holden, E. W., Friedman, R. M., & Santiago, R. L. (2001a). Overview of the national evaluation of the Comprehensive Community Mental Health Services for Children and Their Families Program. *Journal of Emotional and Behavioral Disorders, 9*, 4–12.

Holden, E. W., Friedman, R. M., & Santiago, R. L. (Eds.). (2001b). Special issue: The national evaluation of the Comprehensive Community Mental Health Services for Children and Their Families Program. *Journal of Emotional and Behavioral Disorders, 9*, 1–80.

Holden, E. W., Santiago, R. L., Manteuffel, B. A., Stephens, R. L., Brannan, A. M., Soler, R. et al. (2003). Systems of care demonstration projects: Innovation, evaluation and sustainability. In A. J. Pumariega & N. C. Winters (Eds.), *The handbook of child and adolescent systems of care: The new community psychiatry* (pp. 432–458). San Francisco: Jossey-Bass.

Judge David L. Bazelon Center for Mental Health Law. (2003). *Help or hindrance?: The federal government and interagency systems of care for children with serious emotional disorders.* Retrieved June 15, 2003, from http://www.bazelon.org/issues/children/publications/helporhindrance/intro.htm

Manteuffel, B., Stephens, R. L., & Santiago, R. (2002). Overview of the national evaluation of the comprehensive community mental health services for children and their families program and summary of current findings. *Children's Services: Social Policy, Research, and Practice, 5*, 3–20.

Mason, C. A. (2003). Developmental epidemiology: Issues, application, and relevance for clinical child psychologists. *Journal of Clinical Child and Adolescent Psychology, 32*, 178–180.

Osher, T. W., van Kammen, W., & Zaro, S. M. (2001). Family participation in evaluating systems of care: Family, research, and service system perspectives. *Journal of Emotional and Behavioral Disorders, 9*, 63–70.

Patton, M. Q. (1997). *Utilization-focused evaluation* (3rd ed.). Thousand Oaks, CA: Sage.

Rosenblatt, A., & Woodbridge, M. W. (2003). Deconstructing research on systems of care for youth with EBD: Frameworks for policy research. *Journal of Emotional and Behavioral Disorders, 11*, 27–38.

Running Wolf, P. R., Soler, R. E., Manteuffel, B., Sondheimer, D., Santiago, R. L., & Erickson, J. S. (2002). Cultural competence approaches to evaluation in tribal communities. In J. D. Davis, J. S. Erickson, S. R. Johnson, C. A. Marshall, P. Running Wolf, & R. L. Santiago (Eds.), *Work group on American Indian Research and Program Evaluation Methodology (AIRPEM), Symposium on research and evaluation methodology: Lifespan issues related to American Indians/Alaska Natives with disabilities* (pp. 32–49). Flagstaff: Northern Arizona University, Institute for Human Development, Arizona University Center on Disabilities, American Indian Rehabilitation Research and Training Center.

Schoenwald, S. K., & Hoagwood, K. (2001). Effectiveness, transportability, and dissemination of interventions: What matters when? *Psychiatric Services, 52*, 1190–1197.

Stephens, R. L., Holden, E. W., & Hernandez, M. (2004). System-of-care practice review scores as predictors of behavioral symptomatology and functional impairment. *Journal of Child and Family Studies, 13(2)*, 179–191 .

Stroul, B. A. (Ed.). (1996). *Children's mental health: Creating systems of care in a changing society.* Baltimore: Paul H. Brookes.

Stroul, B. A., & Friedman, R. M. (1986). *A system of care for children and youth with severe emotional disturbances* (Rev. ed.). Washington, DC: Georgetown University Child Development Center, CASSP Technical Assistance Center.

Stroul, B. A., Pires, S. A., Armstrong, M. I., & Zaro, S. (2002). The impact of managed care on systems of care that serve children with serious emotional disturbances and their families. *Children's Services: Social Policy, Research, and Practice, 5*, 21–36.

U.S. Department of Health and Human Services. (1999). *Mental health: A report of the Surgeon General.* Washington, DC: U.S. Government Printing Office.

Tu, S. (2003). Developmental epidemiology: A review of three key measures. *Journal of Clinical Child and Adolescent Psychology, 32*, 187–192.

Vinson, N., Brannan, A. M., Baughman, L., Wilce, M., & Gawron, T. (2001). The system-of-care model: Implementation in twenty-seven communities. *Journal of Emotional and Behavioral Disorders, 9*, 30–42.

Wolff, N. (2000). Using randomized trials to evaluate socially complex services: Problems, challenges and recommendations. *The Journal of Mental Health Policy and Economics, 3*, 97–109.

World Health Organization. (2001). *World Health Report: 2001: Mental Health: New Understanding, New Hope.* Geneva: Author.

26

The Future of Mental Health Service Delivery for Children, Adolescents, and Families[†]

An Agenda for Organization and Research

RIC G. STEELE and MICHAEL C. ROBERTS

As suggested by the breadth of services outlined in this volume, the rubric "mental health service" has come to encompass a wide variety of activities in a number of different settings, with a number of different specific goals and objectives. From the early beginnings of mental health services being delivered in the context of university-based clinics (e.g., the University of Pennsylvania Psychology Clinic with Lightner Witmer in 1896), the field has grown to include services provided in private psychology clinics, community mental health centers, primary medical care settings, hospitals (both general and psychiatric), residential centers, schools, summer and wilderness camps, and across considerable distances via teletechnology.

Equally impressive is the spectrum of conditions for which services are now provided. Rather than services only for children evidencing significant psychopathology (i.e., diagnosable conditions), programs have been developed for children who are at risk for emotional and behavioral problems, including those at risk due to physical, medical, and socioeconomic

RIC G. STEELE and MICHAEL C. ROBERTS • Clinical Child Psychology Program, University of Kansas, Lawrence, Kansas 66045.

[†] The second author was supported by a grant from the U.S. Department of Education (#R305T010147) during the preparation of this chapter. The views expressed are those of the authors.

conditions. Further, mental health service provision has come to include programs designed to enhance or protect physical as well as mental health among children with no specific identifiable risk factors (e.g., promotion of safer sexual practices among healthy teenagers).

Developments along these two dimensions (i.e., setting and population) represent significant steps toward the fulfillment of several mandates and calls for action for improving the mental health of children and adolescents (e.g., Joint Commission on the Mental Health of Children [JCMHC], 1969; Knitzer, 1982; President's Commission on Mental Health, 1978). Generally, these reports have called for an increased range of services at both the severe and mild ends of the emotional and behavioral disorder spectrum, better integration of mental and physical health, and more preventive mental health services. To varying degrees, the services described in this volume suggest movement in these directions. In addition, recommendations for better means of evaluating and insuring accountability in mental health services (e.g., Knitzer, 1982; President's Commission on Mental Health, 1978) have been answered by both large- and small-scale program evaluations as well as changes in the methods that some states assess programmatic success.

However, despite these positive steps toward addressing some of the limitations in the mental health service delivery system, a number of areas highlighted several decades ago are still in need of attention. Most notably, the World Health Organization (WHO, 2001) estimated that between 17% and 22% of children and adolescents exhibit emotional or behavioral problems, and many more are at risk for additional problems, such as substance abuse, school drop-out, unsafe sexual practices, and delinquency. Of those with diagnosable mental disorders, approximately two-thirds remain without appropriate mental health services each year (U.S. Department of Health and Human Services [US DHHS], 1999), and, related to this concern, funding sources are not uniformly supportive of preventive services or mental health promotion in the absence of a diagnosable disorder. Thus, the need for psychological services, broadly defined, remains substantial.

Adding to the continued need for mental health services, are the complexities related to mental health service provision among individuals of racial or ethnic minority status. Currently, a disproportionate number youth with unmet mental health needs are children of ethnic minority groups, or are from socioeconomically disadvantaged families (Shaffer et al., 1996; US DHHS, 2001; Vega, Kolody, Aguilar-Gaxiola, & Catalano, 1999). In addition to a lower rate of service provision, the research base on mental health services for individuals of ethnic minority status remains underdeveloped (US DHHS, 2001). This deficit in the literature occasions a number of potentially negative consequences for the quality and efficacy of services provided to members of ethnic minority groups, and should continue to be considered a priority for research.

To a large extent, the inter-related forces that have wrought many positive changes in the delivery and evaluation of mental health services (e.g., public and federal discourse, professional input, funding sources and market pressures) are the same forces that continue to exert their influence. This fact is both comforting and disconcerting. Whereas the positive changes that have occurred may be seen as promising, the lack of progress in other areas (e.g., services to ethnic and racial minority groups, coverage of preventive services) gives pause to wonder whether and when these forces will address the as yet unmet needs.

Among the most obvious concerns facing the future of mental health service provision is that of the further impact of managed care. A number of recent commentaries have forecast various scenarios regarding the future of psychological services in the managed care environment (Drotar, 2004; Mitchell & Roberts, 2004; Rae, 2004; Sanchez & Turner, 2003). Whereas these opinions and observations have varied with regard to their level of optimism and the projected place that psychological services will have in future health care, most seem to recognize the likelihood of additional changes in the way services will be conceptualized and rendered. Perhaps more important than "*what will services look like?*" or "*how will services be funded?*" are the questions of "*are services working?*" and "*are services being provided to those in need?*"

Inherent in the first question (i.e., "Are services working?") is the expectation that services *should* have a measurable positive impact on the recipients. In the past several years, this expectation has been increasingly voiced by the public sector and in other health care professions (viz., medicine, nursing), as well as from within the mental health professions (viz., psychiatry, social work). Although perhaps not uniformly, mental health service professional organizations have begun to respond to this call for evidence-based practices.

One question that remains to be fully investigated, however, is whether managed care (or any funding arrangement, for that matter) has a positive or negative influence on the quality of services. So, beyond "are services working?" is the question of "Does (*fill in your funding source*) have a measurable impact on the effectiveness of services?" Some investigators (e.g., Buckloh & Roberts, 2001; Stroul, Pires, Armstrong, & Meyers, 1998) have begun to address such questions, but more work is certainly warranted.

Some evidence suggests that the answer to the second question (i.e., "*Are services being provided to those in need?*") is a resounding "no," given that approximately only one third of the children who are in need of services actually receive them (US DHHS, 1999). However, rather than a static snapshot of services currently provided, the more pressing question may be "*what is the impact of current fiscal trends on the distribution of psychological services to youth and families?*" As we discussed in Chapter 1 (this volume) current research in this area is mixed, with some studies suggesting increased mental health services among some samples, and others reporting decreased coverage and services. Since the existing evidence suggests that distribution of mental health services is not uniform across samples (see Dickey, Normand, Norton, Rupp, & Azeni, 2001; Stroul et al., 1998), more work is clearly needed to identify samples that are underserving under the current and evolving fiscal policies.

Particularly germane to the topic of this volume is the concern that current trends in mental health funding will have an adverse affect on the development and implementation of new services. As we noted in Chapter 1, Stroul and colleagues (1998) provided some evidence of the perception that managed care organizations (MCOs), while not averse to the development of new services, were also not particularly encouraging of them. We see this as a particularly important area to be addressed, and one that has significant consequences for mental health providers. As we discuss in more detail below, at least part of the solution likely requires that mental health professionals demonstrate that such services will have a measurable positive impact not only on the recipients, but also on the funding agencies' financial balance sheets. Whereas this conclusion may seem mercenary to some, it does represent the most probable route to insuring that psychological services are provided—particularly those services that are seen as preventative in nature. Sanchez and Turner (2003) have noted that such demonstration projects have already resulted in the integration of mental health services into primary care settings by insurance companies.

As is evident from some of the chapters in this volume, program evaluations will likely play a large role in the demonstration of clinical and cost effectiveness, and may take a number of different forms. One of the authors (R.G.S.) recently attended a meeting of representatives of city governments in which innovative programs to reduce school violence were shared and discussed. One of the presenters, a School Resource (Police) Officer, lamented the difficulty in demonstrating the effectiveness of his program, when the base rates of school violence were relatively low to begin with (but where *any* incidents are harmful). This comment serves as a reminder that program evaluations of field research are inevitably complicated and should be approached with creativity and in consultation with consumers (i.e., those to whom the evaluation will be presented, such as city or state governments, MCOs), recipients of the services, as well as technical experts in program evaluation (e.g., university and professional researchers).

Not inconsistent with the School Resource Officer's observation, a common frustration for researchers and practitioners alike is the unnecessary and potentially dangerous disconnect between mental health research and service provision. How does one translate the empirical research into viable "real-world" interventions, and, conversely, how does one demonstrate to policy makers, MCO administrators, and the public that an intervention works? As we noted in Chapter 23 (this volume) the National Institute of Mental Health (Clinical Treatment and Services Research Workgroup, 1998) produced a document that provides a potentially useful continuum from which to view program evaluations. Fundamentally, this continuum allows the evaluation of "what works?", "for whom?", and "in what settings?" Adaptation of this continuum perspective allows for a professional space that can bring together the service application and empirical research arms of mental health. From this framework, the research-oriented mental health service provider can examine where on the continuum a particular program is, and work with stakeholders to determine what the next steps in the continuum should be. Similarly, the researcher who is sensitive to practice concerns (e.g., generalizability, transportability) can examine a potential service program in light of the "next steps" to demonstrating real-world effectiveness.

Unfortunately, even university-based clinical training programs are not uniformly supportive of integrating evidence-based services into their curricula. Although part of the accreditation criteria for professional psychology states that students should receive "training in empirically supported procedures" (American Psychological Association [APA], 2002), specific courses on empirically supported (evidence-based) practices appear to be less than optimally provided. This training gap suggests an area in which to focus more efforts to integrate science and practice in mental health service provision. For example, in Canada, rather than protesting or rejecting the evidence-based practice movement, the practitioner-oriented Canadian Register of Health Service Providers in Psychology (CRHSPP) developed a project of enhancing its registrants' practices through an education or information package. A set of materials entitled "Evidence-Based Practice, Empirically Supported Interventions and Behavioral Health Services" was disseminated to the CRHSPP registrants. This package was prepared by John Hunsley, who was subsequently available for online consultations over an extended period of time. A series of continuing education workshops have also been offered, such as "Developing an Evidence-Based Psychological Practice," conducted by Dr. Hunsley at the Psychologists' Association of Alberta in 2003. These workshops were intended to help practitioners maintain knowledge of the scientific research most germane to clinical practice. According to the Executive Director of CRHSPP, Pierre Ritchie, the materials, consultation, and workshops were positively evaluated, and the project was considered successful (CRHSPP, 2004). We view this activity as a model for integration, service-oriented science, and a more harmonious way to implement needed change without the dissension that has marked evidence-based practice elements in the United States.

We began this handbook with a review of the various influences that have shaped mental health service provision for children, youth, and families. Such influences have included empirical reports documenting the need for children's services (e.g., *Unclaimed Children*, Knitzer, 1982), American federal initiatives calling for the provision of such services (e.g., the *Mental Health Systems Act of 1980*), professional initiatives related to what and how services are to be provided (Chambless & Hollon, 1998; Chambless et al., 1996), and the sometimes related considerations of how those services are to be funded. As we reflect over the history of mental health services for children and adolescents, we experience alternating feelings of pessimism and optimism. Our pessimism results from the recognition that children's needs are greater than ever before and the consequences of not providing services appear to be more severe. Additionally, the fact that seeming gains in providing better services are all too frequently counteracted by a variety of forces and actions, such as ideology shifts and budget cuts at all levels. Like the metaphorical inch worm climbing out of a well, there has been sliding back 2 feet for every 4 feet movement upward. Ultimately, however, we sense (and hope) greater success can be reached.

We place our trust in the continuing examination of therapeutic interventions, programs, and services in a variety of evaluations. The professionals, advocacy organizations, and private and public entities should invest good effort in fixing what does not work to create interventions, programs, and infrastructures to support effective, organized service delivery. We also trust application of the scientific method to develop effective interventions through the careful study of human development, psychopathology and related problems, and designate principles of change for therapeutic benefit. We place our qualified faith in psychological scientist-practitioners (and other providers in psychiatry, medicine, and social work) to rationally apply effective techniques and services, while continuing to innovate and educate for future developments. We say "qualified" only because some of the obstacles to adequate development have been professional biases, application of tired old concepts, and "turf" protectionism. We expect professional psychology training programs, in particular, to provide more training, education, and experience in terms of evidence-based practices and services, rather than repeat old and unproven techniques and service delivery modalities that might have been current when the trainers were trained, but are no longer supported by improved methodologies. Whereas the past can guide the future to some extent, past practices should not block improvements in the development and provision of quality care. We have to trust (having no alternatives) in our policymakers to make informed decisions free of political ideology, based on objective examinations of what works and what does not.

Of course, until the science of psychology catches up with the serious and complex problems presented by humans in need, we acknowledge that all too often there are limitations to what is empirically supported for implementation in clinical practice. Mental health providers will have to continue to innovate and reorganize services even in the absence of adequate scientific base. An orientation to systematic evaluation of services will also advance the field and improve what is provided.

We are heartened by the types of services and programs presented in this volume. Of course, we selected these services and authors based on a set of criteria: the need to be comprehensive in our coverage, but each approaching service delivery in an evidence-based mind set. Although there are others we could have selected, but did not have enough space to include, there are some that we "deselected" because they could not provide minimal evidence of meeting the needs, despite multiple years of opportunities to prove their worth.

One source of our pessimism comes from the fact that funding and organization for mental health services in the United States are fragmented, which almost guarantees a noncomprehensive analysis of needs and nonintegrated development of services to meet the needs. The variety of settings and range of services described in this volume illustrate some of the difficulties. Each developed in particular settings to meet particular identified needs by specific professionals, but they often do not combine together in a cohesive way and are rarely available to all children.

We expect that funding for mental health services for children and adolescents will continue to change. "Managed care" in its complexity will evolve into new patterns. The remaining issues that require sustained attention will be organization, staffing, access to care, and quality of services. We hope that the models and issues presented in this volume will advance the cause of improving these services.

Recently, the American Psychological Association Council of Representatives, on behalf of the largest organization of psychologists, adopted a resolution on children's mental health (February 2004). In the preamble of the resolution, the APA governing body stated,

> The Report of the Surgeon General's Conference on Children's Mental Health: A National Action Agenda states that the "nation is facing a public crisis in mental healthcare for infants, children and adolescents. Many children have mental health problems that interfere with normal development and functioning (U.S. Public Health Service, 2000). Currently, the best epidemiological evidence indicates that between 10 and 15% of children and adolescents in the United States suffer from a mental disorder severe enough to cause some level of functional impairment (Burns et al., 1995; Shaffer et al., 1996; Roberts, Attkisson, & Rosenblatt, 1998) however, only 1 in 5 of these children receive specialty mental health services (Burns et al., 1995). The World Health Organization indicates that by the year 2020, childhood psychiatric disorders will rise proportionately by over 50% internationally, and will become one of the 5 most common causes of morbidity, mortality, and disability among children. The Surgeon General's report highlights the lack of a unified infrastructure nationwide to provide mental health services to children, leading to fragmented treatment services, limited prevention and early identification, and low priorities for resources.
>
> Given the vicissitudes of healthy child development, the complexities of child mental disorders, and the multiple settings in which children, live, grow, and function, there is need for a comprehensive policy to promote child mental health. (APA, 2004)

The resolution also noted that children have "inadequate access to appropriate evidence-based promotion, prevention, and treatment services," that there is a "disparity of access" based on poverty, ethnicity, and race, as well as the types of problems children exhibit, that there is inadequate financing, that there is a need for improved research in several domains, and that there is a shortage of adequately trained providers to meet the needs. The resolution concluded that "it is every child's right to have access to culturally competent, developmentally appropriate, family oriented, evidence-based, high-quality mental health services that are in accessible settings". Although we find it remarkably late in history that this organization finally turned its collective attention to children's mental health issues in this way, we are optimistic that finally not only the organization, but its advocacy for practice and public interest will work with other organizations to foster improved services for children and adolescents.

Earlier, the American Academy of Pediatrics (AAP), in conjunction with mental health organizations such as American Psychological Association, American Academy of Child and Adolescent Psychiatry, and American Psychiatry Association, articulated a consensus statement on the coverage of mental health and substance abuse services for children and adolescents. This position statement held that to improve mental health services, three issues must be addressed: access, coordination, and monitoring from "the standpoint of needs for preventive interventions, direct mental health and substance abuse services, and coordinated multiservice care" (AAP, 2000, p. 860). The statement concluded that:

- Clinician professional organizations and provider plans should be encouraged to better define and use evidence-based care in mental and behavioral health and substance abuse services for children, adolescents, and families. Empirically supported assessments and treatment should include level-of-care criteria, best practices, and monitoring of incremental expectations for progress. Research on quality of care and outcomes effectiveness should also be enhanced by these groups.
- Public and private sectors should develop mechanisms for system accountability in the cost-effectiveness of service calculations, including consideration of administrative costs.
- Mechanisms to provide user-friendly information to families and purchasers regarding the availability, adequacy, and quality of mental and behavioral health and substance abuse services must be developed.
- Simplified and timely internal and independent external appeals processes should be developed by health plans and mental health care management programs. Families should be included on such panels.
- The decreasing availability of health care services to meet the mental health needs of children and adolescents is a serious and worsening problem. Action must be taken to curb this decrease. Issues that negatively impact the access, coordination, and monitoring of such services must be addressed. Improvements in these services will have a positive impact not only on the health and well-being of children and adolescents but on society as well. (AAP, 2000, p. 862)

Given the Surgeon General's Conference on Children's Mental Health (US DHHS, 1999), the position statements of the various professional organizations (AAP, 2000; APA, 2004), and the vital presentations in this volume of excellent services, we should be rather optimistic about the future. Yet, our optimism must be tempered by caution, given the history of mental health services, especially for children and adolescents (Peterson & Roberts, 1991). Over the years, each national comprehensive assessment of needs and services has repeated the failure to meet the needs and called for greater effort. Like the inch worm working up the side of the well, we have to hope for greater continual progress for every setback.

REFERENCES

American Psychological Association. (2002). *Guidelines and procedures for accreditation of programs in professional psychology.* Washington, DC: American Psychological Association.

American Psychological Association. (2004, February). *Resolution on Children's Mental Health approved by Council of Representatives.* Washington, DC: American Psychological Association.

American Academy of Pediatrics. (2000). Insurance coverage of mental health and substance abuse services for children and adolescents: A consensus statement. *Pediatrics, 106,* 860–862.

Buckloh, L. M., & Roberts, M. C. (2001). Managed mental health care: Attitudes and ethical beliefs of child and pediatric psychologists. *Journal of Pediatric Psychology, 26,* 193–202.

Canadian Register of Health Services Provider in Psychology. (2004, January). Annual report to the Psychology Executives Roundtable by Pierre L. J. Ritchie, Exective Director. Ottawa, Ontario, Canada.

Chambless, D. L., & Hollon, S. D. (1998). Defining empirically supported therapies. *Journal of Consulting and Clinical Psychology, 66,* 7–18.

Chambless, D. L., Sanderson, W. C., Shoham, V., Bennett-Johnson, S., Pope, K. S., Crits-Christoph, P. et al. (1996). An update on empirically validated therapies. *The Clinical Psychologist, 49,* 5–18.

Clinical Treatment and Services Research Workgroup of the National Institute of Mental Health, National Advisory Mental Health Council. (1998). *Bridging science and service.* Bethesda, MD: National Institutes of Health. Retrieved July 15, 2003, from http://www.nimh.nih.gov/research/bridge.htm#br8

Dickey, B., Normand, S. L., Norton, E. C., Rupp, A., & Azeni, H. (2001). Managed care and children's behavioral health services in Massachusetts. *Psychiatric Services, 52,* 183–188.

Drotar, D. (2004). Commentary: We can make our own dime or two, help children and their families, and advance science while doing so. *Journal of Pediatric Psychology, 29,* 61–63.

Joint Commission on the Mental Health of Children. (1969). *Crisis in child mental health.* New York: Harper and Row.

Knitzer, J. (1982). *Unclaimed children: The failure of public responsibility to children and adolescents in need of mental health services.* Washington, DC: Children's Defense Fund.

Mitchell, M. C., & Roberts, M. C. (2004). Commentary: Financing pediatric psychology services: "Look what they've done to my song, Ma" or "The sun'll come out tomorrow." *Journal of Pediatric Psychology, 29,* 55–59.

Peterson, L., & Roberts, M. C. (1991). Treatment of children's problems. In C. E. Walker (Ed.), *Clinical psychology: Historical and research foundations* (pp. 313–342). New York: Plenum.

President's Commission on Mental Health. (1978). *Report to the President from the President's Commission on Mental Health,* Vol. 1 (Commission Report) and Vol. 3 (Task Panel Reports). Washington, DC: U.S. Government Printing Office.

Rae, W. A. (2004). 2000 SPP Salk Award Address: Financing pediatric psychology services: Buddy can you spare a dime? *Journal of Pediatric Psychology, 29,* 47–52.

Sanchez, L. M., & Turner, S. M. (2003). Practicing psychology in the era of managed care. *American Psychologist, 58,* 116–129.

Shaffer, D., Fisher, P., Dulcan, M. K., Davies, M., Piacentini, J., Schwab-Stone, M. E. et al. (1996). The NIMH Diagnostic Interview Schedule for Children Version 2.3 (DISC-2.3): Description, acceptability, prevalence rates, and performance in the MECA Study. Methods for the Epidemiology of Child and Adolescent Mental Disorders Study. *Journal of the American Academy of Child and Adolescent Psychiatry, 35,* 865–877.

Stroul, B. A., Pires, S. A., Armstrong, M. I., & Meyers, J. C. (1998). The impact of managed care on mental health services for children and their families. *Future of Children, 8,* 119–133.

U.S. Department of Health and Human Services. (1999). *Mental health: A report of the Surgeon General.* Rockville, MD: U.S. Department of Health and Human Services, Substance Abuse and Mental Health Services Administration, Center for Mental Health Services, National Institutes of Health, National Institute of Mental Health.

U.S. Department of Health and Human Services. (2001). *Mental health: Culture, race, and ethnicity: A supplement to Mental Health: A report of the Surgeon General.* Rockville, MD: U.S. Department of Health and Human Services.

Vega, W. A., Kolody, B., Aguilar-Gaxiola, S., & Catalano, R. (1999). Gaps in service utilization by Mexican Americans with mental health problems. *American Journal of Psychiatry, 156,* 928–934.

World Health Organization. (2001). The world health report: 2001: *Mental health: New understanding, new hope.* Geneva: World Health Organization.

Index